# THE ROLE OF PHARMACOLOGY IN PEDIATRIC ONCOLOGY

# DEVELOPMENTS IN ONCOLOGY

F.J. Cleton and J.W.I.M. Simons, eds., Genetic Origins of Tumour Cells. ISBN 90-247-2272-1

J. Aisner and P. Chang, eds., Cancer Treatment Research. ISBN 90-247-2358-2

B.W. Ongerboer de Visser, D.A. Bosch and W.M.H. van Woerkom-Eykenboom, eds., Neurooncology: Clinical and Experimental Aspects. ISBN 90-247-2421-X

K. Hellmann, P. Hilgard and S. Eccles, eds., Metastasis: Clinical and Experimental Aspects. ISBN 90-247-2424-4

H.F. Seigler, ed., Clinical Management of Melanoma. ISBN 90-247-2584-4

P. Correa and W. Haenszel, eds., Epidemiology of Cancer of the Digestive Tract. ISBN 90-247-2601-8

L.A. Liotta and I.R. Hart, eds., Tumour Invasion and Metastasis. ISBN 90-247-2611-5

J. Bánóczy, ed., Oral Leukoplakia. ISBN 90-247-2655-7

C. Tijssen, M. Halprin and L. Endtz, eds., Familial Brain Tumours. ISBN 90-247-2691-3

F.M. Muggia, C.W. Young and S.K. Carter, eds., Anthracycline Antibiotics in Cancer. ISBN 90-247-2711-1

B.W. Hancock, ed., Assessment of Tumour Response. ISBN 90-247-2712-X

D.E. Peterson, ed., Oral Complications of Cancer Chemotherapy. ISBN 0-89838-563-6

R. Mastrangelo, D.G. Poplack and R. Riccardi, eds., Central Nervous System Leukemia. Prevention and Treatment. ISBN 0-89838-570-9

A. Polliack, ed., Human Leukemias. Cytochemical and Ultrastructural Techniques in Diagnosis and Research. ISBN 0-89838-585-7

W. Davis, C. Maltoni and S. Tanneberger, eds., The Control of Tumor Growth and its Biological Bases. ISBN 0-89838-603-9

A.P.M. Heintz, C.Th. Griffiths and J.B. Trimbos, eds., Surgery in Gynecological Oncology. ISBN 0-89838-604-7

M.P. Hacker, E.B. Double and I. Krakoff, eds., Platinum Coordination Complexes in Cancer Chemotherapy. ISBN 0-89838-619-5

M.J. van Zwieten, The Rat as Animal Model in Breast Cancer Research: A Histopathological Study of Radiation- and Hormone-Induced Rat Mammary Tumors. ISBN 0-89838-624-1

B. Löwenberg and A. Hagenbeek, eds., Minimal Residual Disease in Acute Leukemia. ISBN 0-89838-630-6

I. van der Waal and G.B. Snow, eds., Oral Oncology. ISBN 0-89838-631-4

B.W. Hancock and A.H. Ward, eds., Immunological Aspects of Cancer. ISBN 0-89838-664-0

K.V. Honn and B.F. Sloane, Hemostatic Mechanisms and Metastasis. ISBN 0-89838-667-5

K.R. Harrap, W. Davis and A.H. Calvert, eds., Cancer Chemotherapy and Selective Drug Development. ISBN 0-89838-673-X

C.J.H. van de Velde and P.H. Sugarbaker, eds., Liver Metastasis. ISBN 0-89838-648-5

D.J. Ruiter, K. Welvaart and S. Ferrone, eds., Cutaneous Melanoma and Precursor Lesions. ISBN 0-89838-689-6

S.B. Howell, ed., Intra-arterial and Intracavitary Cancer Chemotherapy. ISBN 0-89838-691-8

D.L. Kisner and J.F. Smyth, eds., Interferon Alpha-2: Pre-Clinical and Clinical Evaluation. ISBN 0-89838-701-9

P. Furmanski, J.C. Hager and M.A. Rich, eds., RNA Tumor Viruses, Oncogenes, Human Cancer and Aids: On the Frontiers of Understanding. ISBN 0-89838-703-5

J. Talmadge, I.J. Fidler and R.K. Oldham, Screening for Biological Response Modifiers: Methods and Rationale. ISBN 0-89838-712-4

J.C. Bottino, R.W. Opfell and F.M. Muggia, eds., Liver Cancer. ISBN 0-89838-713-2

P.K. Pattengale, R.J. Lukes and C.R. Taylor, Lymphoproliferative Diseases: Pathogenesis, Diagnosis, Therapy. ISBN 0-89838-725-6

F. Cavalli, G. Bonadonna and M. Rozencweig, eds., Malignant Lymphomas and Hodgkin's Disease: Experimental and Therapeutic Advances. ISBN 0-89838-727-2

J.G. McVie, W. Bakker, Sj.Sc. Wagenaar and D. Carney, eds., Clinical and Experimental Pathology of Lung Cancer. ISBN 0-89838-764-7

D.G. Poplack, L. Massimo and P. Cornaglia-Ferraris, eds., The Role of Pharmacology in Pediatric Oncology. ISBN 0-89838-795-7

A. Hagenbeek and B. Löwenberg, eds., Minimal Residual Disease in Acute Leukemia: 1986. ISBN 0-89838-799-x

# THE ROLE OF PHARMACOLOGY IN PEDIATRIC ONCOLOGY

*edited by*

D.G. POPLACK
*Leukemia Biology Section, Pediatric Branch*
*National Institutes of Health, Bethesda, Maryland, U.S.A.*

L. MASSIMO and P. CORNAGLIA-FERRARIS
*Istituto Giannina Gaslini*
*Genova, Italy*

1987 **MARTINUS NIJHOFF PUBLISHERS**
a member of the KLUWER ACADEMIC PUBLISHERS GROUP
DORDRECHT / BOSTON / LANCASTER

**Distributors**

*for the United States and Canada*: Kluwer Academic Publishers, P.O. Box 358, Accord Station, Hingham, MA 02018-0358, USA
*for the UK and Ireland*: Kluwer Academic Publishers, MTP Press Limited, Falcon House, Queen Square, Lancaster LA1 1RN, UK
*for all other countries*: Kluwer Academic Publishers Group, Distribution Center, P.O. Box 322, 3300 AH Dordrecht, The Netherlands

**Library of Congress Cataloging in Publication Data**

The Role of pharmacology in pediatric oncology.

   (Developments in oncology)
   Includes bibliographies and index.
   1. Tumors in children--Chemotherapy.  2. Pediatric
pharmacology.  I. Poplack, David G.  II. Massimo,
Luisa.  III. Cornaglia Ferraris, Paolo.  IV. Series.
[DNLM: 1. Neoplasms--drug therapy.  2. Neoplasms--
in infancy & childhood.  W1 DE998N / QZ 267 R745]
RC281.C4R65  1986        618.92'99'2061        86-687
ISBN-13:978-94-010-8395-9      e-ISBN-13:978-94-009-4267-7
DOI: 10.1007/978-94-009-4267-7

ISBN-13:978-94-010-8395-9

**Copyright**

# Preface

The dramatic improvement made in recent years in the treatment of childhood malignancies has been in large part the result of advances in the field of pharmacology. Chemotherapy is the major therapeutic modality used to treat childhood cancer. Rational administration of antineoplastic chemotherapy to the child with cancer requires the pediatric oncologist to have a thorough understanding of the fundamental principles of clinical pharmacology, an intimate knowledge of the specific agents being used, and an awareness of the unique biologic and physiologic features of children.

In mid 1985, a distinguished group of pediatric oncologists and clinical pharmacologists convened in a unique workshop to review the subject of pharmacology in pediatric oncology. A goal of this workshop was to produce a book which would review this topic and present it in a format useful for the clinician.

In this book basic principles of pharmacology, mechanisms of drug resistance, new methods of drug delivery, guidelines for studying new agents in children, new biological response modifiers and the pharmacology of the most commonly used chemotherapeutic agents in children are reviewed in depth. Particular emphasis is given to discussing those topics which uniquely apply to the use of antineoplastic agents in children with cancer.

The Editors

# Contents

**Principles of Antineoplastic Therapy in Children**

**Pharmacologic reasons for treatment failure**

## High dose chemotherapy

## Biological response modifiers

# List of major contributors

Vassilios AVRAMIS, Department of Pediatrics, Children's Hospital at Los Angeles, P.O. Box 54700, Los Angeles, CA 90054-0700, U.S.A.

Frank BALIS, Pediatric Branch, National Cancer Institute, NIH, Building 10, Room 13N240, Bethesda, MD 20205, U.S.A.

W.A. BLEYER, Children's Orthopedic Hospital, P.O. Box C5371, 4800 Sand Point Way, N.E., Seattle, WA 98105, U.S.A.

Jos P.M. BÖKKERINK, Center for Pediatric Oncology S.E. Netherlands, Department of Pediatrics, Catholic University of Nijmegen, P.O. Box 9101, 6500 HB Nijmegen, The Netherlands.

Jerry COLLINS, Clinical Pharmacology Branch, National Cancer Institute, NIH, Building 10, Room 6N119, Bethesda, MD 20205, U.S.A.

P. CORNAGLIA-FERRARIS, Department of Pediatric Oncology, G. Gaslini Institute for Children, I-16148 Genova, Italy.

Kenneth COWAN, Clinical Pharmacology Branch, National Cancer Institute, NIH, Building 10, Room 6N116, Bethesda, MD 20205, U.S.A.

Ronney A. DE ABREU, Center for Pediatric Oncology S.E. Netherlands, Department of Pediatrics, Catholic University of Nijmegen, P.O. Box 9101, 6500 HB Nijmegen, The Netherlands.

G. DINI, Division of Hematology and Oncology, G. Gaslini Institute for Children, I-16148 Genova, Italy.

R. ERTTMANN, Department of Hematology and Oncology, Children's Hospital, University of Hamburg, Martinistrasse 52, D-2000 Hamburg 20, F.R.G.

Williams EVANS, Clinical Pharmacokinetics Laboratory, St. Jude Children's Research Hospital, 332 N. Lauderdale, Memphis, TE 38105, U.S.A.

Felice GAVESTO, Medical Clinic I, Via Genova 3, I-10126, Torino, Italy.

A. GINER-SOROLLA, Program of Immunopharmacology, College of Medicine, University of South Florida, Tampa, FL 33612, U.S.A.

C. GRANDORI, Department of Experimental Medicine and Biochemical Science, Second University of Rome, Via Orazio Raimondo, I-00173 Roma, Italy.

John HOLCENBERG, Division of Hematology and Oncology, Children's Hospital at Los Angeles, P.O. Box 54700, Los Angeles, CA 90054-0700, U.S.A.

L. MASSIMO, Department of Pediatric Hematology and Oncology, G. Gaslini Institute for Children, I-16148 Genova, Italy.

Thierry PHILIP, Centre Léon Bérard, 28 Rue Laennec, F-69008 Lyon Cédex 02, France.

David G. POPLACK, Leukemia Biology Section, Pediatric Branch, National Cancer Institute, NIH, Building 10, Room 13N240, Bethesda, MD 20205, U.S.A.

Carlo RICCARDI, Institute of Pharmacology, University of Perugia, Via del Giochetto, I-06100 Perugia, Italy.

Riccardo RICCARDI, Institute of Clinical Pediatrics, Catholic University of Roma, Largo A. Gemelli 8, I-00168 Roma, Italy.

Gian Paolo TONINI, Pediatric Oncology Research Laboratory, Department of Pediatric and Oncology, G. Gaslini Institute for Children, I-16148 Genova, Italy.

Guiseppe TORELLI, Medical Clinic II — Policlinic, Via del Pozzo 71, I-41100 Modena, Italy.

Richard UNGERLEIDER, Cancer Treatment Evaluation Program, National Cancer Institute, NIH, Landow Building, Room 4A-12, Bethesda, MD 20205, U.S.A.

Solomon ZIMM, Pediatric Branch, National Cancer Institute, NIH, Building 10, Room 13N240, Bethesda, MD 20205, U.S.A.

# Principles of antineoplastic therapy in children

# 1. Clinical Pharmacokinetics for the Pediatric Oncologist

JERRY M. COLLINS

## Abstract

The emphasis of this chapter is upon the fundamental concepts of pharmacokinetics: clearance, half-life, and volume of distribution. As used in pharmacokinetics, clearance encompasses all mechanisms of drug elimination and is the single most important index of drug exposure. Half-life, the interval required to remove half of the drug from the body, is the most familiar of all pharmacokinetic concepts. The half-life for an anticancer drug is usually several hours, but can range from a few minutes to over a month. Volume of distribution is used to scale drug dosages, and is an estimate of drug penetration to different spaces in the body. Its value ranges from 3 liters (or less in small children) to several thousand liters.

The one-compartment model is the most commonly used model in clinical pharmacokinetics. This chapter explains the behavior of a drug which exhibits one-compartment kinetics. Drug administration as a bolus, continuous infusion, or first-order absorption are covered. Saturable (i.e., nonlinear) behavior is also discussed.

The majority of clinically-relevant drugs exhibit kinetics which are best described by the two-compartment model. There is also an increasing use of pharmacokinetic techniques which do not depend upon a specific number of compartments.

## Introduction

Some of the subsequent presentations at this conference will focus on specific issues which involve applications of pharmacokinetics in pediatric oncology. The purpose of this introductory chapter is to provide a common background in the issues, concepts, and terminology of pharmacokinetics.

Although there are many models and equations which could be included in a survey of pharmacokinetics [1–3], there are only three fundamental quantities: clearance, half-time, and volume of distribution. Since these quantities are interrelated, one usually needs to separately determine only two of these quantities for each drug. In this chapter, I will cover the standard pharmacokinetic nomenclature and models, but I want to keep the focus on these three quantities, especially the clinical implications in terms of dose size, dose frequently, and route of administration.

## Clearance

Many investigators tend to consider only the narrow definition of clearance as it applies to renal physiology. A more general definition is that of Total Body Clearance ($CL_{TB}$), which incorporates all mechanisms of drug removal from the body, including renal and biliary excretion or metabolic conversion.

For individual patients, the single most important index of changes in drug exposure will be individual variations in clearance. If an individual rapidly removes drug from the body compared with the average, his drug exposure will be less than average. Similarly, if drug clearance is slower than average, drug exposure will be greater than average. Because of the steep dose-response curves which are characteristic of nearly all anticancer drugs, such changes in drug exposure are likely to lead to either subtherapeutic treatment or excessive toxicity.

Although other organs can be important in specific cases, the liver and kidneys are generally the predominant organs of drug clearance. When a patient has impaired renal or hepatic function, the drug dose must be reduced in order to avoid excessive toxicity. Most standard treatment regimens have 'dose-reduction factors' which make some attempt to select the appropriate dose in these cases. It is difficult to judge the success of such schemes. If patients become excessively toxic, the schemes are inadequate and further dose-reductions are required. If toxicity is not observed, it is assumed that these schemes are successful. However, one can always avoid toxicity by overly conservative doses. The possibility of under-treating the patient becomes substantial.

There have been some attempts to individualize the dose based upon an evaluation of the quantitative pharmacologic impact. Direct pharmacokinetic measurement of a test-dose of the drug [4] can be pursued in some cases, but such approaches are likely to be impractical in most situations. Recently, Egorin *et al.* [5] have elegantly demonstrated the practicality of dose-adjustment for the new drug carboplatinum (CBDCA). This drug appears to be primarily eliminated by renal filtration, and the rate of removal can be ascertained from serum creatinine. Thrombocytopenia is the dose-limiting toxicity. The fall in platelets following a CBDCA dose was shown to be easily standardized by adjusting the dose on the basis of serum creatinine.

## Half-life

The persistence of a drug in the body as a function of time is best denoted by its half-life. In formal terms, the half-life of a drug in the body is the time required to eliminate (by all available mechanisms) one-half of the drug from the body. From a clinical perspective, the most important application of half-life is a determination of the appropriate interval between doses, e.g., b.i.d., t.i.d., q.d., and so forth.

The half-life for drugs used in oncology is usually measured in hours, but there is a wide variation. In my lab, we have recently finished a study of iododeoxyuridine [6] in which we determined the $t_{1/2}$ to be 4 min. This is among the shortest half-life values for any substance given therapeutically. Coincidentally, we are currently studying the pharmacokinetics of suramin. It appears that the $t_{1/2}$ for this drug is 40 days [7], somewhat of a record for the longest persistence.

Short $t_{1/2}$ can be an annoyance, especially for an antimetabolite whose concentration must be kept above a threshold for a prolonged time. Frequent dosing is required in such situations. For truly chronic chemotherapy (6 months or more), a 40-day $t_{1/2}$ is quite convenient, but this type of application is rare in oncology. It is more relevant to supportive measures such as antibiotic administration or the use of drugs such as allopurinol in conjunction with cytotoxics. More frequently, we need to have the drug present for a few days, but then the drug must be removed in order to allow recovery of normal host tissues.

## Volume of distribution

It might be expected that volume of distribution would be one of the easiest kinetic concepts, since it describes 'where the drug goes in the body'. However, a number of misconceptions have arisen which require that we spend some time discussing this concept.

Volume of distribution ($V_d$) is defined as that volume in which the total amount of drug in the body would have to be *uniformly* distributed in order to give the observed plasma concentration. $V_d$ is *not* necessarily a real volume, but rather an *apparent* one. It is a proportionality constant which relates the amount of drug in the body to its concentration in plasma. It has units of ml or liters, and is especially useful when expressed as ml/kg or l/kg.

It is appealing to relate this apparent volume to some physiological space in the body, such as total body water or extracellular fluid, but there can be problems with these comparisons. The *minimum* value for $V_d$ must be plasma volume (3 liters in adults or about 5% of body weight in children), since the drug is being measured in plasma. Although it might seem reasonable to suppose that the maximum value for $V_d$ is 100% of the body size, there is *no maximum* value for $V_d$. If a drug is concentrated in tissue (e.g., by protein binding or partitioning into fat), then distribution volumes much larger than body size will be observed. As an example, doxorubicin has a $V_d$ of about 2000 liters [8].

Although the anatomical significance of $V_d$ may sometimes be obscured, there is practical significance for this term, since it is used to scale drug dosage. Furthermore, we can appreciate that drugs with large distribution volumes may be protected from rapid elimination from the body compared with drugs with smaller $V_d$ values. Finally, changes in $V_d$ can alter the elimination rate and, hence, pharmacologic effect. The most acute change in drug distribution can occur through displacement of one drug from tissue stores by other drugs. Depending upon the mechanism for drug elimination from the body, these competitive displacements may require short-term and/or long-term adjustments in drug dosage [9].

With this quick background regarding the conceptual basis for pharmacokinetic inquiry, we can delve into the often abstract world of modeling.

### One-compartment, linear model

*Bolus drug input*

The one-compartment model is the most commonly used clinical model. Figure 1 shows the concentration-time curve which is observed for a drug which exhibits one-compartment kinetics following bolus injection of drug. The initial concentration, $C(0)$, is dose/$V_d$. The disappearance curve is a straight line on a semilogarithmic plot, and can be summarized:

$$C_p(t) = C(0) \exp(-k_{el}t) \tag{1}$$

where t is time following injection and $k_{el}$ is the elimination rate. There are many mechanisms which eliminate drugs from the body (e.g., renal or biliary excretion, metabolic processes), and $k_{el}$ is the sum of these individual processes. The most familiar pharmacokinetic parameter is half-life, $t_{1/2}$, which is readily calculated from the elimination rate: $t_{1/2} = 0.693/k_{el}$. For a one-compartment, linear pharmacokinetic model, the half-life is independent of concentration. Linearity is a term used frequently by modelers. For pharmacokinetic purposes, it simply means that changes in concentration

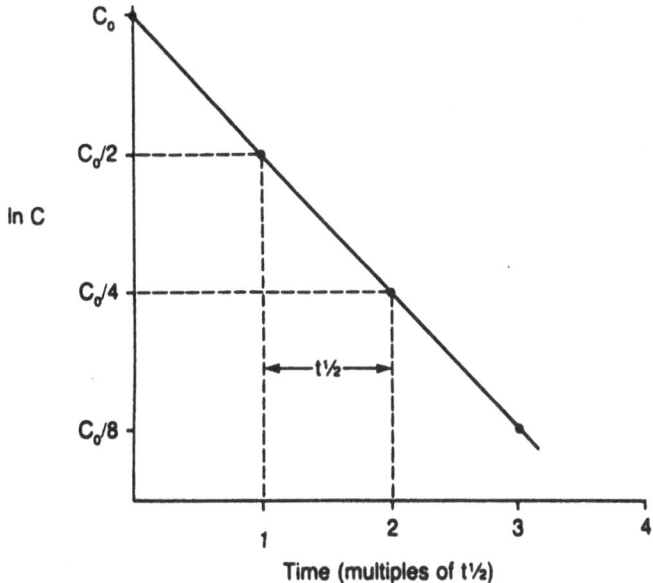

*Figure 1.* Concentration-time profile observed after bolus input to one-compartment model. From Collins and Dedrick [3].

are proportional to changes in dose. Clearance ($CL_{TB}$) is defined as the product of $k_{el}$ and $V_d$.

## Continuous drug infusion

In some situations, it is necessary to maintain the concentration of drug above a threshold value for a prolonged period of time. A variety of technical advances have made continuous infusion therapy more practical. The studies of 6-mercaptopurine by Zimm *et al.* [10] illustrate the rationale for the use of this schedule. Figure 2 shows the pharmacokinetic behavior of a one-compartment, linear system for the case of continuous drug infusion. As for the case of bolus drug input, the half-life (or $k_{el}$) is the key parameter of interest. The drug concentration rises towards a steady-state value. In one half-life, the concentration has reached 50% of its plateau value. In 3 to 5 half-lives, the concentration has effectively reached its plateau. Mathematically, the curve can be described:

$$C_p(t) = C_{ss}(1 - \exp(-k_{el}t)) \tag{2}$$

where $C_{ss}$ is the ratio of infusion rate, G, to elimination rate, $k_{el} V_d$, or $CL_{TB}$. If the infusion is stopped (before or after reaching a plateau), the drug concentration will decline with the same $t_{1/2}$ observed following bolus input.

8

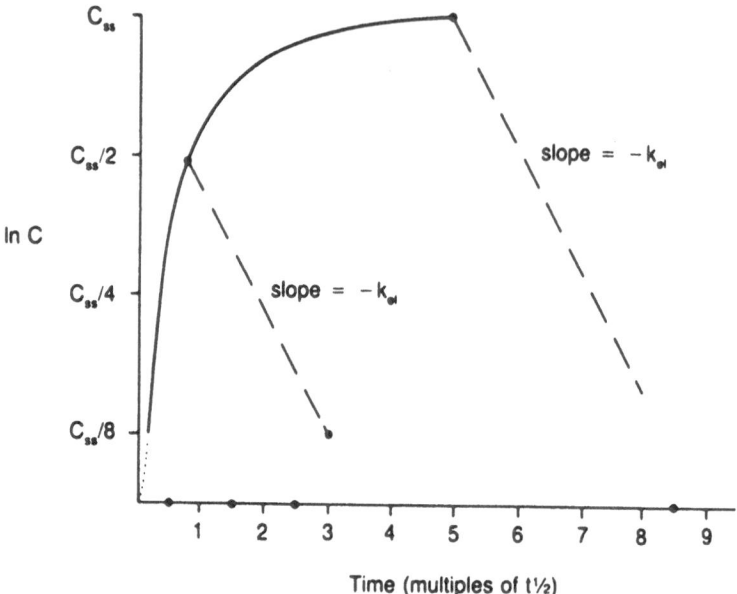

*Figure 2.* Concentration-time profile observed for constant infusion input to one-compartment model. From Collins and Dedrick [3].

Note that the magnitude of $C_{ss}$ is dependent upon the rate of infusion, but the time to reach $C_{ss}$ is *not* dependent upon infusion rate.

Many treatment protocols consist of repetitive drug administration. Combinations of a bolus and infusion, or multiple bolus injections may be described by mathematical combination of Equations (1) and (2). In some cases, the goal is to accelerate the attainment of a desired steady-state concentration. A 'loading dose' is given as a bolus prior to starting an infusion or a series of intermittent injections.

Although infusions are more technically feasible than before, the convenience of bolus drug administration remains an important practical consideration. If the drug $t_{1/2}$ is sufficiently long, then repeated injections may suffice to achieve reasonably 'constant' drug levels. Clearly, drug levels will reach a peak immediately after each bolus injection and fall to a nadir just before each bolus. This oscillation in drug levels from maximum to minimum will be less than a factor of 2 so long as the dose interval is less than the drug $t_{1/2}$.

*First-order absorption*

When the drug is given orally, subcutaneously, intramuscularly, or intraperitoneally, it must be absorbed from the delivery site into the systemic circulation. Generally, it is assumed that the rate of absorption is not instan-

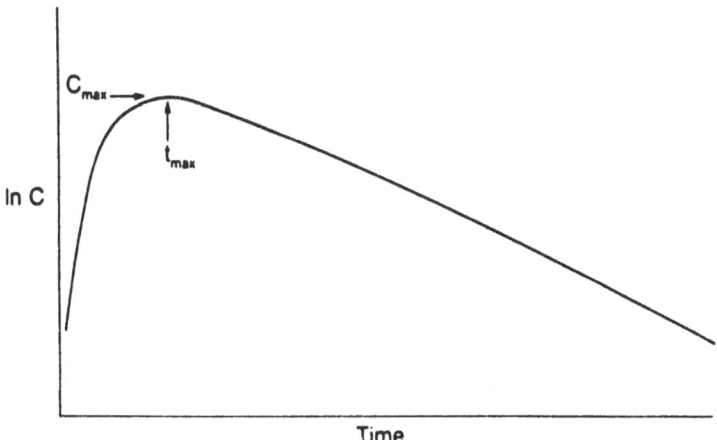

*Figure 3.* Effect of first-order absorption on concentration-time profile for a one-compartment model. Can be used to represent oral, intramuscular, intraperitoneal, or subcutaneous routes of delivery. From Collins and Dedrick [3].

taneous, and that the rate of absorption (e.g., mg/min) is proportional to the amount of drug remaining at the delivery site. Unike either bolus or continuous infusion cases, there is a rise in plasma concentration to a peak value, followed by a decrease in plasma concentration (Figure 3).

The concepts of principal interest are: (1) the magnitude of the peak concentration, (2) the time at which this peak occurs, and (3) the total amount absorbed. The first two parameters depend upon the rate constants for absorption and elimination. The first and third parameters depend upon the drug bioavailability, which is governed by pharmaceutical factors (e.g., ease of dose absorption, stability of dose at site of administration) and 'first-pass' effects. The first-pass effect includes any drug clearance prior to entry into the systemic circulation.

*Nonlinear processes*

If a drug exhibits a deviation from first-order (linear) kinetics, then a non-linear model is required. Nonlinearities may occur in drug excretion, metabolism, or protein binding. All of these processes may be saturable; thus, deviations from linearity occur when the maximum capacity is approached. On the other hand, all of these processes can be approximated by linear kinetics when the concentration is well below saturation. 5-Fluorouracil is the principal example for an anticancer drug [11]; ethanol, salicylate, and phenytoin are other well-known examples.

For a bolus injection, nonlinear behavior can be detected on a semilogarithmic plot by a rapidly increasing slope (Figure 4a) or as a straight-line

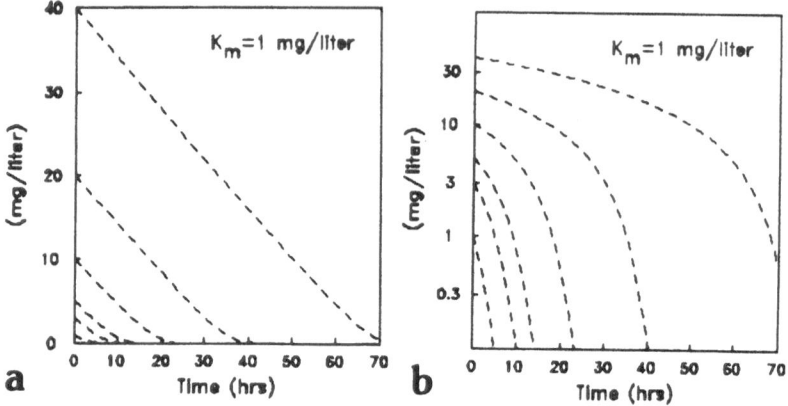

*Figure 4.* Nonlinear, one-compartment model with bolus input; (A) Rectilinear plot; (B) Semilogarithmic plot.

segment on a rectilinear plot (Figure 4b). For continuous infusion, the steady-state concentration depends upon the maximum elimination capacity, $V_{max}$, and the half-saturating concentration, $K_m$:

$$C_{ss} = G\,K_m/(V_{max} - G) \tag{3}$$

### Two-compartment linear model

There are many conceptual advantages to the one-compartment model, but it has been empirically found that most drugs require two compartments in order to adequately describe the observed pharmacokinetic behavior [12]. Figure 5 illustrates typical two-compartment kinetics following a bolus dose. There are many synonyms which are used interchangably: biphasic, biexponential, two spaces, two pools, and two compartments.

In addition to the empirical demonstration that most drugs have two-compartment kinetics, we need to consider the two-compartment model because we are ultimately faced with decisions such as dose size and dose interval which must be based upon a more realistic view of drug distribution. Finally, there is the possibility that the cells which we are trying to treat can be situated outside the region of the body which is easily sampled (namely, peripheral blood). Examples include 'sanctuaries' such as the central nervous system and testes.

In the terminology of pharmacokinetics, the first part of the curve shown in Figure 5 is called the alpha, or distributive phase. During this time, drug which has entered the first (central) compartment circulates to other areas of the body (lumped into the peripheral, or second compartment), which equilibrate with the central (first) compartment.

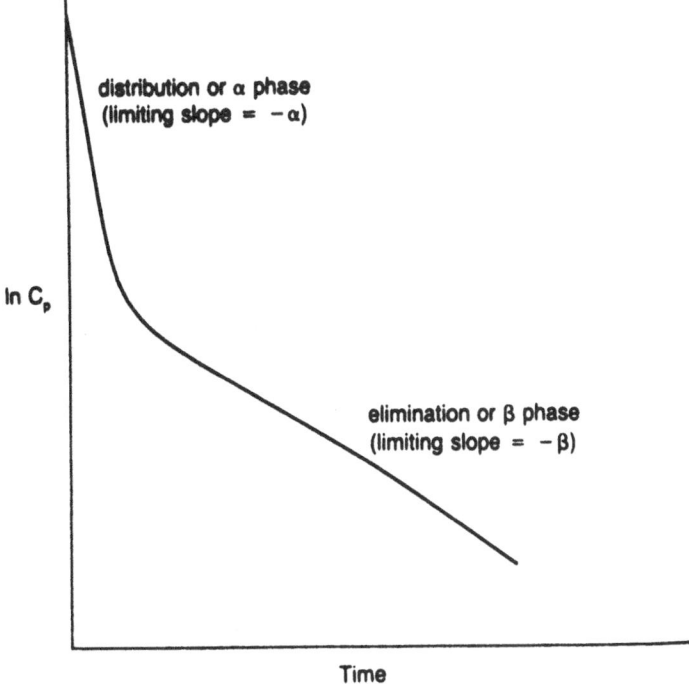

*Figure 5.* Concentration-time profile observed after bolus input to two-compartment model. From Collins and Dedrick [3].

The second part of the curve in Figure 5 is called the beta phase, the post-distributive phase, or the elimination phase. It is a bit misleading to use the term 'elimination phase', since drug elimination occurs from the first moment that a drug enters the body.

Analysis of *infusion* input to a two-compartment system is more complex than for the one-compartment model. The time to steady-state depends upon two half-times instead of one, and the type of behavior observed when the infusion is stopped depends upon how long the infusion was running. Finally, there is no simple loading dose which readily facilitates attainment of steady-state. However, the calculation of steady-state concentration is identical to that for the one-compartment case: $C_{ss} = G/CL_{TB}$.

## Compartmental vs. noncompartmental analysis

Once the two-compartment model made inroads into pharmacokinetics, models with three or more compartments were close behind. Such models have a place in some research settings, but are beyond the scope of practical clinical utility. Nonetheless, their existence does warrant a few comments.

It should be realized that there is a continuous spectrum of blood:tissue exchange rates in the body. Therefore, the separation of tissues into various boxes will always be somewhat arbitrary. There are techniques available to decide which model structure is most preferred (these techniques are largely statistical in nature), but the *application* of the pharmacokinetic exercise should determine the minimum complexity needed to reach a certain goal. In the focus of this presentation, those goals will be defined in terms of: (1) total exposure (clearance), (2) drug persistence in the body (half-life), or (3) distribution throughout the body (volume of distribution).

The methods of moment analysis ('noncompartmental methods') have emerged as an alternative to a specific characterization of drug kinetics in terms of identifiable compartments [13]. Clearance is calculated from dose divided by area under the plasma curve, as with compartmental methods. The calculation of a mean residence time by moment analysis replaces the multiple half-lives (alpha, beta, etc.) used in compartmental analysis. Finally, volume of distribution at steady-state is calculated from clearance and mean residence time.

## Other perspectives

Pharmacokinetics can sometimes appear to be exclusively concerned with modeling or the analysis of data in terms of models. There are other types of applications of pharmacokinetics. Sometimes, the goal is to describe the pharmacokinetic behavior of a drug in a patient population, including estimates of variance within the population or between groups. Clearly, this is a field in which statistics and pharmacokinetics interrelate strongly.

In some studies, the emphasis is upon the relationship between pharmacokinetics and drug effects. The correlation of plasma levels and thrombocytopenia [5] is an example of such a study. For drugs with extensive protein binding, pharmacologic effect should correlate with free drug concentration.

When a drug is first introduced into the clinic, pharmacokinetic studies are often performed to assist initial toxicity and efficacy evaluations.

## References

1. Gibaldi M, Perrier D: Pharmacokinetics, 2nd Edition. Marcel Dekker, New York, 1982.
2. Wagner JG: Fundamentals of clinical pharmacokinetics. Drug Intelligence Publications, Hamilton, II, 1975.
3. Collins JM, Dedrick RL: Pharmacokinetics of anticancer drugs. In: Pharmacologic principles of cancer treatment. Chabner BA (ed). W.B. Saunders, Philadelphia, PA 77–99, 1982.

4. Kerr IG, Jolivet J, Collins JM, Drake J, Chabner BA: Test dose for predicting high-dose methotrexate infusions. Clin Pharmacol Ther 33:44–51, 1903.

5. Egorin MJ, Van Echo DA, Tipping SJ, Olman EA, Whitacre MY, Thompson BW, Aisner J: Pharmacokinetics and dosage reduction of cis-diammine (1,1-cyclobutanedicarboxylato) platinum in patients with impaired renal function. Cancer Res 44:5432–5438, 1984.

6. Klecker RW, Jenkins JF, Kinsella TJ, Fine RL, Strong JL, Collins JM: Iododeoxyuridine and iodouracil: Clinical pharmacology and modulation of endogenous pyrimidines. Clin-Pharmacol Ther, accepted 1–9–85.

7. Collins JM, Klecker RW, Broder SA, Yarchoan Y, Lane HC, Fauci AS: Clinical pharmacology of suramin, a reverse transcriptase inhibitor with potential application for the treatment of AIDS patients. Proc Amer Soc Clin Oncol 4:2, 1985.

8. Greene RF, Collins JM, Jenkins JF, Speyer JL, Myers CE: Plasma pharmacokinetics of adriamycin and adriamycinol: Implications for the design of in vitro experiments and treatment protocols. Cancer Res 43:3417–3421, 1983.

9. Koch-Weser J, Sellers EM: Binding of drugs to serum albumin. New Engl J Med 294:526–531, 1976.

10. Zimm S, Ettinger L, Holcenberg J, Kamen BA, Vietti TJ, Belasco J, Shutta N, Balis F, Collins JM, Poplack DG: Pediatric phase I and clinical pharmacologic study of mercaptopurine administered as a prolonged intravenous infusion. Cancer Res, April issue, 1985.

11. Collins JM, Dedrick RL, King FG, Speyer JL, Myers CE: Nonlinear pharmacokinetic models for 5-fluorouracil in man: Intravenous and intraperitoneal routes. Clin Pharmacol Ther 28:235–246, 1980.

12. Oates JA, Wikinson GR: Principles of drug therapy, in Harrison's Principles of Internal Medicine, 8th ed. Mc Graw-Hill, New York, 1977.

13. Benet LZ, Galeazzi RL: Noncompartmental determination of the steady-state volume of distribution. J Pharm Sci 68:1071–1074, 1979.

# 2. The pharmacology of antineoplastic agents in children

FRANK M. BALIS

## Introduction

The greatest impact of cancer chemotherapy has been in the treatment of the malignant diseases of childhood. Diseases such as Wilms' tumor, acute lymphoblastic leukemia and lymphoma, which were uniformly fatal in the pre-chemotherapy era, now have complete remission rates of greater than 90%, and a majority of children with these disorders will be cured. Because of the successes in the treatment of these and other childhood cancers, the field of pediatric oncology has contributed significantly to the development of many of the principles of modern chemotherapy [1], including:

### Adjuvant chemotherapy

The addition of chemotherapy to surgery or radiation (multimodal approach) for the treatment of 'localized' tumors has been demonstrated to dramatically improve the prognosis of many common pediatric solid tumors, such as Wilms' tumor, rhabdomyosarcoma, retinoblastoma, lymphoma, and Ewing's sarcoma [2]. This approach, which was first used for Wilms' tumor, has now become standard therapy for most pediatric solid tumors and many adult malignancies, and is based on the recognition that 'localized' cancer is, in fact, a systemic disease [3].

### Combination chemotherapy

The concurrent administration of two or more antineoplastic agents evolved primarily in the treatment of acute lymphoblastic leukemia, where drug combinations improved both remission rate and remission duration compared to single agent therapy [4]. Although the concept arose from empirical observations, the effectiveness of combination chemotherapy has a scientific rationale [5]. The different sites of action of the drugs in the biochemical pathways of tumor cells can result in additive or synergistic cytotoxic effects and slow or prevent the emergence of clinical resistance.

### Intensive, intermittent therapy

Because of the steep dose-response curves for most antineoplastic agents, administration of maximally tolerated doses with intervening intervals off therapy to allow for recovery from toxicity appears to be more efficacious than continuous low dose therapy [6]. Clinical confirmation of the importance of administering full doses of these agents has been reported in acute lymphoblastic leukemia [7].

### Sanctuary therapy

The concept that tumor cells can be sequestered in an anatomic site that protects the cells from the cytotoxic effects of chemotherapy due to poor penetration of drugs into that tissue, was first recognized when CNS relapses occured in children with acute lymphoblastic leukemia in systemic remission. Intrathecal therapy was initiated to specifically treat cells in this sanctuary, first in patients with overt CNS leukemia and eventually in all newly diagnosed patients to prevent relapses [8].

### Preoperative chemotherapy

The value of chemotherapy as initial treatment for the primary tumor as well as micrometastases has been recently demonstrated in osteosarcoma [9]. The advantages of this approach include shrinking the primary tumor prior to surgery and, therefore, decreasing the extent of the surgical resection required to remove the primary tumor (in some instances allowing limb salvage procedures in place of amputation) and *in vivo* sensitivity testing of the drugs given preoperatively through histologic study of the resected primary tumor.

### Role of clinical pharmacology in cancer chemotherapy

Although the discovery and application of the above principles have led to a more rational approach to the treatment of childhood malignancies, the drug therapy of cancer remains empirical when compared to drug dosing and monitoring techniques utilized in other medical specialties. With exception of methotrexate, therapeutic drug monitoring has not been used in the management of cancer patients, despite the drugs' pharmacologic characteristics, such as low therapeutic index, potentially life-threatening toxicities, and wide individual variability in drug disposition, that would be strong indications for closely monitoring plasma drug concentration. Instead, antineoplastic agents are administered in a standard starting dose with subsequent dose modifications determined only by ensuing toxicities. The routine use of therapeutic drug monitoring has not been feasible because therapeutic and toxic levels of anticancer drugs have not been defined.

However, comprehensive pharmacokinetic studies of the commonly used antineoplastic agents have helped define the optimal dose, schedule, route of administration and dose modifications in patients with organ dysfunction [10]. In addition, the effective use of these toxic agents requires a fundamental knowledge of each drug's mechanism of action, absorption, distribution, metabolism, route of elimination and toxicities [10]. Since most pediatric malignancies are treated with a combination of these agents, potential drug interactions must also be anticipated. By investigating and defining these parameters the clinical pharmacologist attempts to make cancer chemotherapy safer and more efficacious.

*Mechanism of action*

Basic research into tumor cell biochemistry and the effects of the various antineoplastic agents on these metabolic pathways has led to a better understanding of how most of the commonly used anticancer drugs produce their cytotoxic effects and the mechanisms for the development of resistance to these agents. Ideally, drugs selected for combination regimens should produce complementary biochemical lesions and not be subject to same mechanisms of resistance. In addition, many drug interactions in antineoplastic therapy are at a biochemical level and some can be predicted from a knowledge of each drug's mechanism of action.

The biochemical interaction between methotrexate and 5-fluorouracil has generated interest and led to several ongoing clinical trials evaluating this drug combination. Methotrexate administered prior to 5-fluorouracil results in enhanced conversion of 5-fluorouracil to its active intracellular metabolite 5-FdUMP, but with the opposite sequence, 5-fluorouracil followed by methotrexate, the depletion of reduced folates by methotrexate is blocked. The methotrexate/5-fluorouracil sequence is synergistic *in vitro* and the 5-fluorouracil/methotrexate sequence is antagonistic [11, 12].

*Absorption*

Studies of the bioavailability of drugs help determine the most appropriate route of administration. For orally administered drugs, cytotoxic effect depends on adequate and consistent absorption into the systemic circulation.

Several anticancer drugs commonly used in the treatment of pediatric cancers have been routinely administered by the oral route, including methotrexate and 6-mercaptopurine. However, recent re-evaluations of the bioavailability of these two agents question the appropriateness of the oral route of administration for these drugs. Methotrexate absorption in children with acute lymphoblastic leukemia has been reported to be highly variable with no correlation found between dose and plasma levels achieved [13–15]. This variability appears to be primarily due to differences in drug bioavailability which ranged from 23 to 95% in one study [13]. Similarly, 6-mercatopurine bioavailability was also recently studied in children with acute lymphoblastic leukemia using a newly developed, specific high-pressure liquid chromatography assay. Plasma levels were highly variable and unpredictable and the fraction of drug absorbed was low (16%) [16]. The poor systemic availability is apparently the result of extensive pre-systemic metabolism of the drug in the liver or gut mucosa [17].

Since neither of these drugs is routinely monitored following oral dosing, it seems likely that some patients with acute lymphoblastic leukemia on maintenance therapy relapse because they do not achieve therapeutic levels of these drugs following an oral dose. This hypothesis is currently the subject of a prospective cooperative study involving the Childrens Cancer study group and the Pediatric Branch of the National Cancer Institute.

Other agents with highly variable oral absorption include melphalan [18] and 5-FU [19], while cyclophosphamide [20] and the nitrosoureas [21] are reported to be well absorbed.

*Distribution*

The distribution of a drug determines the amount that reaches the primary tumor or its metastases. Of particular interest to the pediatric oncologist is the distribution or penetration of the various antineoplastic agents into the CNS, since brain tumors are the most common solid tumor in children and other diseases like acute lymphoblastic leukemia and rhabdomyosarcoma can spread to the meninges. A number of factors influence the degree of penetration of a drug into the CNS, including the physico-chemical properties of the drug (lipophicity, degree of ionization, molecular weight), plasma protein or tissue binding of the drug, and the affinity for the drug of the various transport systems that facilitate the passage of endogenous molecules into the CNS. Table 1 lists the degree of CSF penetration for the antineoplastic drugs commonly used in pediatric oncology. In recent years an effort has been made to rationally design drugs that would readily penetrate the blood-brain barrier and be useful in the treatment of brain tumors. AZQ and spiromustine are two such agents currently undergoing clinical trials.

Another strategy used to overcome poor CNS penetration is to give higher systemic doses of the drug. Methotrexate penetrates into the CNS poorly but, because of the availability of leucovorin rescue, can be safely given in high-dose infusions with tolerable toxicity. We recently reported on 20 children with acute lymphoblastic leukemia who developed meningeal leukemia and were treated with a high-dose intravenous infusion regimen of methotrexate which was designed to achieve and maintain therapeutic methotrexate concentrations within the CSF without the need for concomitant intrathecal therapy. All 20 patients responded and 80% achieved a complete remission [32]. High-dose infusions of cytosine arabinoside and 6-mercatopurine also result in cytotoxic levels within the CSF [24, 25].

Alternatively, drugs can be administered directly into the CSF. When chemotherapy is administered intrathecally, the volume of CSF becomes the initial volume in which the drug is distributed and, therefore, determines the concentration of drug in the CSF. In the growing child CSF volume increases much more rapidly than body surface area, reaching the adult volume by three years of age [33]. Calculating intrathecal dose based on body surface area will underdose young children. Therefore, dosage schedules based on age have been recommended for methotrexate (Table 2).

*Table 1.* Penetration of the commonly used antineoplastic agents into the Cerebrospinal fluid.

| Agent | CSF: plasma ratio | Reference |
|-------|-------------------|-----------|
| Nitrosoureas | .30–.97 (Metabolite) | 21, 22 |
| Cytosine arabinoside | .40 (Std. dose) | 23 |
|  | .12 (High dose) | 24 |
| 6-Mercaptopurine | .27 | 25 |
| Vincristine | .04 | 26 |
| Methothrexate | .03 | 27 |
| Actinomycin D | <.10 | 28 |
| Cisplatin | .03 | 29 |
| Cylophosphamide | ND[a] (Parent drug) | 30 |
|  | .10 (Active metabolites) | 30 |
| Adriamycin | ND | 31 |

[a] ND: Not detectable in CSF.

This dosage regimen has been shown to be less neurotoxic [33]; and since incorporating this dosing scheme into their protocols, the Children's Cancer Study Group has noted a statistically significant decline in the CNS relapse rate in acute lymphoblastic leukemia from 12.5 to 6.9% [34].

Plasma protein binding of a drug can have a marked effect on the drug's distribution and can also effect the rate of elimination. Table 3 lists the published values of protein binding for the commonly used antineoplastic drugs. Of special interest is the interaction of cisplatin with plasma proteins. The interaction is a time-dependent one with the bound fraction increasing over 2 to 4 h to 90% [36] and having the characteristics of a first order process [43]. Once protein bound, the cisplatin is transformed to an inactive form [43]. The active (unbound) species of cisplatin can be separated from the bound form by ultrafiltration and have quite different disposition kinetics with much more rapid plasma clearance, primarily by renal excretion [43, 44].

*Table 2.* Dosing schedule for intrathecal methotrexate based on age/CSF volume relationship [33].

| Age (yr) | Dose (mg) |
| --- | --- |
| <1 | 6 |
| 1 | 8 |
| 2 | 10 |
| ≥3 | 12 |

*Table 3.* Protein binding of the commonly used antineoplastic agents.

| Agent | % Protein bound | Reference |
| --- | --- | --- |
| Methotrexate | 95[a] | 35 |
| Cisplatin | 90[b] | 36 |
| Adriamycin | 75 (Parent drug) | 37 |
| | 75 (Active metabolite) | 37 |
| Vincristine | 75 | 38 |
| Nitrosoureas | 50[b] | 39 |
| Cyclophosphamide | 15 (Parent drug) | 40 |
| | 60 (Active metabolite) | 40 |
| 6-Mercaptopurine | 20 | 41 |
| Cytosine arabinoside | <10 | 42 |

[a] Decreases to 60% with increasing methotrexate concentration.

[b] Nonspecific chemical interaction with protein leads to decomposition or inactivation.

*Metabolism*

Drug metabolism is not only a means of inactivating or detoxifying many antineoplastic agents but is also required for activation of several drugs. Cyclophosphamide, for example, is an inactive prodrug that requires hydroxylation by hepatic mixed function oxidases to express its cytotoxic effects [45]. These metabolites of cyclophosphamide can then be inactivated by further enzymatic oxidation. The requirement for hepatic activation obviously precludes the use of cyclophosphamide in regional chemotherapy such as intrathecal therapy or arterial infusions. Another type of activation is illustrated by several of the antimetabolites, particularly the purine and pyrimidine analogues (e.g., 6-mercaptopurine and cytosine arabinoside) which must be converted intracellularly to their corresponding nucleotide to exert their antitumor effect. With these agents intracellular pharmacokinetics should be considered along with plasma pharmacokinetics to optimize dose and schedule [46, 47].

Methotrexate also undergoes intracellular metabolism to form polyglutamated derivatives. The formation of these important metabolites is dependent on drug concentration and duration of exposure. These polyglutamated metabolites can not diffuse out of the cell allowing accumulation of much higher intracellular concentrations of methotrexate during drug exposure. In addition, they are retained in the cell after extracellular drug is removed, thus prolonging the cell's exposure to methotrexate [48]. Polyglutamates of methotrexate are apparently more potent inhibitors of the target enzyme of methotrexate, dihydrofolate reductase, and are also capable of inhibiting other enzymes in the thymidine and purine synthetic pathways not inhibited by methotrexate [48]. Dosing schedules that result in higher extracellular methotrexate concentration for prolonged periods of time will enhance the formation of these metabolites intracellularly.

Metabolism or biotransformation to pharmacologically less active compounds is the primary route of elimination for several anticancer drugs. Since drug metabolism is usually carried out by enzymes, disposition kinetics can be dose-dependent if the catabolic enzymes become saturated with increasing dose. Once saturation occurs, logarithmic rather than linear increases in plasma level may be observed with increasing dose. This phenomenon has been observed with 5-fluorouracil [49]. Another antimetabolite, cytosine arabinoside, which is cleared by enzymatic deamination, does not exhibit dose-dependent kinetics over a broad dosage range of 100 mg/sq m to 3000 mg/sq m [50].

The disposition kinetics of drugs cleared by metabolism can also be altered by other agents that compete for, inhibit or induce the enzymes responsible for biotransformation. 6-Mercaptopurine is cleared primarily by catabolism to thiouric acid by the enzyme xanthine oxidase. Allopurinol, an

22

inhibitor of xanthine oxidase, administered prior to treatment with oral 6-mercaptopurine will result in a 5-fold increase in peak concentration and area under the plasma concentration time curve of the 6-mercaptopurine [17]. Conversely, the chronic administration of phenobarbital to rats has been shown to reduce the antitumor activity of lomustine (CCNU) apparently through increased metabolism of the drug by hepatic microsomal enzymes [51].

*Route of elimination*

The duration of drug exposure is primarily determined by the rate of drug elimination. Most anticancer drugs are eliminated by renal excretion, biotransformation (usually by hepatic enzymes), or biliary excretion. Table 4 lists the primary route of elimination for most of the commonly used anticancer agents. Patients undergoing treatment for cancer often suffer from other illnesses or are receiving other drugs that can lead to hepatic or renal dysfunction and result in altered disposition kinetics of a variety of anticancer drugs [52]. These alterations in kinetics often lead to an increase in toxicity. Knowledge of the route of elimination of the anticancer drugs is essential in predicting and preventing potentially serious toxicity in patients

*Table 4.* The route of elimination and recommended dosage modifications with organ dysfunction for the commonly used antineoplastic agents.

| Agent | Route of elimination | Recommended dose modification | Reference |
|---|---|---|---|
| Methotrexate | R [a] | Low dose – ↓ dose 50% for creat. of 1.2–2.0 mg%. Hold if creat. >2.0 mg% High dose – Hold if creat. cl. <50 to 75% of normal | 53 |
| Actinomycin D | B, R | | 28 |
| Cyclophosphamide | M* | ↓ Dose for creat. cl. <20 ml/min | 54 |
| 6-Mercaptopurine | M, R [b] | | 55, 25 |
| Cisplatin | M, R | ↓ Dose for low creat. cl. | 52 |
| Nitrosoureas | M* | | 56 |
| Vincristine | M, B | ↓ Dose 50% for bili. >3.0 mg% | 57 |
| Adriamycin | M*, B | ↓ Dose 50% for bili. 1.2–3.0 mg% ↓ Dose 75% for bili. >3.0 mg% | 31 |
| Cytosine arabinoside | M | | 23 |

[a] R: renal excretion; B: biliary excretion; M: metabolism; M*: metabolism to both active and inactive metabolites.
[b] For i.v. dose 30% excreted unchanged in the urine.

with organ dysfunction. Recommended dosage modifications for these patients are also given in Table 4.

*Toxicity*

Most oncologists are all too familiar with the toxicities produced by the antineoplastic agents. Because of the low therapeutic index of this class of drugs, the oncologist and cancer patient often have to accept certain side effects associated with the dose of an anticancer drug required to produce a significant oncolytic effect. In designing drug combinations, overlapping toxicities should be avoided so that maximally effective doses of each drug can be administered. In addition, organ dysfunction caused by one drug can alter the elimination of other agents. For example, the clearance of methotrexate, which is dependent on renal excretion, can be altered by nephrotoxic drugs like cisplatin or high-dose methotrexate [52].

The long-term side effects of antineoplastic therapy must also be of concern to the pediatric oncologist, since more children are now surviving longer and many are probably cured. Late effects on growth and development, the reproductive system and nervous system and the occurrence of second malignacies will require further study in long-term survivors of childhood cancer.

**Future role of clinical pharmacology**

The goal of the clinical pharmacologist is to make cancer chemotherapy less toxic and more efficacious, either through the development of new agents with greater selectivity or the more effective use of existing ones. This could be accomplished with several of the established anticancer drugs by defining toxic and therapeutic drug levels and closely monitoring patients on therapy. The value of therapeutic drug monitoring in the management of patients receiving high-dose methotrexate has been clearly established [58]. The identification of patients with delayed clearance and institution of more intensive leucovorin rescue can lessen or prevent severe or potentially fatal toxicities. In addition, discontinuation of leucovorin rescue as soon as plasma methotrexate levels fall below nontoxic levels may lessen the possibility of rescuing the tumor that could occur with excessive or more prolonged empirical leucovorin rescue.

A more rational approach to designing treatment regimens should incorporate knowledge gained from *in vitro* experiments. Tumor cell biochemistry and growth kinetics should be considered when selecting the dose and schedule of anticancer drugs. Such a timed-sequential regimen, based on a knowledge of when maximal tumor regrowth occurs, appears to be effective in producing long-term remissions in patients with acute nonlymphocytic leukemia [59].

It is likely that in some patients, one or more agents in empirical drug combinations are ineffective against that individual's tumor and, therefore, only add to toxicity and may prevent the patient from receiving full doses of the effective drugs. Sensitivity testing, which revolutionized antimicrobial therapy, would allow the oncologist to tailor therapy to the individual patient as is currently done in treating serious infections. Recent reports of correlations between drug sensitivity in an *in vitro* human tumor stem cell assay and clinical tumor response (or lack of response) are encouraging [60, 61], but the current limitations to the use of such an assay, including the low cloning efficiency [61] and the two to three week wait from biopsy until results are available [60], will have to be overcome before it is practical.

The clinical pharmacologist must also solve the problem of clinical drug resistance, both acquired and naturally occurring. Once the mechanisms of resistance [62] and patterns of cross-resistance [63] are defined for individual agents, more effective drug combinations can be designed to prevent the development of clinical resistance or even exploit drug resistance in the situation where resistant tumors are collaterally sensitive to other agents [62].

## References

1. Bleyer WA: Antineoplastic agents. In: Pediatric Pharmacology: Therapeutic Principles in Practice. Yaffe S (ed). Grune & Stratton, Inc., New York, 349–377, 1980.
2. Hammond GD, Bleyer WA, Hartman JR, Hays DM, Jenkins DT: The team approach to the management of pediatric cancer. Cancer 41:29–35, 1978.
3. Martin DS: The scientific basis for adjuvant chemotherapy. Cancer Treat Rev 8:169–189, 1981.
4. Henderson EH, Samaha RJ: Evidence that drugs in multiple combinations have materially advanced the treatment of human malignancies. Cancer Res 29:2272–2280, 1969.
5. DeVita VT, Schein PSÇ: The use of drugs in combination for the treatment of cancer, rationale and results. N Engl J Med 288:998–1005, 1973.
6. Frei E, Canellos GP: Dose: a critical factor in cancer chemotherapy. Am J Med 69:585–594, 1980.
7. Pinkel D, Hernandez K, Borella L, Holton C, Aur R, Samoy G, Pratt C: Drug dosage and remission duration in childhood lymphocytic leukemia. Cancer 27:247–256, 1971.
8. Pochedly C: Prophylactic CNS therapy in childhood acute leukemia. Am J Pediatr Hematol Oncol 1:119–126, 1979.
9. Rosen G, Caparros B, Huvos AG, Kosloff C, Nirenberg A, Marcove RC, Lane JM, Mehta B, Urban C: Preoperative chemotherapy for osteogenic sarcoma. Cancer 49:1221–1230, 1982.
10. Erlichman C, Donehower RC, Chabner BA: The practical benefits of pharmacokinetics in the use of antineoplastic agents. Cancer Chemother Pharmacol 4:139–145, 1980.

11. Cadman E, Heimer R, Davis L: Enhanced 5-fluorouracil nucleotide formation after methotrexate administration: explanation for drug synergism. Science 205:1135–1137, 1979.

12. Bowen D, White JC, Goldman ID: Basis for fluoropyrimidine-induced antagonism to methotrexate in Ehrlich ascites tumor cells in vitro. Cancer Res 38:219–222, 1978.

13. Balis FM, Savitch JL, Bleyer WA: Pharamcokinetics of oral methotrexate in children. Cancer Res 43:2342–2345, 1983.

14. Kearney PJ, Light PA, Preece A, Mott MG: Unpredictable serum levels after oral methotrexate in children with acute lymphoblastic leukemia. Cancer Chemother Pharmacol 3:117–120, 1979.

15. Pinkerton CR, Welshman SG, Dempsey SI, Bridges JM, Glasgow JFT: Absorption of methotrexate under standardized conditions in children with acute lymphoblastic leukemia. Br J Cancer 42:640–645, 1980.

16. Zimm S, Collins JM, Riccardi R, O'Neill D, Barang PK, Chabner BA, Poplack DG: Variable bioavailabilty of oral 6-mercaptopurine: Is maintanence chemotherapy in acute lymphoblastic leukemia being optimally delivered? N Engl J Med 308:1005–1009, 1983.

17. Zimm S, Collins JM, O'Neill D, Chabner BA, Poplack DG: Inhibition of first-pass metabolism in cancer chemotherapy: Interaction of 6-mercaptopurine and allopurinol. Clin Pharmacol Ther 34:810–815, 1983.

18. Alberts DS, Chang SY, Chen HS, Evans TL, Moon TE: Oral melphalan kinetics. Clin Pharmacol Ther 26:737–745, 1979.

19. Fraile RJ, Baker LH, Buroker TR, Horwitz J, Vaitkevicius VK: Pharmacokinetics of 5-fluorouracil administered orally, by rapid intravenous and by slow infusion. Cancer Res 40:2223–2228, 1980.

20. D'Incalci M, Bolis G, Facchinetti T, Mangioni C, Morasca L, Morazzoni P, Salmona M: Decreased half life of cyclophosphamide in patients under continual treatment. Europ J Cancer 15:7–10, 1979.

21. DeVita VT, Denham C, Davidson JD, Oliverio VT: The physiological disposition of the carcinostatic 1,3-bis (2-chloroethyl)-1-nitrosourea (BCNU) in man and animals. Clin Pharmacol Ther 8:566–577, 1967.

22. Sponzo RW, DeVita VT, Oliverio VT: Physiologic disposition of 1-(2-chloroethyl)-3-cyclohexyl-1-nitrosourea (CCNU) and 1-(2-chloroethyl)-3-(4-methyl cyclohexyl)-1-nitrosourea (MeCCNU) in man. Cancer 31:1154–1159, 1973.

23. Ho DHW, Frei E: Clinical pharmacology of 1-$\beta$-D-arabinofuranosyl cytosine. Clin Pharmacol Ther 12:944–954, 1971.

24. Slevin ML, Piall EM, Aherne GW, Harvey VJ, Johnston A, Lister TA: Effect of dose and schedule on pharmacokinetics of high-dose cytosine arabinoside in plasma and cerebrospinal fluid. J Clin Oncol 1:546–551, 1983.

25. Zimm S, Ettinger LJ, Holcenberg JS, Kamen BA, Vietti TJ, Belasco J, Cogliano-Shutta N, Balis F, Lavi LE, Collins JM, Poplack DG: Phase I and clinical pharamcologic study of mercaptopurine administered as a prolonged intravenous infusion, Cancer Res, 1985 (in press).

26. Jackson DV, Sethi VS, Spurr CL, McWhorter JM: Pharmacokinetics of vincristine in the cerebrospinal fluid of humans. Cancer Res 41:1466–1468, 1981.

27. Bleyer WA, Poplack DG: Clinical studies on the central-nervous-system pharmacology of methotrexate. In: Clinical Pharmacology of Anti-neoplastic Drugs. Pinedo, Boelsma (eds). Elsevier/North Holland Biomedical Press, Amsterdam, 115–131, 1978.

28. Tattersall MHN, Sodergren JE, Sengupta SK, Trites DH, Modest EJ, Frei E: Pharmacokinetics of actinomycin D in patients with malignant melanoma. Clin Pharmacol Ther 17:701–707, 1975.

29. Higby DJ, Buchholtz L, Chary K, Avellanosa A, Henderson ES: Kinetics of cis-platinum (DDP) with intensive diuresis. Proc Am Assoc Cancer Res 18:110, 1977.

30. Jardine I, Fenselau C, Appler M, Kan M-N, Brundrett RB, Colvin M: Quantitation by gas chromatography-chemical ionization mass spectrometry of cyclophosphamide, phosphoramide mustard, and nornitrogen mustard in the plasma and urine of patients receiving cyclophosphamide therapy. Cancer Res 38:408–415, 1970.

31. Benjamin RS, Wiernik PH, Bachur NR: Adriamycin chemotherapy – efficacy, safety, and pharmacologic basis of an intermittent single high-dosage schedule. Cancer 33:19–27, 1974.

32. Balis FM, Savitch JL, Bleyer WA, Reaman GH, Poplack DG: Remission induction of meningeal leukemia with high dose intravenous methotrexate. J Clin Oncol, 1985 (in press).

33. Bleyer WA: Clinical pharmacology of intrathecal methotrexate II. An improved dosage regimen derived from age-related pharmacokinetics. Cancer Treat Rep 61:1419–1425, 1977.

34. Bleyer WA, Level C, Sather HN, Niebrugge DJ, Coccia PF, Siegel S, Littman PS, Leikin SL, Miller DR, Chard RL Hammond GD: Reduction in central nervous leukemia with a pharmacokinetically derived intrathecal-methotrexate dosage regimen. In: Mastrangelo R, Poplack DG, Riccardi R (eds). Martinus Nijhoff Pulishers, Boston, 27–37, 1983.

35. Steele WH, Lawrence JR, Stuart JFB, McNeill CA: The protein binding of methotrexate by the serum of normal subjects. Europ J Clin Pharmacol 15:363–366, 1979.

36. DeConti RC, Toftness BR, Lange RC, Creasy WA: Clinical and pharmacological studies with cis-diamminedichloroplatinum (II). Cancer Res 33:1310–1315, 1973.

37. Greene RF, Collins JM, Jenkins JF, Speyer JL, Myers CE: Plasma pharmacokinetics of adriamycin and adriamycinol: implications for the design of in vitro experiments and treatment protocols. Cancer Res 43:3417–3421, 1983.

38. Donigian DW, Owellen RJ: Interaction of vinblastine, vincristine and colchicine with serum proteins. Biochem Pharmacol 22:2113–2119, 1973.

39. Weinkam RJ, Liu T-YJ, Lin H-S: Protein mediated chemical reactions of chloroethylnitrosoureas. Chem-Biol Interactions 31:167–177, 1980.

40. Bagley CM, Bostich FW, Devita VT: Clinical pharmacology of cyclophosphamide. Cancer Res 33:226–233, 1973.

41. Loo TL, Luce JK, Sullivan MP, Frei E: Clinical pharmacologic observations on 6-mercaptopurine and 6-methylthiopurine ribonucleoside. Clin Pharmacol Ther 9:180–194, 1960.

42. Haskell CM: Cancer Treatment. W.B.Saunders Co, Philadelphia, 55, 1980.

43. Gormley PE, Bull JM, LeRoy AF, Cysyk R: Kinetics of cis-dichlorodiammineplatinum. Clin Pharmacol Ther 25:351–357, 1979.

44. Himmelstein KJ, Patton TF, Belt RJ, Taylor S, Repta AJ, Sternson LA: Clinical kinetics of intact cisplatin and some related species. Clin Pharmacol Ther 29:658–664, 1981.

45. Fenselau C, Kan M-NN, Subba Rao S, Myles A, Friedman OM, Colvin M: Identification of aldophosphamide as a metabolite of cyclophosphamide in vitro and in vivo in humans. Cancer Res 37:2538–2543, 1977.

46. Iacoboni S, Plunkett W, Danhauser L, Estey E, Walters R, Keating M, McCredie K, Freireich EJ: Clinical results of pharmacologically directed schedules of high dose Ara-C for relapsed acute leukemia. Proc Am Soc Clin Oncol 3:200, 1984.

47. Zimm S, Johnson GE, Chabner BA, Poplack DG: Cellular pharmacokinetics of 6-mercaptopurine in human leukemia and lymphoma cells. Proc Am Assoc Cancer Res 25:349, 1984.

48. Jolivet J, Cowan KH, Curt GA, Clendenin NJ, Chabner BA: The pharmacology and clinical use of methotrexate. n Engl J Med 309:1094–1104, 1983.

49. Collins JM, Dedrick RL, King FG, Speyer JL, Myers CE: Nonlinear pharmacokinetic models for 5-fluorouracil in man. Clin Pharmacol Ther 28:235–246, 1980.

50. Hande KR, Stein RS, McDonough DA, Greco FA, Wolff SN: Effects of high dose cytarabine. Clin Pharmaxol Ther 31:669–674, 1982.

51. Levin VA, Sterns J, Byrd A, Finn A, Weinkam RJ: The effect of phenobarbital pretreatment on the antitumor activity of 1,3-bis(2-chloroethyl)-1-nitrosourea (BCNU), 1-(2-chloroethyl)-3-cyclohexyl-1-nitrosourea (CCNU) and 1-(2 chloroethyl)-3-(2,6-dioxo-3-piperidyl)-1-nitrosourea (PCNU), and the plasma pharmacokinetics and biotransformation of BCNU. J Pharmacol Exp Ther 208:1–6, 1979.
52. Powis G: Effect of human renal and hepatic disease on the pharmacokinetics of anticancer drugs. Cancer Treat Rev 9:85–124, 1982.
53. Balis FM, Holcenberg JS, Bleyer WA: Clinical pharmacokinetics of commonly used anticancer drugs. Clin Pharmacokinet 8:202–232, 1983.
54. Bramwell V, Calvert RT, Edwards G, Scarffe H, Crowther D: The disposition of cyclophosphamide in a group of myeloma patients. Cancer Chemother Pharmacol 3:253–259, 1979.
55. Elion GB: Biochemistry and pharmacology of purine analogues. Fed Proc 26:898–904, 1967.
56. Schein PS, Heal J, Green D, Wolley PV: Pharmacology of nitrosourea antitumor agents. Antibiot Chemother 23:64–75, 1978.
57. Bender RA, Chabner BA: Tubulin binding agents. In: Pharmacologic Principles of Cancer Treatment. Chabner BA (ed). W.B. Saunders Vo, Philadelphia, 256–268, 1982.
58. Chabner BA: Methotrexate. In: Pharmacologic Principles of Cancer Treatment. Chabner BA (ed). W.B. Saunders Co, Philadelphia, 229–255, 1982.
59. Vaughan WP, Karp JE, Burke PJ: Long chemotherapy free remissions after single-cycle timed-sequential chemotherapy for acute myelocytic leukemia. Cancer 45:859–865, 1980.
60. Salmon SE, Hamburger AW, Soehnlen B, Durie BGM, Alberts DS, Moon TE: Quantitation of differential sensitivity of human tumor cells to anticancer drugs. N Engl J Med 298:1321–1327, 1970.
61. Von Hoff DD, Casper J, Bradley E, Sandbach J, Jones D, Makuch R: Association between human tumor colony-forming assay results and response of an individual patient's tumor to chemotherapy. Am J Med 70:1027–1032, 1981.
62. Bertino JR, Skeel RT: Resistence to chemotherapeutic agents. In: Pharmacology and the Future of Man. Karger, Basel, 376–392, 1973.
63. Schabel FM, Skipper HE, Trader MW, Laster WR, Griswold DP, Corbett TH: Establishment of cross-resistance profiles for new agents. Cancer Treat Rep 67:905–922, 1903.

# 3. Clinical pharmacology of anticancer drugs in children: differences and similarities between children and adults

WILLIAM E. EVANS, CLINTON F. STEWART,
MICHAEL L. CHRISTENSEN and WILLIAM R. CROM

## Introduction

Chemotherapy is currently a major component of the therapy for most disseminated pediatric cancers. Through the development of effective drugs and the optimal utilization of these agents, major advances have been achieved in the response rate, disease-free survival, and cure of several pediatric cancers, including acute lymphocytic leukemia and Hodgkin's disease. Since improvement in the efficacy of cancer chemotherapy can result from better utilization of currently available drugs, in addition to the development of new agents, knowledge of these drugs' pharmacokinetics in children is important for the design of optimal dosage schedules. As with many therapeutic classes of drugs, the pharmacokinetics of antineoplastic drugs have not been studied extensively in children, compared to adults. Before the 1970s, very little had been published about drug disposition in children, leading Shirkey to coin the appropriate term 'therapeutic orphan' [1] to describe the fact that many drugs are usually not evaluated in children until well after they have been investigated and approved for use in adults. Since 1968, much work has been published describing drug disposition, but mainly in the period of rapid maturational change, from birth to infancy (1 year). There is still a paucity of data describing drug disposition in children greater than one year of age. As a preface to the review of selected anticancer drugs, age-related changes in the four major determinants of drug disposition (absorption, distribution, metabolism and elimination) are briefly reviewed to familiarize the reader with the concepts of drug disposition in children. For further information the reader is referred to one of the many excellent reviews on the topic [2–5].

There are many physiochemical and physiological factors that may affect drug absorption in children. Physiochemical determinants include molecular size and shape, solubility at the site of absorption, degree of ionization, relative lipid solubility of the ionized versus nonionized form, and formu

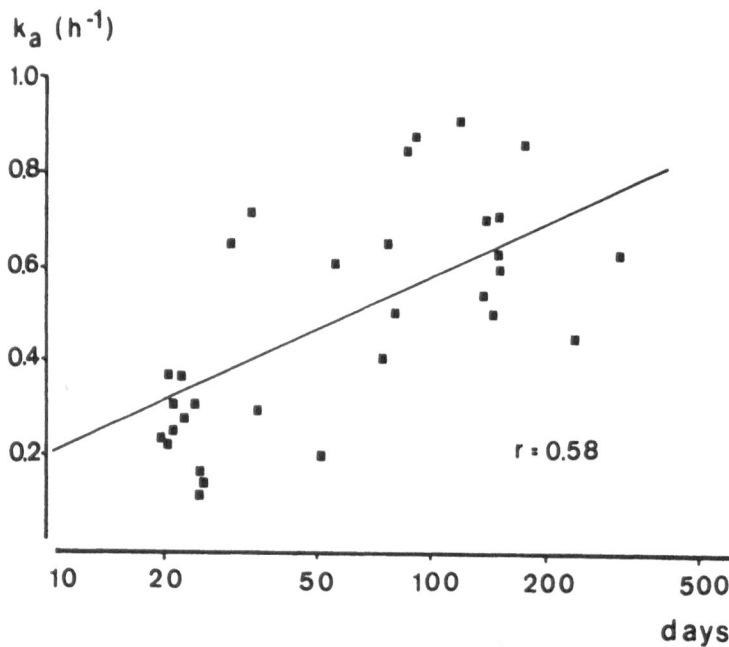

*Figure 1.* Rate constant of enteral absorption (Ka) of phenobarbital in relation to age after a single oral dosage of 5–10 mg phenobarbital per kg bodyweight. Reproduced with permission from reference 10.

lation of the pharmaceutical preparation. These factors are drug specific and are therefore relatively fixed; whereas, the physiological factors, which include circulation to the site of absorption, surface area of the site of absorption, gastric and intestinal transit time, gastric and intestinal pH and gastrointestinal contents (such as microflora and enzymes) are subject to maturational changes [6].

Relatively little has been published regarding drug bioavailability and the rate of absorption of drugs in children over one year old. Disregard for the determinants of drug absorption (e.g., absorption rate, volume of distribution, elimination) may lead to wrong conclusions, as in the case of the studies of nafcillin, penicillin G, and ampicillin where increased dose-adjusted concentration and area under the concentration time curve were attributed to increased absorption [7–9]. These studies were not designed to exclusively evaluate the rate or extent of absorption, and as the authors observed the differences were probably a result of changes in renal elimination, not absorption. The appropriately designed study of Heimann and associates found that the *amount* of phenobarbital, digoxin, and β methyl digoxin absorbed was not correlated with age, but the *rate* of absorption was significantly slower in neonates [10]. Figure 1 demonstrates the relationship observed by Heiman between age and rate of absorption for phenobarbital. Additional studies in children are necessary in order to specifically assess age-related changes in the absorption of most anticancer drugs.

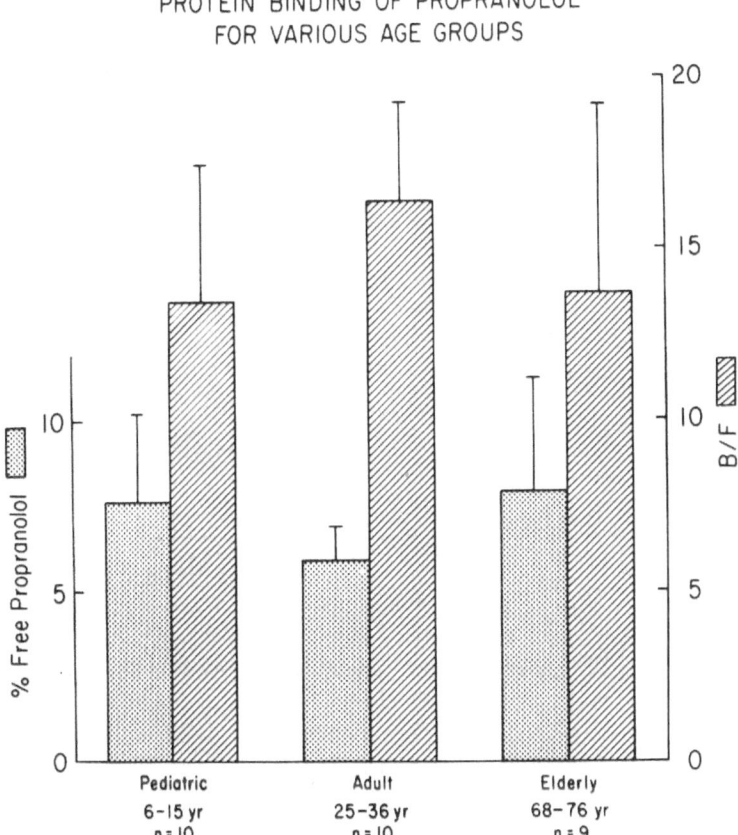

PROTEIN BINDING OF PROPRANOLOL
FOR VARIOUS AGE GROUPS

Bendayan Eur. J Clin Pharmacol 1984; 26:251-254.

*Figure 2.* Protein binding of propranolol (as expressed by % free) for pediatric (6–16 yr), adult (25–36 yr), and elderly (68–76 yr) patients. Adapted from reference 13.

Drug distribution in children is also affected by physiochemical and physiological factors. The physiological factors which undergo maturational changes include vascular perfusion, body composition, tissue binding characteristics, and the extent of plasma and protein binding [11]. While the neonate experiences extreme changes in body composition, the child (greater than one year) undergoes relatively minor changes, which consist of a decrease in total body water and extracellular water as a percentage of total body weight [12]. There are, however, major changes in percentage of adipose tissue that occur after infancy in both genders. The varying affinities that tissues have for binding to drugs as well as the maturational changes in the amount and composition of such tissues may significantly alter drug distribution. Finally, protein binding may be altered in children by the presence of pathologic conditions, changes in the amount and type of protein

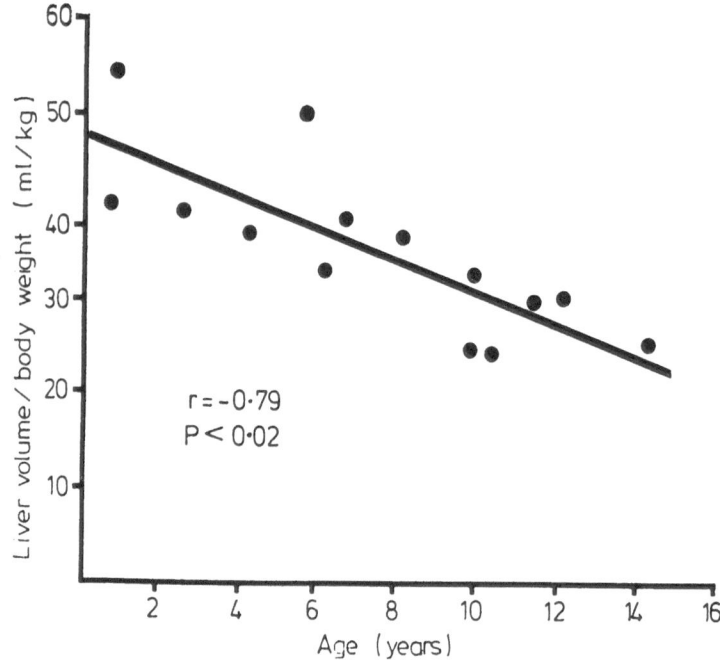

*Figure 3.* Plot of liver volume per body weight versus age in years. Reproduced with permission from reference 16.

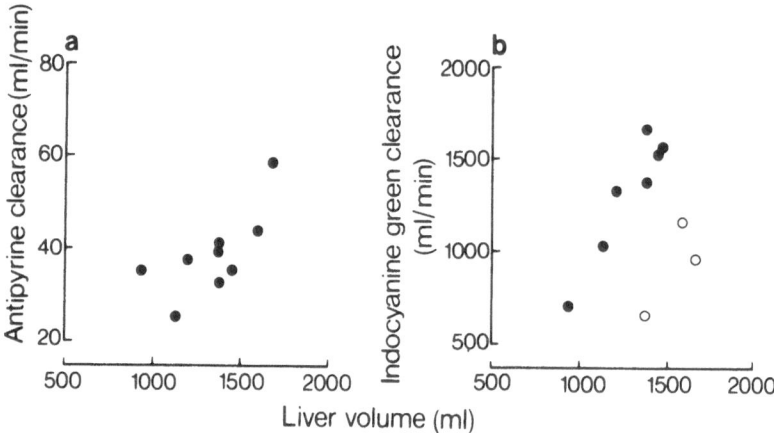

*Figure 4.* The relationships (A) between liver volume and autipyrine clearance (nine healthy subjects) and (B) between liver volume and indocyanine green clearance (ten healthy subjects) before enzyme induction. Open circles identify subject with an apparently low indocyanine green clearance for their liver volume. For (A) r = 0.69, p<0.05. Reproduced with permission from reference 17.

present and changes in the affinity of the drug-protein complex. These alterations have been observed mainly in the neonate, and protein binding in the child greater than one year seems to be roughly equivalent to that of an

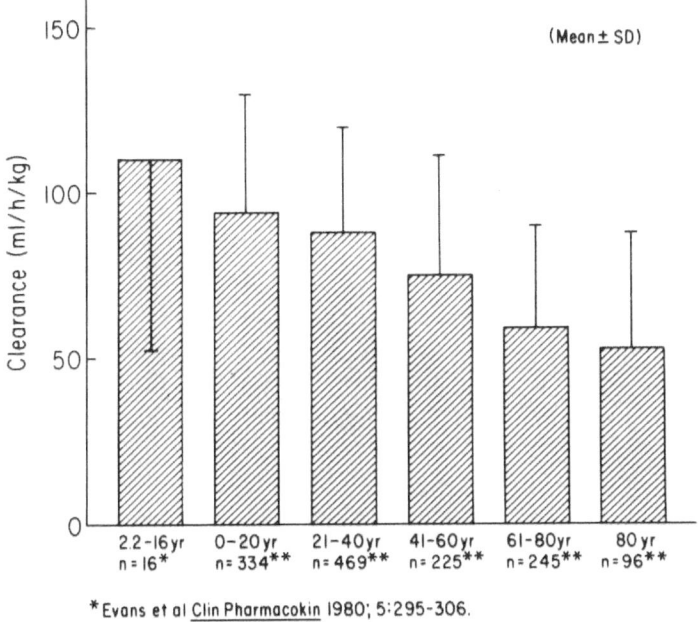

GENTAMICIN CLEARANCE FOR VARIOUS AGE GROUPS

*Evans et al Clin Pharmacokin 1980; 5:295-306.

**Zaske et al Antimicrob Ag Chemo 1982; 21:407-411.

*Figure 5.* Bar graph of gentamicin clearance demonstrating the relationship between clearance and age.

adult [13–15] (see Figure 2). In general, major alterations in drug distribution appear to occur in the first year of life, however wide inter- and intra-patient variability in body composition, tissue binding and protein binding may occur in infants and older children.

The rates of maturation of the two major categories of drug metabolism – Phase I and Phase II – vary from one child to another. In addition, various metabolic pathways in each of these processes mature at different rates. Thus, it is almost impossible to predict the effect of maturation on drug metabolism [4]. Quantitative electron microscopy has documented that there is an increase in hepatocyte membrane area from one to four years and that after four years the hepatocyte membrane area approaches adult levels [16]. Morselli and associates have long observed a lower steady-state peak concentration of anticonvulsants per mg/kg dose in children compared to adults, suggesting more rapid clearance in children [17]. Other studies have demonstrated that liver volume (relative to body weight) correlates with age [18, 19], and that antipyrine clearance and indocyanine green clearance correlated with liver volume (Figures 3 and 4). It is interesting that these studies found no significant age-related change when liver volume was

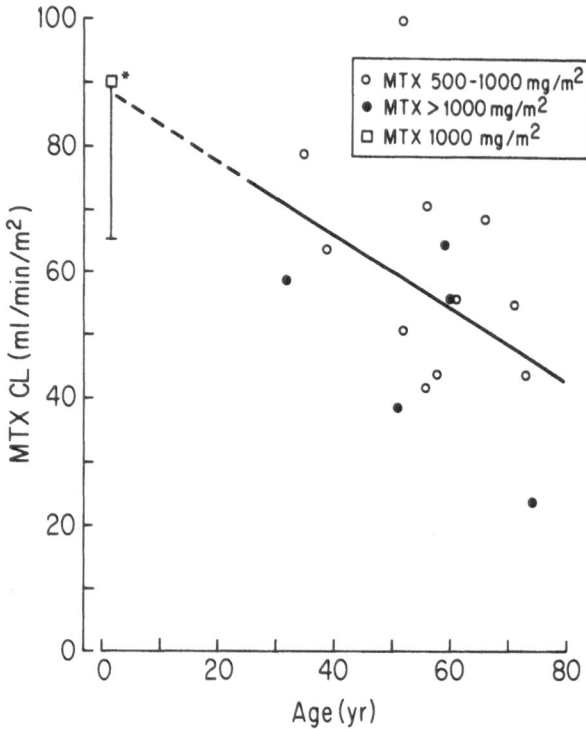

*Figure 6.* MTX systemic clearance versus age in years. Solid line represents data from Kerr et al [23]. Dashed line connects the solid line with the mean (□ *) MTX systemic clearance from the study of Evans et al. (229).

expressed as a function of body surface area. These data suggest that when drug clearance is related to liver volume, clearance normalized to body weight (ml/m/km) may change with age, whereas, clearance normalized to body surface area (ml/m/m²) may not change with age.

The processes that affect renal elimination of drugs include renal blood flow, glomerular filtration, tubular reabsorption and secretion. These processes undergo extensive maturational changes both in utero and during the first few weeks of life [20]. The clearance of drugs may be greater in infants and young children than in adults, due to greater GFR and more developed renal filtration and secretion, relative to reabsorption. An example of this can be found in the studies of aminoglycoside and methotrexate disposition in children, where clearances (or half-lives) are significantly faster than in adults [21–23] (Figures 5 and 6).

When searching for age-related pharmacokinetic differences between children and adults, it is important to rule out variables other than age (i.e., disease status, prior or concomitant therapy, etc.) before concluding that observed differences are related to age. Likewise, when age-related differences are observed, it is important to determine what age-related physiological changes are responsible for pharmacokinetic differences. It is also possible that more than one pharmacokinetic parameter may change with age (i.e., clearance and distribution volume), and that correlated age-related changes in these two parameters may occur yielding no age-related change in half-life. This possibility is understood best when one considers the following relationship between clearance (CL), volume of distribution (V) and half-life ($T_{1/2}$) in a first-order one-compartment model;

$$T_{1/2} = \frac{0.693}{Ke} \tag{1}$$

where Ke is the first-order elimination rate constant and 0.693 is the natural logarithm of 2. It follows that,

$$T_{1/2} = \frac{0.693}{Ke} \cdot \frac{V}{V},$$

which yields,

$$T_{1/2} = \frac{0.693 \cdot V}{Ke \cdot V}. \tag{2}$$

Since CL = Ke $\cdot$ V, Equation 2 can be rearranged to yield;

$$T_{1/2} = \frac{0.693 \cdot V}{CL}.$$

Therefore, if one considers the following example, where for patient A (age 4) CL = 100 ml/min/m$^2$ and V = 1000 ml/m$^2$, and for patient B (age 50) CL = 50 and V = 500, the $T_{1/2}$ for both is 6.93 min, despite a two-fold difference in clearance and volume of distribution. The serum concentration-time curves for these two hypothetical patients is simulated in Figure 7, depicting identical half-lives but clearly different concentrations following a 250 mg/m$^2$ intravenous bolus dose.

This simple example demonstrates the need to thoroughly examine the pharmacokinetics of a drug before excluding the possibility of age-related differences in the disposition of drugs.

The following sections of this chapter attempt to identify and critique pediatric pharmacokinetic and pharmacodynamic studies which have been published, using the more extensive adult studies for comparison or as a source of reference when pediatric data are not available.

## Anthracyclines (Doxorubicin and Daunorubicin)

Doxorubicin (Adriamycin, Adria Laboratories) and daunorubicin (Cerubidine, Ives) are anthracycline antibiotics which have each demonstrated anti-

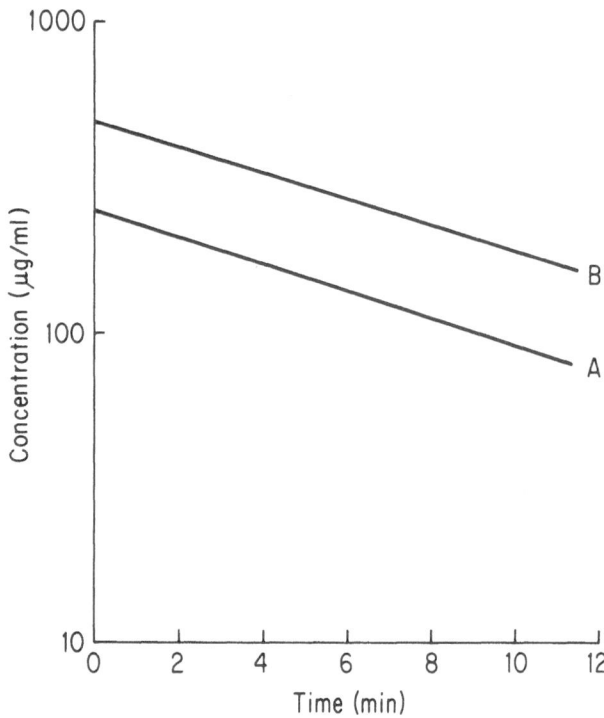

*Figure 7.* Simulation of a concentration-versus-time plot of two patients given the same dose of drug 250 mg/m$^2$ IV bolus; patient A has a clearance of 100 ml/min/m$^2$ and a volume of 1000 ml/m$^2$, whereas Patient B has a clearance of 50 ml/min/m$^2$ and a volume of 500 ml/m$^2$. Both patients have a half-life of 6.9 min, assuming a one-compartment first-order pharmacokinetic model.

neoplastic activity in several malignant diseases in children [24]. Doxorubicin is active in the treatment of acute leukemia (both lymphocytic and non-lymphocytic), lymphomas (Hodgkin's and non-Hodgkin's), embyronal rhabdomyosarcoma, Ewing's sarcoma, Wims' tumor, neuroblastoma, ovarian tumors, embryonal carcinomas, malignant teratomas, osteosarcoma and hepatoblastoma [24]. It is one of the most widely used and important drugs in the treatment of childhood cancer. Daunorubicin has a more limited spectrum of activity [25], but it is active in the treatment of acute leukemia and is used widely in remission-induction regimens for acute nonlymphocytic leukemia [25].

No published adult studies have reported apparent volumes of distribution for doxorubicin, either central volume (Vd$_c$) or steady-state volume (Vd$_{ss}$). However, the low serum concentrations reported (peak ≈ 1 µg/ml or less) in all studies [26–34], following dosages of 50–75 mg/m$^2$, indicate that the apparent volume of distribution of doxorubicin is large, with the bulk of the drug rapidly distributing into tissues. Our studies in children also indicate a large central volume of distribution averaging ≈ 632 l/m$^2$ [35]. Alberts *et al.* [36] reported a mean volume of distribution of daunorubicin of 619 l/m$^2$, based on a total fluorescence assay, in seven adult patients.

Although published data on the metabolism of anthracyclines in children are limited, both drugs have been extensively studied in adults, and a number of metabolites, both active and inactive, have been identified. Anthracyclines undergo extensive metabolism and subsequent biliary elimination [37]. These drugs contained a reducible carbonyl in their C-9 side chain which yields an alcohol metabolite (doxorubicinol or daunorubicinol) as the product of the intracellular cytoplasmic aldo-ketoreductases. These metabolites are active cytotoxic agents, and increased aldo-ketoreductase activity in myeloblasts has been associated with improved response to daunomycin therapy of acute myelocytic leukemia [38]. It is of particular interest that increased enzyme activity and response rates were observed in *younger* patients.

The anthracyclines and their alcohol metabolites also undergo metabolic conversion by microsomal reductive glycosidase to relatively inactive anthracycline aglycones. The enzyme responsible for this reaction has been identified as NADPH cytochrome P-450 reductase. This reductive glycosidase catalyzes the formation of a free-radical semiquinone form of the anthracycline by transfer of a single electron from NADPH to a microsomal flavoprotein and subsequently to doxorubicin. When this semiquinone form of the anthracycline is produced, it readily transfers its single electron to oxygen to form superoxide and thereby cycles back to the stable quinone form. If the supply of oxygen is limited, this semiquinone form apparently cannot donate its electron rapidly enough to other electron acceptors. The anthracycline semiquinone then undergoes a rearrangement whereby the glycoside bond is cleaved. This reaction is apparently due to the electron-withdrawing effect of the oxygen-containing ether linkage, which attracts the unpaired electron and cleaves the glycosidic bond. Hydrogen abstraction replaces the sugar, yielding 7-deoxyaglycone. This metabolic conversion requires the first step to be enzymatic formation of the free-radical semiquinone. The presence of deoxyaglycone metabolites in bile, urine, and tissue indicates that anthracyclines exist in a free-radical state *in vivo*. The formation of free radicals may be directly related to both the anti-cancer activity of the anthracyclines and their cardiotoxicity [37].

Anthracycline elimination is almost entirely nonrenal, with only about 5–15% of a dose excreted in the urine [32, 37]. Doxorubicin disappears from serum in a triphasic manner following a short intravenous infusion. The initial distribution half-life has been reported [33] as 12 ($\pm$8) min, followed by a second phase with a half-life of 3.3 ($\pm$2.2) h and a third phase ($\approx$12 h after drug administration) half-life of 29.6 ($\pm$13.5) h. The half-lives of the various metabolites appear to be longer than that of the parent drug, as the disappearance of total fluorescence from the serum is slower than the disappearance of parent drug [28]. An earlier report by Creasey *et al.* [30] revealed an initial half-life of 1.5 h followed by a secondary half-life of 14–21 h.

In patients with decreased hepatic function, Benjamin [39] has recommended dosage reductions based on total bilirubin serum concentrations. In patients with moderately abnormal hepatic function (bilirubin = 1.2–3.0 mg/dl), the dosage is reduced by 50%. In patients with bilirubin greater than 3.0 mg/dl, the dosage is reduced by 75%.

In an early study of daunomycin pharmacokinetics, Alberts *et al.* [36] evaluated 11 patients given either 80 mg/m$^2$ or 120 mg/m$^2$ and described a biphasic plasma concentration curve with an initial half-life of about 0.7 h and a terminal half-life of about 55 h. In a recent paper Nilsson *et al.* [40] described the pharmacokinetics of daunorubicin following either a 45-min or a 240-min infusion of free daunorubicin, or an infusion of daunorubicin-DNA complex over 150–300 min. A biphasic disposition curve was identified for all three treatment protocols, with a $t_{1/2}$ of 60–75 min for all three groups. However, these investigators did not characterize the true terminal phase half-life of daunomycin, since data beyond 3–6 h postinfusion were not assessed.

In our ongoing study of doxorubicin pharmacokinetics in children, preliminary data are similar to results of adult studies [35]. Doxorubicinol was the major metabolite found in serum, with lower concentrations of 7-deoxyaglycones detected. The apparent central volume of distribution ($Vd_c$) was large, with a mean ($\pm$SEM) of 632 ($\pm$59.4) l/m$^2$ in 60 patients receiving 10–75 mg/m$^2$. Plasma clearance of doxorubicin was rapid (1,443$\pm$113.9 ml/min/m$^2$) and not dose-dependent. This average clearance value is about twice the average value reported for adults [41], suggesting possible age-related differences. These findings are also consistent with animal studies demonstrating age-related differences in aldo-ketoreductase activity (N. Ahmed, personal communication). In addition, within our pediatric-adolescent population, there was a significant (p = 0.0059) relationship between age and systemic clearance standardized for body weight (ml/min/kg), as shown in Figure 8. Although this regression was significant, it is clearly not predictive ($r^2$ = 16.6%). Interestingly, this age-related correlation was not significant when doxorubicin clearance was normalized for body surface area (m$^2$) instead of body weight.

Also in our studies, the doxorubicinol area under the concentration-time curve (AŪC) was significantly greater in patients who had received cyclophosphamide for 7 consecutive days before doxorubicin, than in patients who received simultaneous or no cyclophosphamide. These results suggest that hepatic microsomal metabolism of doxorubicinol (and doxorubicin) to aglycones may have been inhibited by cyclophosphamide or its metabolites, whereas conversion of doxorubicin to doxorubicinol (by cytoplasmic aldo-

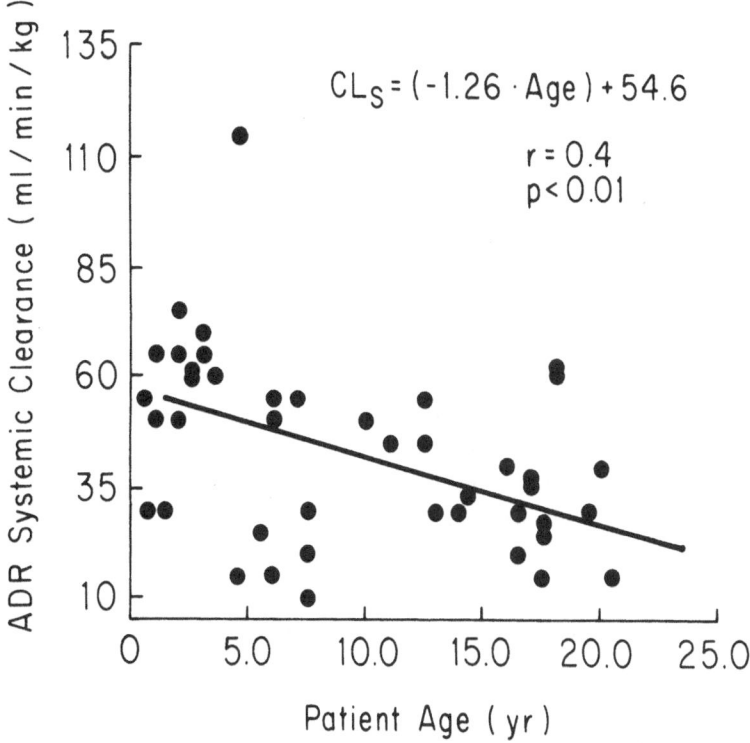

*Figure 8.* Relationship of doxorubicin (Adriamycin) systemic clearance normalized to body weight (ml/min/kg) and patient age in 43 children and adolescents with cancer. Reprinted with permission from Evans WE et al.: Pharmacokinetics of anticancer drugs in children. Drug Metabolism Rev 14:847–886, 1983.

keto reductases) was not significantly affected. Subsequent *in vitro* metabolism studies in our laboratory and by others have verified that the cyclophosphamide metabolite acrolein inhibits the ability of hepatic microsomal enzymes to convert doxorubicin and doxorubicinol to 7-deoxyaglycones [42].

Our clinical study is continuing to accumulate data which will allow further characterization of the influence of various population variables on doxorubicin pharmacokinetics in children.

## AMSA

The acridine derivative m-AMSA [14'-(9-acridinylamino)-methanesulfon-m-amisidide] is one of a series of derivatives synthesized by Cain and others in an effort to find new antitumor agents [43]. The drug is currently investigational and is undergoing phase II/III clinical trials. Although its spectrum of antitumor activity is not yet defined, phase I and II studies in children indicate activity in acute lymphocytic leukemia and acute myelogenous leukemia [44, 45]. Preliminary studies indicate that m-AMSA is less active in childhood solid tumors [45]. However, m-AMSA is an active single agent in acute leukemic and has been included in combination chemotherapy of untreated poor-risk leukemia patients [46].

Several preclinical studies indicate that the pharmacokinetics of m-AMSA is complex, with metabolism to both active and inactive metabolites. Rodent studies indicate that following oral and intravenous administration [47], AMSA is selectively localized and metabolized in the liver. The primary metabolic pathway is believed to be nucleophilic attack by endogenous thiols on the 9 or 5′ position of the AMSA molecule which results in the formation of inactive thioethers of acridine [48, 49]. However, highly reactive quinoidal intermediates are formed prior to inactivation with thiols, and these intermediates are more cytotoxic *in vitro* in L1210 cell cultures than is the parent drug [50].

Since m-AMSA has only recently entered clinical investigation, pharmacokinetic data are limited. Analysis by high-performance liquid chromatography (HPLC) indicates that, in adults, the apparent volume of distribution during the terminal elimination phase is 126 $l/m^2$ [51]. The total body clearance for parent drug was calculated to be 216 $ml/min/m^2$ in one patient. As expected from animal studies, patients with hepatic dysfunction cleared m-AMSA more slowly than patients with normal hepatic function [47, 52]. Hall et al. [53] have described the elimination of m-AMSA as biphasic with an initial half-life of about 20 min and a terminal half-life of 7.4 h in patients with normal hepatic and renal function. Patients with severe liver and renal disease had decreased clearance of m-AMSA, and the investigators recommended decreasing the dose by 30% to 40% in the patients.

To date, our laboratory has conducted the only published pediatric pharmacokinetic study, which was part of a phase I clinical trial [45]. Using a relatively nonspecific fluorescence assay [54], total m-AMSA concentrations in the serum declined with initial and terminal phase half-lives of 2.9 and 17.8 h, respectively. Free or unbound m-AMSA concentrations declined more rapidly, as evidenced by initial and terminal phase half-lives of 1.5 and 5.6 h, respectively. The latter results are almost identical to the decline in m-AMSA serum concentrations measured by HPLC in adults [51]. There are insufficient data in children to assess possible age-related differences in pharmacokinetics.

## Bleomycin

The bleomycins are a highly water-soluble group of complex glycopeptides produced from *Streptomyces verticillus*. The commercially available preparation consists of 13 different bleomycin species. The drug's cytotoxic activity is primarily related to its excising effect on free bases after binding to DNA, which results in single strand breaks [55].

Bleomycin is incorporated into combination regimens for the therapy of selected childhood solid tumors. As expected from its relative lack of bone marrow toxicity, the drug does not possess significant antileukemic activity [24]. Bleomycin is active as a single agent in Hodgkin's disease, non-Hodgkin's lymphoma, and germ cell tumors [56–58]. Whereas bleomycin-containing combination regimens are usually reserved as second-line therapy for Hodgkin's disease and non-Hodgkin's lymphoma, they are frequently used as initial therapy for older children with testicular cancer and other germ cell tumors [59].

Very few data on bleomycin pharmacokinetics in children have been published, because of its infrequent use in these patients. We concluded a pharmacokinetic study of bleomycin in ten children (median age, 14.5 yr) with solid tumors treated at St. Jude Children's Research Hospital [60]. Bleomycin concentrations were measured in plasma and urine by radioimmunoassay [61]. Following intravenous bolus administration, plasma bleomycin concentrations declined rapidly, with mean $t_{1/2\alpha}$ and $t_{1/2\beta}$ values of 0.3 and 3.2 h, respectively. The apparent volume of distribution for the central compartment and the volume of distribution at steady-state averaged 4.3 ($\pm$0.5) $l/m^2$ and 9.9 ($\pm$1.1) $l/m^2$. Previous studies have demonstrated that bleomycin is eliminated by both renal and nonrenal processes. In our study, renal clearance averaged 33 ($\pm$2.4) ml/min/$m^2$, a value which was 65% of the systemic clearance. The analytical method did not allow identification or quantitation of bleomycin metabolites. Data from two children indicated that concurrent administration of cisplatin, a known nephrotoxin, may reduce the renal clearance of bleomycin [62].

*Table 1.* Bleomycin kinetics (mean $\pm$ SEM) after intravenous bolus doses.

| Parameter | Cumulative cisplatin dosage of <300 mg/m² | | | Cumulative cisplatin dosage >300 mg/m² |
|---|---|---|---|---|
| | All patients (n = 11) | Patients <3 yr old (n = 3) | Patients >8 yr old (n = 8) | (n = 3) |
| $t_{1/2\alpha}$ (h) | 0.3$\pm$0.1 | 0.2$\pm$0.1 | 0.3$\pm$0.1 | 0.4$\pm$0.2 |
| $t_{1/2\beta}$ (h) | 3.2$\pm$0.7 | 3.5$\pm$2.2 | 3.1$\pm$0.6 | 6.0$\pm$1.0 |
| $V_c$ (L/m²) | 4.3$\pm$0.5 | 4.7$\pm$1.0 | 4.1$\pm$0.6 | 3.7$\pm$0.8 |
| $V_{ss}$ (L/m²) | 9.9$\pm$1.1 | 10.6$\pm$3.2 | 9.7$\pm$1.0 | 8.1$\pm$0.7 |
| $Cl_T$ (ml/min/m²) | 51.8$\pm$6.1 | 70.5$\pm$15.1[a] | 44.8$\pm$4.0 | 18.0$\pm$3.3[a] |
| $Cl_R$ (mL/min/m²) | 33.5$\pm$2.4 | 26.2[b] | 34.7$\pm$2.4 | 8.2[b] |

[a] $P < 0.05$.
[b] Measured from one patient.

Continuous intravenous bleomycin infusions have been advocated because of the drug's cell kinetic properties [63]. We have studied the pharmacokinetics of bleomycin in four pediatric patients given 24- to 48-h continuous intravenous infusions. Following administration of 30 mg/m$^2$/day in children with normal renal function, steady-state plasma concentrations of 200–300 ng/ml were maintained. As with intravenous bolus administration, plasma concentrations rapidly declined after the end of the infusion. Systemic clearance ranged from 62 to 99 ml/min/m$^2$ during the continuous infusion.

As summarized in Table 1, comparison of our data in children (median age, 14.5 yr) to data from studies in adults indicates that adults and older children eliminate bleomycin similarly following intravenous bolus [64] and continuous intravenous infusion administration [65]. However, children less than 3 years of age had a significantly faster rate of systemic clearance $(70 \pm 15$ ml/min/m$^2)$ [63].

## Cisplatin

Cisplatin (Platinol, Bristol) is a platinum coordination compound which has been shown to be active in a number of pediatric solid tumors [66, 67]. It has activity against neuroblastoma, germ cell tumors, and osteosarcoma [65, 67], and has also been evaluated at our institution in the treatment of nasopharyngeal carcinoma in children. Its activity appears to be limited to solid tumors, and therefore cisplatin has no apparent role in the treatment of leukemia.

Cisplatin is not administered by the oral route, since it is not absorbed intact following oral administration. There are data [68–71] which suggest that cisplatin and other platinum-containing metabolites are excreted in the bile. However, the possible reabsorption of platinum compounds (enterohepatic circulation) has not been adequately studies. The appearance of a second peak in the serum concentration versus time curve of some patients has lead to speculation that enterohepatic circulation of cisplatin, or a platinum-containing metabolite, does take place [70, 72, 73].

The biotransformation of cisplatin is apparently complex and not completely understood. The parent drug is unstable in aqueous solution and readily undergoes conversion to the aquated form by stepwise replacement of the chloride ligands by water molecules [74]. The equilibrium constants for the first and second replacements are $3.36 \times 10^{-3}$ M and $1.1 \times 10^{-4}$ M, respectively. The rate of these reactions is influenced by chloride concentrations in the aqueous solution, since addition of chloride stabilizes cisplatin by shifting the equation equilibrium to the left. This aquated form of the cisplatin molecule is very reactive. Since the intracellular chloride concentration is low, it has been suggested [74] that conversion of cisplatin to the aquated form takes place intracellularly and is necessary for the therapeutic activity of the drug. Further evidence for this process will have to await development of more specific analytical methods for detection of intracellular parent cisplatin.

The highly reactive aquated forms appear to bind readily to proteins in plasma and serum, and are not readily transported across cell membranes. About 90% of the total platinum in serum is protein-bound [75–77]. However, it appears that the parent drug is not highly protein-bound, and that conversion to the aquated form is necessary before protein binding occurs [68].

Other biotransformations of cisplatin may take place as well. Using gel filtration chromatography, Repta and Long [78] have detected up to seven distinct platinum species in plasma ultrafiltrate (protein-free plasma). However, these species have not been identified, and their anticancer activity is unknown.

Elimination of total platinum, both in plasma and in plasma ultrafiltrate has been evaluated in a number of studies [70, 72, 76, 77, 79–82], which indicate that platinum is eliminated from serum in a biphasic manner. These studies agree that the initial half-life is less than 1 h and that it is followed by a slower terminal half-life of 1–3 days. In early studies, $^{193m}$Pt-labeled cisplatin was used to determine platinum pharmacokinetics. In the earliest such study, by Deconti et al. [76], the initial half-life was 25.0–49.0 min, followed by a slower half-life of 58.5–73.0 h.

In more recent studies, atomic absorption spectrophotometry has been used to determine total platinum concentrations. Gormley et al. [77] determined mean initial and terminal half-lives of 23 min and 67 h, respectively, following doses of 70 mg/m$^2$ infused over 1 h. Frick et al. [80] measured urinary excretion rates of platinum and determined mean initial and terminal half-lives of 76 min (range, 37.8–1 03.8 min) and 26.8 h (range, 14.4–57.7 h), respectively. The terminal half-life reported by Frick et al. is shorter than those reported by other investigators and is probably due to the relatively short (24-h) evaluation interval. Studies from our laboratory [72] yielded mean ($\pm$SEM) half-lives of 0.4 ($\pm$0.10) and 44.4 ($\pm$8.2) h following dosages of 90 mg/m$^2$ administered over 6 h to nine children. Additional studies in 17 other patients suggest that those who have a greater accumulation of platinum following cisplatin therapy may be more likely to develop significant hearing loss, particularly in the higher frequency ranges [72].

Several investigators [68, 72, 73, 81–83] have studied the clearance of non-protein-bound platinum from humans receiving cisplatin, by a procedure involving ultrafiltration and atomic absorption spectroscopy. The significance of following non-protein-bound platinum species is predicated on the basis that protein-bound platinum appears to possess no anticancer

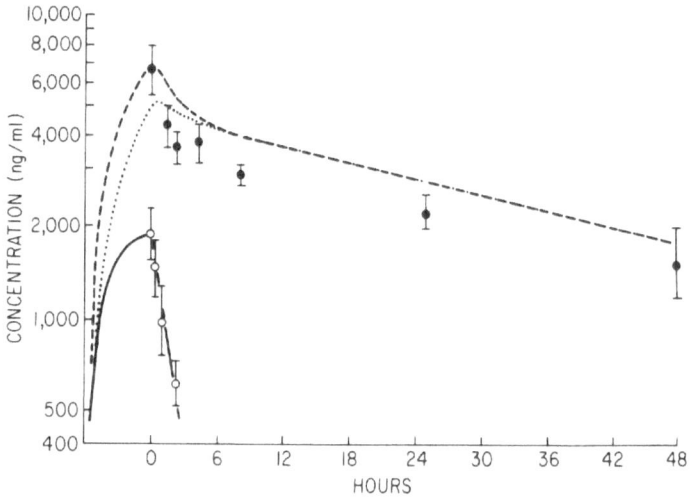

*Figure 9.* Semilogarithmic plot of total platinum (▮) and free platinum (▯, cisplatin) in nine children and adolescents given 90 mg/m² of cisplatin as a 6-h intravenous infusion. Vertical bars represent standard deviations of mean values, solid and broken lines represent computer-simulated curves using a multicompartment pharmacokinetic model.

activity as determined by cell culture studies, and that non-protein-bound platinum is a good approximation of parent cisplatin. Patton *et al.* [83] detected a biphasic decline in plasma concentrations of filterable platinum, with a terminal half-life of 32–53.5 min. In a later report by this group, Belt *et al.* [81] reported mean terminal half-lives for filterable platinum of 48 min following rapid (15-min) infusion of 100 mg/m², and 26 min following 6-h infusions of the same dose. Gullo *et al.* [73] reported a mean half-life of 22 min following a 1-h infusion of 50 or 100 mg/m². Platinum was not detected in plasma ultrafiltrate following 20-h infusions. Himmelstein *et al.* [82] reported half-lives for both filterable platinum and intact cisplatin ranging from 0.3 to 0.5 h for both species. This study separated intact cisplatin from plasma ultrafiltrate by high-performance liquid chromatography and quantitated the platinum content by atomic absorption spectrophotometry. The fact that total filterable platinum and intact cisplatin concentrations declined at the same rate supports the previous assumption that measurement of total platinum in the ultrafiltrate is a good estimate of parent drug. Our laboratory has reported [72] a mean half-life of 1.3 h for filterable platinum following 6-h infusions of 90 mg/m² in children. It therefore appears that the filterable platinum species (i.e., parent cisplatin) disappears more rapidly from the serum than total platinum (Figure 9); this finding is not unexpected since the filterable species is available for renal clearance and cellular uptake, in addition to conversion to aquated platinum species.

Studies [72, 73, 76, 77, 80, 81, 83] of renal excretion of platinum show incomplete (25–75%) urinary recovery of total platinum. Belt *et al.* [81] recovered a greater proportion of the dose of cisplatin as filterable platinum in the urine after 24 h, following 6-h infusions (75%) than after 15-min infusions (40%). LeRoy *et al.* [84] reported that several different but as yet unidentified platinum species are excreted in urine and that their individual rates of elimination are different. Platinum has also been detected in the bile of patients treated with cisplatin [69, 71]. In addition, several investigators [66, 69, 70] have reported the appearance of a second (later) plasma concentration peak, particularly following long infusions of cisplatin. Some [70, 73] have speculated that this second peak may be due to enterohepatic recycling of platinum. The significance of the enteric route of elimination has not been determined. The incomplete urinary recovery of platinum, and detectable concentrations of platinum 3 or more weeks following a dose [77; Crom and Evans, unpublished data], suggest that platinum may remain highly distributed into tissues and be very slowly removed from the body, once cisplatin has been converted to other platinum species.

The metabolism and elimination of cisplatin are complex and incompletely understood at this time. Our data [72] do not reveal significant differences between children and adults in the disposition of cisplatin. The recent development [74, 85] of more specific assays for cisplatin and its metabolic products may allow more precise determination of the pharmacokinetic parameters for this agent.

### Cyclophosphamide

Cyclophosphamide is a widely used alkylating agent that requires metabolic conversion to its active form. The drug has been incorporated into many pediatric cancer treatment protocols, including those designed to treat osteosarcoma, acute lymphocytic leukemia, Hodgkin's and non-Hodgkin's lymphomas, Burkitt's lymphoma, germ cell tumors, Ewing's sarcoma, and rhabdomyosarcoma. Doses used at our institution range from 50 to 1200 mg/m$^2$.

Analysis of cyclophosphamide and its metabolites has been hampered by indirect assay methods. In most cases, the presence of the parent drug is differentiated from its metabolites by the extraction and removal of the parent drug into an organic solvent such as methylene chloride [86, 87]. Thereafter, the amount of $^{14}$C can be measured, if radiolabeled cyclophosphamide is used, or the alkylation of 4-(4-nitrobenzyl)-pyridine (NBP) can be measured spectrophotometrically [88]. More specific quantitative measurement of cyclophosphamide and its metabolites has been accomplished with the use of gas chromatography with preliminary extractions and derivitization [89–92].

Most studies of cyclophosphamide disposition in humans have dealt with adults. The bioavailability of orally administered cyclophosphamide has been estimated at 74–97% [93]. The relative AUC for the alkylating substances is three times greater for an oral dose than for an equal dose administered intravenously [94].

Cyclophosphamide has been shown to distribute first into a central compartment with an apparent volume ($Vd_c$) of 0.32–0.34 l/kg, followed by an apparent steady-state distribution volume ($Vd_{ss}$) of 0.64–0.71 l/kg [93–95]. Parent drug has been detected in saliva, cerebrospinal fluid, sweat, synovial fluid, and breast milk, but the concentrations relative to that of plasma were not determined [96]. Rat studies have shown that the highest tissue concentrations occur in the kidney, liver, spleen, and heart [97].

The apparent half-life of cyclophosphamide is 4–10 h in adults [90, 91] and 2.5–6.5 h in children [86] and does not appear to be dose dependent. Peak alkylating activity occurs within 1–2 h of a dose, and the apparent half-life of the alkylating substances approximates that of the parent drug [90, 93, 94].

Two to twenty-one percent of the dose of cyclophosphamide is excreted unchanged in the urine [86, 93, 94]. Using $^{14}$C-labeled cyclophosphamide, Bagley *et al.* [94] found that 62% of the administered radioactivity was excreted within 48 h, and 58% within 96 h. Stools and expired air accounted for only 4% of the total labeled drug administered. Cyclophsophamide has been found to be from 12% to 24% protein-bound [89, 94, 98]. In contrast, non-cyclophosphamide-alkylating metabolites were approximately 56% protein-bound [94].

Mouridsen and Jacobsen [99] studied five adult patients with severe renal disease (creatinine clearance of less than 10 ml/min/1.73 m$^2$) and found a beta half-life of 6–11.5 h (mean, 8.5 h) and a gamma half-life of 11.7–15 h (mean, 14 h), when the data were fitted to a three-compartment first-order model. The fact that most of the $^{14}$C-labeled substances were not cyclophosphamide indicates the importance of renal excretion in the elimination of metabolites. The renal clearance of intact cyclophosphamide is approximately 11 ml/min [95] in patients with normal renal function.

Metabolism accounts for 90–95% of the elimination of available cyclophosphamide and is required for the desired cytotoxic effect. The rate-limiting step is the hydroxylation of cyclophosphamide by cytochrome-P-450-dependent mixed-function oxidases in the liver. Although the rate-limiting process of cyclophosphamide activation is enzymatic, no dose-dependent kinetics have been observed at clinically utilized doses [94, 100]. The metabolite 4-hydroxycyclophosphamide is in equilibrium with its tautomer aldophosphamide, and it is postulated that after these two compounds enter cells, they decompose into the primary cytotoxic or immunosuppressive agents phosphoramide mustard and acrolein [101]. Despite nitrogen mustard's potential for alkylation at acidic pH, the antineoplastic effect of cyclophosphamide is thought to arise primarily from the action of phosphoramide mustard. Acrolein and the enzymatically formed metabolites 4-ketocyclophosphamide and carboxyphosphamide are not considered antineoplastic.

The presence of acrolein in bladder urine may be causally related to the development of hemorrhagic cystitis [102]. Good hydration (1–3 $l/m^2/day$) and frequent voiding have been encouraged to decrease this toxicity. Recent research has shown that sulfhydryl-containing compounds such as N-acetylcysteine prevent cystitis without decreasing the antitumor effect [103, 104].

The data on cyclophosphamide metabolism and disposition in children are quite limited, and many of the questions raised about the effect of drug interactions, enzyme induction, absorption, and metabolites have been answered by inference from animal or adult studies. It has been shown that the apparent volume of distribution of cyclophosphamide and percent of parent drug excreted unchanged are similar to those seen in adults. Children apparently have a shorter cyclophosphamide half-life than do adults (2.5–6.5 h vs. 4–10 h); the difference has been postulated to be due to the higher activity of the microsomal mixed-function oxidases per kilogram in children versus adults [86]. There has been no clinical significance placed on these apparent differences in the rate of cyclophosphamide metabolism and activation.

## Vinca Alkaloids

Vincristine (VCR), vinblastine (VBL), and vindesine (VDS) are structurally related dimeric alkaloids derived from the periwinkle plant *(Vinca rosea)*. Although the vinca alkaloids' spectra of clinical activity and toxicity differ [105–107], these dimeric (indole-dihydroindoline) alkaloids are structurally similar compounds. The formyl group on the dihydroindoline nitrogen atom of VCR is replaced by a methyl group in VBL and VDS. Desacetyl vinblastine carboxamide, vindesine, which is the new semisynthetic derivative of VBL, differs from VBL at carbons 3 and 4 of the dihydroindoline moiety.

Vincristine is used extensively in combination with other drugs to treat several pediatric malignancies, including acute lymphocytic leukemia, acute myelogenous leukemia, Hodgkin's and non-Hodgkin's lymphoma, Wilms' tumor, Ewing's sarcoma, embryonal rhabdomyosarcoma, hepatoblastoma, neuroblastoma, osteosarcoma, and other soft-tissue sarcomas [108–113]. In combination with prednisone, remission of acute lymphocytic leukemia is achieved in 85–90% of newly diagnosed patients [108]. Because VCR is not highly myelosuppressive, it is an attractive agent for use in combination chemotherapy. The dose-limiting toxicity of VCR is usually its neurotoxicity and gastrointestinal side effects.

Vinblastine is also used in combination-drug therapy to treat Hodgkin's and other lymphomas and is one of the agents that produce long-term remission in infants with histiocytosis X (Letterer-Siwe disease) [114]. The combination of vinblastine, bleomycin, and cisplatin produces a complete response in nearly 100 % of patients with testicular cancer [115, 116]. Other malignant disorders which may respond to vinblastine include neuroblastoma and gestational choriocarcinoma. The dose-limiting side effect of VBL is usually myelosuppression.

Vindesine was recently synthesized in an attempt to alter or enlarge the spectrum of antitumor activity, increase the therapeutic index, reduce toxicity, and overcome clinical cross-resistance with VCR and VBL [116-118]. VDS is reported to have essentially the same spectrum of activity as VCR and VBL [119], at 2-3 times the maximum tolerable dose of VCR. The most common toxicities are dose-related myelosuppression, gastrointestinal toxicities which include constipation and paralytic ileus, and a VCR-like clinical manifestation of peripheral neuropathy [120].

The pharmacokinetics of VCR and VBL have not been studied in infants and small children, and only recently has a brief report on the disposition of VDS in children appeared in the literature [121]. Mean half-lives for the initial and terminal phase were 14 min and 10 h. Comparative studies in adults [122-124] show appreciable differences in their pharmacokinetic parameters (i.e., $t_{1/2}$, Vd, $Vd_{ss}$, $AUC_0^\infty$, and $Cl_p$). VDS has a central compartment distribution volume approximately equal to the plasma volume, while the values for VCR and VBL are much larger. These larger volumes probably reflect rapid tissue uptake and extensive binding of VCR and VBL to both blood components and protein [122-124].

The vinca alkaloids are poorly absorbed and are therefore given intravenously as a bolus dose or by prolonged infusion. The serum concentration-time curves of vincristine, vinblastine, and vindesine after i.v. bolus doses have been adequately described by triexponential equations [122, 125]. The initial and second-phase half-lives are similar for all three drugs. The terminal-phase half-lives for VBL and VDS are essentially the same, 22-24 h, while VCR has a much longer terminal half-life of about 84 h [125].

About 11 % of the VCR dose is excreted in the urine by 72 h, more than half of which is excreted within the first 3 h [122]. Nearly 33 % of the drug is excreted in the feces by 24 h, and 68.9-76 % is excreted in 72 h [122, 126]. Approximately 50 % of the radioactivity is excreted in the bile as metabolite (intact dimeric structure with side-chain alterations), suggesting possible glucuronide conjugation [112, 118]. A recent study [127] suggests an increased toxicity of VCR in infants and small children when dosed using body surface area calculations. The authors relate these age-dependent toxicities to delayed hepatic conjugation and clearance of VCR in younger children, and to the relatively large ratio of body surface area to weight in infants. This report of a small number of children is provocative but is not conclusive because it did not include any pharmacokinetic studies.

There are reports of VCR and VDS metabolites, but their structures remain unidentified [122, 125, 126]. Deacetylvinblastine has been identified as a metabolic product of VBL and is reportedly more biologically active than the parent drug [128]. Nelson and associates [125] have reported significant differences in plasma clearance among the vinca alkaloids. These investigators [125] have postulated that these differences in VCR's pharmacokinetic properties (low plasma clearance and very long terminal half-life) reflect rapid tissue uptake and slow redistribution back into the central volume; these characteristics could account for the drug's greater potency and neurotoxicity.

As newer, more specific, and nonradioactive methods [129] are developed for the separation and quantitation of the vinca alkaloids and their metabolites in biological fluids (i.e., HPLC), comparative studies in infants and children should be conducted to better elucidate the pharmacokinetics of these drugs.

## Etoposide and Teniposide: Epipodophyllotoxin Derivatives

Etoposide (VP16) recently approved by the USFDA for germ-cell tumors, and teniposide (VM26), an investigational drug, have established antineoplastic activities in a variety of childhood cancers. Etoposide and teniposide are structurally related semisynthetic derivatives of podophyllotoxin. Podophyllotoxin is synthesized from the plant *Podophyllum pellatum,* commonly known as the American mandrake or May apple. Podophyllotoxin is a potent mitotic inhibitor, binding to the same receptor site on tubulin subunits as colchicine and the vinca alkaloids. This reversible binding to tubulin inhibits microtubular assembly and causes accumulation of cells in mitosis [130]. Etoposide and teniposide do not bind to tubulin [131] but cause a blockade of cells in the premitotic phase of the cell cycle and induced DNA strand breaks. The accumulation of cells in the $G_2$ phase may be due to the drug's lethal effects in S and $G_2$, but the mechanism has not been precisely defined [132, 133].

The epipodophyllotoxin derivatives are active against acute leukemias, Hodgkin's and non-Hodgkin's lymphoma, histiocytic lymphoma, neuroblastoma, Wilms' tumor, Ewing's sarcoma, germ-cell tumors, brain tumors, and adult small-cell lung cancer and breast cancer [134–141].

Pharmacokinetic differences between these two structurally similar analogs have been reported in adults and children. Teniposide and etoposide are most frequently given by the intravenous route, although oral dosage forms of etoposide are available. The oral bioavailability is 30–63% for the soft gelatine capsule and 50–90% for the drink ampule [140, 141]. The time to peak blood concentrations after an oral dose is from 1 to 4 h. Etoposide and teniposide are usually administered by infusion over 30–60 min, although continuous infusion may prove to be valuable because of the drug's schedule-dependent effects [142, 143].

Clinical pharmacokinetic studies of teniposide and etoposide have been conducted in children [144–146, 149] and adults [144, 147, 148]. Results of pediatric studies from our laboratory are summarized in Table 2 [145, 150]; these demonstrate that the biological half-lives, steady-state volumes of distribution, and systemic clearances for etoposide and teniposide are more similar than previously thought. The lower teniposide systemic clearance observed in our previous study [150] of six children may have been related to high alkaline phosphatase values in half of these patients, since our recent studies show a significant correlation between alkaline phosphatase and teniposide clearance ($r = 0.64$, $p < 0.05$). Our studies were conducted with an HPLC assay which quantitates parent drugs, their picroisomers and hydroxy acid metabolites. Previous studies have established that these two drugs are extensively metabolized, with renal clearance accounting for only about half of total systemic clearance [148].

These data also indicate that the pharmacokinetics of VP16 and VM26 in children are similar to those in adults given comparable dosages. Allen and Creaven [148] have studied the pharmacokinetics in six patients given

*Table 2.* Summary of VM26 and VP16 pharmacokinetic parameters (mean $\pm$ SD) in children.

| | Non-compartmental[a] | | Model dependent[b] | | | |
|---|---|---|---|---|---|---|
| | Systemic clearance (ml/min/m$^2$) | $Vd_{ss}$ (l/m$^2$) | $Vd_c$ (l/m$^2$) | $K_{el}$ (h$^{-1}$) | $t_{1/2\alpha}$ (h) | $t_{1/2\beta}$ (h) |
| VM26 | 13.8 | 7.9 | 3.1 | 0.36 | 0.86 | 8.95 |
| (n = 21) | ($\pm 6.9$) | ($\pm 4.9$) | ($\pm 2.9$) | ($\pm 0.18$) | ($\pm 0.64$) | ($\pm 3.7$) |
| VP16 | 17.2 | 6.1 | 4.1 | 0.33 | 0.95 | 5.7 |
| (n = 12) | ($\pm 5.6$) | ($\pm 1.1$) | ($\pm 1.9$) | ($\pm 0.16$) | ($\pm 0.34$) | ($\pm 0.8$) |

[a] Non-compartmental: Systemic clearance $(Cl_s) = Dose/AUC_0^\infty$;

$$VD_{ss} = Dosage \times \frac{AUMC}{AUC_0^\infty} - \frac{K_0 \cdot t}{Dosage} \cdot \frac{t}{2}.$$

[b] Model-dependent parameters derived from NONLIN best fit of two-compartment model.

tritiated teniposide and 10 patients given tritiated etoposide. The terminal half-life of teniposide ranged from 11 to 38 h. After 72 h, 44% of the radioactivity was eliminated in the urine, with 9% unchanged and 35% as metabolite. Recovery of radioactivity in the feces varied from 0 to 10%. Penetration of VM26 into the cerebrospinal fluid varied from 1 to 27%. VP16 plasma decay followed a biexponential function, with a terminal phase half-life of about 11 h. After 72 h, 44% of the dose was eliminated in the urine, with 29% unchanged and 15% as metabolized drug. The major metabolite was later identified as the hydroxy acid of the parent drug, which appears to be biologically inactive [150, 151]. Recovery of radioactive VP16 in the feces ranged from 2 to 16%. Concentrations of VP16 in the cerebrospinal fluid varied from less than 1 to 10% of the concurrent plasma levels at 2 and 26 h postinfusion, respectively. The plasma clearance for VP16, when compared to VM26, was three times greater (47.1 ml/min vs. 16 ml/min), and renal clearance was six times greater (13.6 ml/min vs. 2.2 ml/min). Recent studies (in adults) using HPLC methods have shown shorter half-lives of 1.7 to 5.2 h, a Vd of 0.19–0.51 l/kg, and a plasma clearance of 23–45 ml/min [144, 147] for VP16 (100–200 mg/m$^2$).

Preliminary data of D'Incalci et al. [152], in a small number of children, suggest that the half-life (and clearance) of VP16 may be dose-related. Their studies of individual patients at two dosage levels (100 and 200 mg/m$^2$) demonstrated a longer $t_{1/2\beta}$ at the higher dosage; and systemic clearances measured at a dosage of 95–108 mg/m$^2$ (40–72 ml/min/m$^2$) were consistently higher then values observed in their patients given 200 mg/m$^2$ (20–46 ml/min/m$^2$) and in our patients given 200–250 mg/m$^2$ (16.2 ± 5.5 ml/min/m$^2$). However, the more recently published studies of Hande et al. [153] indicate that systemic clearance of etoposide is similar over a dosage range of 200 to 800 mg/m$^2$, hence not saturable in the clinical dosage range.

We have recently studied adult patients given etoposide and have found no difference in the systemic clearance when patients with total bilirubins ≤ 1.5 mg/dl were compared to patients with bilirubins ranging from 1.9 to 23 mg/dl (21.4 ml/min/m$^2$ versus 22.4 ml/min/m$^2$) [154]. It is apparent that the metabolic fate and disposition of etoposide and teniposide remain to be clearly defined in both children and adults.

## Cytarabine

Cytarabine (ara-C) is a cytidine nucleoside analog that is primarily used in the treatment of acute leukemia. Ara-C has been administered at conventional doses (100–200 mg/m$^2$/d) in children with acute nonlymphocytic leukemia and at high doses (1.0–3.0 mg/m$^2$/d) in children with leukemia refractory to standard chemotherapeutic regimens [155–157].

Ara-C is administered intravenously or subcutaneously because of extensive and rapid deamination within the gastrointestinal tract. Only about 20% of the inact drug is absorbed following oral administration [158].

Ara-C is widely distributed into body tissues. Approximately 10–15% is bound to plasma proteins [157, 159]. Concentrations in the CSF have been reported to range from about 8% [160] to 40% [158]. The lower CSF:plasma ratios have been observed under steady-state continuous-infusion conditions, whereas the relatively higher ratios have generally been observed several hours after short IV infusions and may have not been reflective of the true distribution equilibrium ratio. The high CSF concentrations may also be due in part to the slow CSF clearance of ara-C because of low deaminase activity. Ara-C has significant antitumor activity when administered intrathecally and is considered an alternative to, or administered in combination with, methotrexate for intrathecal prophylaxis and treatment of CNS leukemia [161].

Ara-C must be transported intracellularly and phosphorylated to the active form, ara-C-triphosphate (ara-CTP), which functions as a competitive inhibitor of DNA polymerase [162]. To a lesser extent, ara-C is also incorporated into DNA and causes premature nucleic chain termination [163]. Ara-C is sequentially phosphorylated to ara-CTP by the enzymes deoxycytidine kinase (ara-CMP), cytosine monophosphate kinase (ara-CDP) and, finally, nucleoside diphosphate kinase (ara-CTP). Deoxycytidine kinase is found in low concentrations in human leukemic cells, but has a relatively high affinity for the drug; its absence may be one mechanism for drug resistance in animal tumor systems [164, 165].

Ara-C is rapidly and extensively (about 80%) metabolized to *uridine arabinoside (ara-U),* primarily by hepatic, gastrointestinal, and leukocyte deaminase. At high doses of ara-C there appears to be saturation of the deaminase enzyme, with an increase in the ara-C:ara-U ratio [158]. Variability in deaminase activity may be important in the mechanism of resistance to ara-C [166]. Other factors that have been implicated in resistance of experimental tumors include the amount of competitive substrate (deoxycytidine triphosphate) and altered affinity of DNA polymerase to ara-CTP [154].

Approximately 90% of the ara-C dose can be recovered in the urine in 24 h, the majority as the ara-U metabolite [158, 167]. To a lesser extent, ara-C is also eliminated in the bile [168]. Conventional doses of ara-C disappear in a biphasic manner, with an initial half-life of about 15 min and a terminal half-life of about 2 h [158]. The metabolic clearance is about 850 ml/min, with a renal clearance of about 80 ml/min [154].

Chou *et al.* [169] have studied the relationship between intracellular ara-CTP and inhbition of DNA synthesis and reported more pronounced inhibition in DNA synthesis with higher intracellular concentrations of ara-CTP. Recent computer simulation and clinical studies have supported

Chou's *in vitro* findings that ara-C exhibits dose-dependent elimination and that high extracellular concentrations of ara-C will result in increased intracellular levels of ara-CTP and greater cell kill [166,167]. These conclusions have prompted clinical trials of high-dose ara-C, as a bolus dose or continuous infusion, in patients refractory to conventional doses. Our own study of high-dose ara-C (3.5 or 5 mg/m$^2$/d) administered to children as a continuous infusion for four consecutive days demonstrated a mean systemic clearance of 555 and 430 ml/min/m$^2$ for 3.5 and 5 mg/m$^2$/d doses, respectively [170]. These results indicate lower systemic clearance for higher doses of ara-C and suggest saturation of the elimination mechanisms. Of particular interest is the report of Rustum and Preisler [171], who observed significantly longer remission durations in ANLL patients whose leukemia cells had relatively good relation of ARA-CTP under standardized conditions *in vitro*.

## 6-Mercaptopurine

The metabolite 6-mercaptopurine (6-MP) was first synthesized in 1952 by Elion, Burgi, and Hitching [172] and in 1953 was demonstrated by Burchenal [173] to have activity in treatment of childhood leukemia. Since then, 6-MP has contributed significantly to the treatment of acute lymphocytic leukemia, primarily in combination with methotrexate as remission maintenance therapy. In the treatment of chronic granulocytic leukemia, maintenance therapy with 6-MP may be useful, but it is not the first drug of choice [174].

Although 6-MP has been used clinically since 1953, relatively little is known about its pharmacokinetics in man. Data that are available have been derived from studies using small numbers of patients and nonspecific assay techniques.

Absorption of 6-MP after oral administration is incomplete and variable, ranging from 12% [175] of the administered dose in rhesus monkeys to about 60% of the administered dose in an adult clinical study [176]. In seven children with ALL [177], the mean oral bioavailability of 6-MP (75 mg/m$^2$) was only 16% (range, 5–37%). Peak serum concentrations ranged from 0.29 to 1.82 µM. The factors which influence oral absorption are unknown.

The mean volume of distribution for the central compartment and the mean steady-state volume of distribution determined in adults given 6-MP intravenously were 0.46 ($\pm$0.8) l/kg (mean $\pm$ SEM) and 1.2 ($\pm$0.3) l/kg, respectively [178]. This is in good agreement with a more recently published study which utilized a more specific assay (high-performance liquid chromatography) and found a steady-state volume of distribution in monkeys of

1.76 ($\pm$0.64) l/kg. In seven children with ALL, Zimm *et al.* [177] reported a mean elimination half-life of 0.9 h (range, 0.5–1.3 h) and a mean distribution volume of 0.9 l/kg (range, 0.2–2.2 l/kg). 6-MP tissue-plasma ratios in rats revealed the liver as the primary site of distribution, with the gut lumen, kidney, spleen, and muscle as the other sites in descending order of extent [179]. These authors took this information and with other published data, developed a physiologically based pharmacokinetic model. Simulated concentrations of 6-MP were predicted and, when compared with clinical data, demonstrated reasonable agreement. 6-MP reportedly is bound to plasma protein on an average of 19% over the concentration range of 10–50 µg/ml (a concentration only achieved by intravenous administration of 6-MP at dosages exceeding 5–10 mg/kg) [176].

6-MP is extensively metabolized, but the relative conversion to each of the reported metabolites has not been quantitated in man. 6-MP is initially activated to 6-thioinosinate (6-TI) via hypoxanthine-guanine phosphoribosyltransferase. This metabolite causes only minor inhibition of various enzymes involved in purine metabolism. 6-TI is further metabolized to 6-thioxanthylic acid (6-TX acid) and subsequently incorporated into DNA and RNA as the 6-thioquanylate derivate [180]. 6-MP is metabolized to 6-methylthioionosinate (6-MeTI), which is a major metabolite of 6-MP in certain cell types. 6-MP is also metabolized to 6-thiouric (6-TU) acid by xanthine oxidase. In man, unchanged 6-MP, 6-TU, and inorganic sulfate are considered the primary urinary excretory products [173].

At present it is thought that the primary mechanisms involved in the production of cellular cytotoxicity is incorporation of 6-MP metabolites into DNA. At least one investigator has suggested that 6-MeTI is the metabolite responsible for most, if not all, of the inhibition of the purine de novo pathway following treatment with 6-MP [175]. The cytotoxicity of 6-MP, however, probably does not depend upon a single mechanism in all sensitive cells. Rather, 6-MP inhibits many different reactions, and cell death may result from combinations of different events, depending upon the type of tumor cell involved. Thus, the major active species, as well as the exact details of cytotoxicity, remain to be elucidated.

Very little is known about the distribution or clearance of the metabolites of 6-MP. An early report described quantitative but not qualitative differences between metabolite production after oral and intravenous administration of 6-MP [181]. In man, 6-MP persists somewhat longer following an oral dose than would be expected (not including absorption time), and the proportion of sulfate generated, presumably by dethiolation, is much higher following an oral dose. The clinical significance of these findings is uncertain at present.

Unchanged 6-MP and some of its metabolites are excreted renally [174]. No well-controlled published studies have quantitated clearance values (renal, systemic, or metabolic) for man. Reports vary on the amount of 6-MP excreted unchanged in the urine, with anywhere from 3 to 50% of the total dose of radioactivity appearing in the urine at up to 48 h [178, 182]. Biliary secretion of 6-MP in man exists, but has not been quantitated experimentally. In rhesus monkeys, 6-MP systemic clearance is 48.4 ($\pm$15.4) ml/min/kg, but no estimates of renal or metabolic clearance in animals have been described [175].

Plasma half-life of distribution ($t_{1/2\alpha}$) for 6-MP is reported to be 7.1 ($\pm$1.3) min in man [178] and 6.3 ($\pm$3.6) min in rhesus monkeys [175]. The half-life of elimination ($t_{1/2\beta}$) for 6-MP is reported to be 10.3 ($\pm$4.2) min in man [178] and 41.6 ($\pm$12.1) min in rhesus monkeys [175]. Loo and associates [176] reported plasma half-times for 6-MP after intravenous administration of 21 min for the four children in their study, and 47 min for the seven adults. These half-lives were determined using only four data points (0.5, 1,2, and 4 h) and do not adequately characterize either the alpha or beta half-life.

Interpretation of the pharmacokinetic studies of 6-MP must be done cautiously and must include consideration of the various dosage regimens of 6-MP, routes of administration, and assay systems which have been used. A definitive study of the pharmacokinetics of 6-MP in adults and children is not yet available.

## Methotrexate

In 1955 Goldin and his associates [183] demonstrated that the folic acid antagonist methotrexate (MTX) was more effective than aminopterin in mice bearing L1210 leukemia. Since this discovery, MTX has been used extensively in treating pediatric malignancies. MTX is used in a wide range of dosages, from 25 mg/m$^2$ up to >30,000 mg/m$^2$. Dosages greater than about 100 mg/m$^2$ are usually followed by leucovorin rescue. MTX is active against acute lymphocytic leukemia, acute nonlymphocytic leukemia, malignant lymphomas, epidermoid carcinoma of the head and neck, osteogenic sarcoma, and other malignancies [184].

Although the oral absorption of MTX is not well elucidated, it is apparently dose-dependent [185, 186], with low dosages of MTX (<30 mg/m$^2$) reported to be well absorbed (70–80%) [187, 188], while absorption of doses in excess of 80 mg/m$^2$ is lower (50–70%) [186–188]. However, these studies were based on absorption characteristics in only 11 patients given 80 mg/m$^2$ or more of MTX. More recent studies by Balis et al. [189] found doses of MTX above 12 mg/m$^2$ had a more prolonged absorption phase and a decreased fraction absorbed. Table 3 summarizes published studies of MTX bioavailability, listed according to the dosage administered. It is evident that oral bioavailability decreases as the dosage is increased. MTX is rapidly

*Table 3.* Summary of MTX oral absorption studies.

| Dosage (mg/m$^2$) | Biovailability (F)% mean (range) | Time of peak (hr) | Number of patients | Investigator (ref) |
|---|---|---|---|---|
| 3 | 69–70 | NR | 2 | 187 |
| 6–10 | 87 (76–93) | 1–2.2 | 5 | 189 |
| 15 | 69 ($\pm$8) | NR | 10 | 190 |
| 15 | 42 (16–91) | 0.7–4 | 28 | 191 |
| 13–28 | 51 (23–95) | 1–5 | 10 | 189 |
| 30 | 62 (36–83) | $\approx$1.7 | 6 | 192 |
| 30 | $\approx$70 | $\approx$1.5 | 7 | 188 |
| 34–110 | 32 (19–39) | 1–4 | 6 | Evans/Choi (unpublished) |
| 50 | 26 (15–54) | 1.2–2.5 | 6 | 193 |
| 80 | 31 | NR | 1 | 188 |
| 200[a] | 28 (14–44) | NR | 8 | 194 |
| 300 | $\approx$48 | NR | 1 | 187 |
| 444[b] | 88 (82–92) | NR | 5 | 195 |
| 800[c] | 16–20 | 2–4 | 2 | 186 |

[a] Divided into 4 doses given Q1H × 4 or, into 8 doses given Q1/2H × 8.
[b] Divided into 16 doses given Q1H × 16.
[c] Divided into 4 doses given Q6H × 4.
NR = not reported.
[Reproduced with permission from Evans WE, Crom WR, Yalowich J: Methotrexate. In: Applied Pharmacokinetics: Principles of Therapeutic Drug Monitoring, 2nd edition. Evans WE, Schentagg JJ, Jusko WJ (eds). Applied Therapeutics, Inc., San Francisco CA, 1986.]

and completely absorbed after intramuscular administration [196], although the clinical usefulness of intramuscular MTX remains to be defined. After intravenous administration, MTX has an initial volume of distribution of approximately 18% (0.18 l/kg) of body weight [197] and has a steady-state volume of distribution of approximately 75–80% of body weight [187, 198]. In man, 45–57% of MTX is bound to plasma protein, primarily albumin, at serum concentrations ranging from 0.1 to 1,000 μM [187, 188]. Highest tissue concentrations are produced in the kidney and liver, with somewhat lower concentrations found in the gastrointestinal (GI) tract and skeletal muscle [199, 200]. Although lower concentrations of MTX are found in the GI tract, this site is important for both distribution and metabolism, as is discussed below. MTX also distributes into pleural fluid and ascites, where maximum concentrations of MTX are about 10% of maximum serum concentrations [201] but decline more slowly. MTX distribution into the central nervous system is poor, with cerebrospinal fluid (CSF) concentrations from continuous infusions being correlated with the steady-state MTX serum concentration [202]. Studies from our laboratory indicate that CSF

MTX concentrations are approximately 2.3% of concurrent serum MTX concentrations immediately after a 24-h infusion of intermediate-dose MTX. Furthermore, our work has shown a significant correlation between CSF MTX concentrations and free (non-protein-bound) MTX serum concentration [203].

Although, initially, MTX was thought not to be metabolized, subsequent work has established that MTX is metabolized in both the liver and the gastrointestinal tract. Intestinal bacteria are capable of metabolizing orally administered as well as parenterally administered (through enterohepatic recycling) MTX to 4-amino-4-deoxy $N^{10}$-methylpteroic acid (DAMPA). This metabolite is apparently not clinically significant, since it is usually not detectable in patients; and DAMPA has only about 1/200th the activity of MTX to inhibit dihydrofolate reductase (DHFR). MTX is also oxidized by a hepatic metalloflavoprotein, aldehyde oxidase, to 7-hydroxymethotrexate (7-OH MTX) [203]. This metabolite is about two orders of magnitude less effective than MTX as an inhibitor of DHFR [204]. Initial reports indicated that this metabolite accounted for only 1–11% of the administered dose in the first 24 h after high-dose MTX [205]. However, more recent studies [206], including pediatric studies from our laboratory, have demonstrated that serum concentrations of 7-OH MTX commonly exceed concurrent serum concentrations of MTX. The overall clinical significance (efficacy and toxicity) of these two extracellular metabolites (DAMPA and 7-OH MTX) has not been determined. Since the aqueous solubility of 7-OH MTX is three- to fivefold less than that of MTX, it has been suggested that this metabolite may contribute to the renal toxicity of high-dose MTX, but this is apparently not a problem in patients adequately hydrated and given sodium bicarbonate or alternative urinary alkalinization.

MTX has been shown to undergo intracellular metabolism to MTX-polyglutamates in animal and human malignant and nonmalignant cell cultures, as well as animal and human tissues [207–220]. It is now recognized that folate polyglutamates are the natural coenzyme forms of folate [221]. Four to seven glutamates bind in a γ-linkage to the glutamate moiety of folate. Similarly, MTX is converted to polyglutamates, which remain as potent an inhibitor of the enzyme DHFR as MTX itself [209]. The formation of MTX-polyglytamates is both time- and dose-dependent, with larger doses resulting in greater formation of MTX-polyglutamate [216, 222, 223]. MTX-polyglutamates may be more toxic to cells, because they are retained by the cells for longer periods of time than MTX as the extracellular concentration of MTX falls [222]. MTX-polyglutamates are potent inhibitors of DHFR and therefore appear to have a major role in the cytotoxicity of MTX. Recent in vitro studies [224] have demonstrated that 7-OH can compete with MTX for membrane transport and for polyglutamylation by folyl polyglutamate synthetase (FPGS).

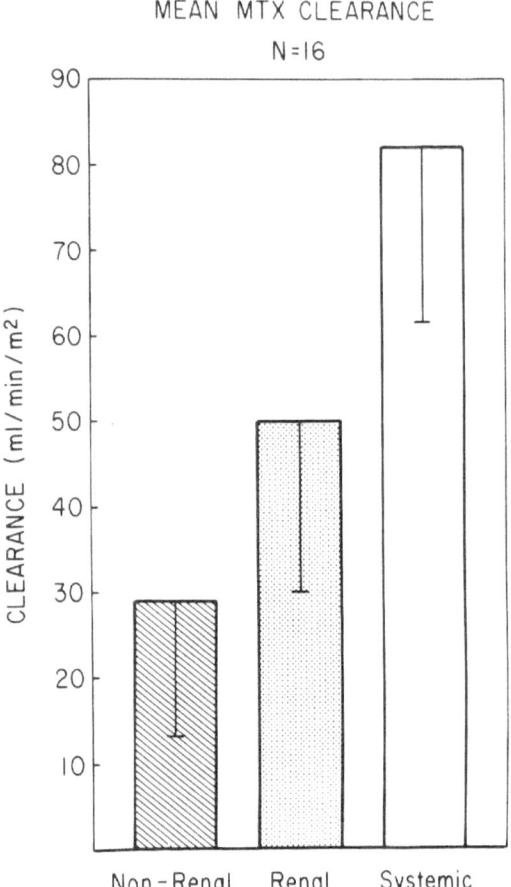

MEAN MTX CLEARANCE

N=16

*Figure 10.* Mean (±SD) of the total systemic, renal, and nonrenal clearances of methotrexate measured in 16 children administered 1,000 mg/m² infused intravenously over 24 h.

Active biliary excretion is a relatively minor excretory pathway and accounts for less than 10% of excretion [225]. However, partial GI obstruction may perturb the enterohepatic cycling of MTX and lead to sustained MTX serum concentrations following high-dose MTX administration [226].

Renal excretion constitutes the major route of MTX elimination (Figure 10), with renal clearance accounting for 60–90% of total body clearance of MTX [202, 227]. Following intravenously administered high-dose MTX, between 40% and 90% may be recovered unchanged in urine [202]. At MTX serum concentrations of ≈0.1–1.0 µM, MTX renal clearance exceeds glomerular filtration as measured by inulin clearance; consistent with active tubular secretion [228]. Shen and Azarnoff's findings of lower net renal clearance at lower serum concentrations suggest extensive tubular reabsorption of MTX. Recent work from our laboratory [229] in 16 children given intermediate-dose MTX (200 mg/m$^2$ i.v. bolus, followed by 800 mg/m$^2$ i.v. over 24 h) has demonstrated a mean ($\pm$SD) renal clearance *during the 24-h infusion* of 1000 mg/m$^2$ ($Cp_{ss} = 19 \pm 5.8$ µM) 0f 50.7 ($\pm 14$) ml/min/m$^2$. During the same time interval, the mean systemic clearance was $81.7 \pm 19$, and nonrenal clearance was 31.1 ($\pm 11.8$) ml/min/m$^2$. Methotrexate systemic clearance is comprised of both non-renal (i.e., metabolic) and renal processes (i.e., glomerular filtration, active tubular secretion, and tubular reabsorption), providing a physiological basis for the observed inter- and intrapatient changes and age-related changes in MTX disposition.

Possible differences in MTX disposition in adults and children have been reported, but are not yet clearly defined. Wang and associates [230] have suggested that the pharmacokinetics of high-dose MTX may be different in children 10 years of age or less. In their study of only three children and six adults, lower serum concentrations at 6 and 24 h, shorter initial half-lives, larger volumes of distribution, and greater urinary recovery of MTX during the infusion were seen for children when compared to adults. It is difficult to compare published adult and pediatric MTX renal clearance studies which used various dosage regimens, since net MTX renal clearance is apparently influenced by the MTX serum concentration. Kerr *et al.* [23] found a significant age-related difference in MTX systemic clearance in a group of patients ranging in age from 28 to 74 years, with older patients having lower clearance. Interestingly, when the regression line for this relationship is back extrapolated, the value estimated for age 4 years is 91 ml/min/m$^2$, which in excellent agreement with the value of $\approx 92$ ml/min/m$^2$, which we measured in a group of children with a median age of 4.2 years (Figure 6). These studies demonstrate faster clearance of MTX in children, consistent with that reported for other drugs (i.e., aminoglycosides) primarily excreted unchanged by the kidney.

The influence of methotrexate systemic clearance on the probability of relapse in children with standard-risk acute lymphoblastic leukemia was evaluated in 108 children [231]. These patients received 15 doses of 1 gm/m$^2$ of methotrexate as a 24-h continuous infusion every 6 weeks over 75 weeks with conventional low-dose mercaptopurine and MTX. Among the 108 patients, methotrexate clearance ranged from 44.7 to 132 ml/min/m$^2$. When the group was divided into three groups according to their rates of methotrexate clearance, the probability of complete remission showed significant differences (p = 0.016) among the subgroups. Patients with faster MTX clearance (Figure 11) had a higher probability of relapse. Multivariant Cox regression analysis was used to assess the influence of MTX systemic clearance and other prognostic variables on the probability of relapse. Factors that were identified in addition to MTX systemic clearance were hemoglobin and white blood cell count at diagnosis. Since recent

60

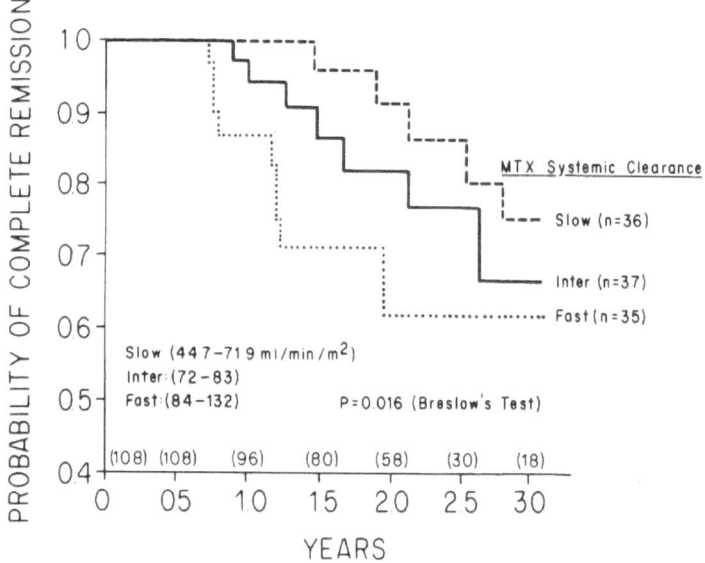

*Figure 11.* Kaplan-Meier curves of complete remission in standard-risk ALL patients sub-grouped according to their median methotrexate clearance. Reproduced with permission from reference 231.

studies have established the prognostic importance of cytogenetic character-istics of leukemic cells at diagnosis [232], the prognostic significance of MTX clearance was reassessed with cytogenetic data [233]. Cytogenetic information (DNA index) was available in 78 of the 108 children, and a similar analysis indicated that DNA index, white cell count, MTX clearance and hemaglobin were significant variables related to the probability of early relapse. This study indicates that interindividual variability in MTX clea-rance can have a significant influence on the probability of relapse early in the course of therapy; those patients with a faster rate of MTX clearance have a higher probability of early relapse. Because higher doses of MTX can be given, disease-specific clinical trials should be undertaken to establish the dosages of MTX that would ensure adequate exposure even in patients with fast clearance.

## Acknowledgements

The authors acknowledge Drs Joseph A. Sinkule, Gary C. Yee, and Paul R. Hutson for their contribution in preparation of this manuscript. This work was supported in part by Cancer Center CORE grant CA 21765, Leukemia Program project grant CA 20180, Solid Tumor project grant CA 23099, grant RO1 CA36401-01A, and the American Lebanese Syrian Associated

Charities (ALSAC). Parts of this review were adapted from Evans, W.E. *et al.*: Clinical pharmacokinetics of anticancer drugs in children. Drug Metabolism Reviews 14:847–886, 1983.

## References

1. Shirkey H: Editorial comment: therapeutic orphans. J Pediatr 72:119–120, 1960.
2. Assael BM: Pharmacokinetics and drug distribution during post-natal development. Pharmac Ther 18:159–197, 1982.
3. Done AK, Cohen SN, Strebel L: Pediatric Clinical pharmacology and the 'therapeutic orphan'. Ann Rev Pharmacol 17:561–573, 1977.
4. Klinger W: Biotransformation of drugs and other xenobiotics during post-batal development. Pharmac Ther 16:377–429, 1982.
5. Morselli PL, Franco-Morselli R, Bossi L: Clinical pharmacokinetics in newborns and infants. Age-related differences and therapeutic implications. Clin Pharmacokin 5: 428–527, 1980.
6. Deren JS: Development of structure and function in the fetal and newborn stomach. Am J Clin Nutr 24:144–159, 1971.
7. Huang NN, High RH: Comparison of serum levels following the administration of oral and parenteral preparations of penicillin to infants and children of various age groups. J Pediatr 42:657–668, 1953.
8. O'Connor WJ, Warren GH, Edrada LS, Mandala PS, Roseman SB: Serum concentrations of sodium nafcillin during the perinatal period. In: Antimicrobial Agents and Chemotherapy. Hobby G (ed). Bethesda, MD, American Society of Microbiology, 220–222, 1965.
9. Silverio J, Poole JW: Serum concentrations of ampicillin in newborn infants after, oral administration. Pediatrics 51:578–580, 1973.
10. Heimann G: Enteral absorption and bioavailability in children in relation to age. Eur J Clin Pharmacol 18:43–50, 1980.
11. Mirkin BL: Drug disposition and therapy in the developing human being. Pediatr Ann 9:542–557, 1976.
12. Friis-Hansen B: Body water compartments in children: changes during growth and related changes in body composition. Pediatrics 28:169–181, 1961.
13. Bendayan R, Pieper J, Stewart RB, Cavanasos GJ: Influence of age on serum protein binding of propranolol. Eur J Clin Pharmacol 26:251–254, 1984.
14. Kurz H, Mauser-Ganshorn A, Sticked HH: Differences in the binding of drugs to plasma proteins from newborn and adult man. I. Eur J Clin Pharmacol 11:463–467, 1977.
15. Koup J, Giacoia GP, Yaffe SJ: Drug-protein binding in the newborn infant. Ann NY Acad Sci 226:101–114, 1973.
16. De le Iglesia FA, Sturgess JM, McGuire EJ, Feuer G: Quantitative microscopic evaluation of the endoplasmic reticulum in developing human liver. Am J Path 82:61–70, 1976.
17. Morselli PL: Clinical pharmacokinetics in neonates. Clin Pharmacokinet 1:81–98, 1976.
18. Rylance GW, Moreland TA, Cowan MD, Clark DC: Liver volume estimation using ultrasound scanning. Arch Dis Child 57:283–286, 1982.
19. Roberts CJC, Jackson L, Halliwell M, Branch RA: The relationship between liver volume, antipyrine clearance and indocyanine green clearance before and after phenobarbitone administration in man. Br J Clin Pharmac 3:907–913, 1976.
20. Arant BS: Developmental patterns of renal functional maturation compared in the human neonate. J Pediatr 92:705–712, 1978.
21. Evans WE, Feldman S, Barker LF et al.: Use of gentamicin serum levels to individualize therapy in children. J Pediatr 93:133–137, 1978.

22. Evans WE, Taylor RH, Feldman S et al.: A model for dosing gentamicin in children and adolescents that adjusts for tissue accumulation with continuous dosing. Clin Pharmacokinet 5:295-306, 1980.

23. Kerr IG, Jolivet J, Collins JM, Drake JC, Chabner BA: Test-dose for predicting high-dose methotrexate infusions. Clin Pharmacol Ther 33:44-51, 1983.

24. Wang JJ, Holland JF, Sinks lf: Phase II study of adriamycin (NSC-123127) in childhood solid tumors. Cancer Chemother Rep 6 (part 3):267-270, 1975.

25. Davis HL, Davis TE: Daunorubicin and adriamycin in cancer treatment: An analysis of their roles and limitations. Cancer Treat Rep 63:809-815, 1979.

26. Rosso R, Ravazzoni C, Esposito M et al.: Plasma and urinary levels of adriamycin in man. Eur J Cancer 8:455-459, 1972.

27. Langone JJ, Vunakis HV, Bachur NR: Adriamycin and metabolites: Separation by high-pressure liquid chromatography and quantitation by radioimmunoassay. Biochem Med 12:283-289, 1975.

28. Benjamin RS, Wiernik PH, Bachur NR: Adriamycin chemotherapy efficacy, safety and pharmacologic basis of an intermittent single high-dosage schedule. Cancer 33:19-27, 1974.

29. Benjamin RS, Riggs CE, Bachur NR: Pharmacokinetics and metabolism of adriamycin in man. Clin Pharmacol Ther 14:592-600, 1973.

30. Creasey WA, McIntosh LS, Brescia T et al.: Clinical effects and pharmacokinetics of different dosage schedules of adriamycin. Cancer Res 36:216-221, 1976.

31. Bachur NR, Riggs CE, Green MR et al.: Plasma adriamycin and daunorubicin levels by fluorescence and radioimmunoassay. Clin Pharmacol Ther 21:70-77, 1977.

32. Riggs CE, Benjamin RS, Serpick AA, Bachur NR: Bilary disposition of adriamycin. Clin Pharmacol Ther 22:234-241, 1977.

33. Benjamin RS, Riggs CE, Bachur NR: Plasma pharmacokinetics of adriamycin and its metabolites in humans with normal hepatic and renal function. Cancer Res 37:1416-1420, 1977.

34. Chan KK, Chelbowski RT, Tong M et al.: Clinical pharmacokinetics of adriamycin in hepatoma patients with cirrhosis. Cancer Res 40:1263-1268, 1980.

35. Crom WR, Riley CA, Green AA et al.: Doxorubicin disposition in children and adolescents with cancer. Drug Intell Clin Pharm (abstract) 17:448, 1983.

36. Alberts DS, Bachur NR, Holtzman JL: The pharmacokinetics of daunomycin in man. Clin Pharmacol Ther 12:96-104, 1972.

37. Bachur NR: Anthracycline antibiotic pharmacology and metabolism. Cancer Treat Rep 63:817-820, 1979.

38. Huffman DH, Bachur NR: Daunorubicin metabolism in acute myelocytic leukemia. Blood 39:637-643, 1972.

39. Benjamin RS: A practical approach to adriamycin (NCS-123127) toxicology. Cancer Chemother Rep 6 (part 3): 191-194, 1975.

40. Nilsson S-O, Andersson B, Eksbert S et al.: Pharmacokinetics of daunorubicin after administration as free drug or as DNA complex in leukemia patients. Cancer Chemother Pharmacol 5:261-266, 1981.

41. Greene RF, Collins JM, Jenkins JF, Speyer JL, Meyers LE: Plasma pharmacokinetics of adriamycin and adriamycinol: implications for the design of in vitro experiments and treatment protocols. Cancer Res 43:3417-3421, 1983.

42. Evans WE, Williams D, Forrester L et al.: Inhibition of adriamycin microsomal metabolism in vitro by the cyclophosphamide metabolite acrolein. Drug Intell Clin Pharm (abstract) 14:634, 1980.

43. Atwell GJ, Cain BF, Seelye RN: Potential antitumor agents. 12. 9-anilinoacidines. J Med Chem 15:611-615, 1972.

44. Arlin ZA, Sklaroff RB Gee TS, Kempin SJ, Howard J, Clarkson BD, Young CW: Phase I and II trial of 4'-(9-acridinylamino) Methanesulfon-m-anisidide inpatients with acute leukemia. Cancer Res 40:3304–3306, 1980.

45. Rivera G, Evans WE, Dahl GV, Yee GC, Pratt CB: Phase I clinical and pharmacokinetic study of 4'-(9-acridinylamino)-methanesulfon-m-anisidide in children with cancer. Cancer Res 40:4250–4253, 1980.

46. McCredie KB, Keating MJ, Estey EH, Zander A, Bodey GP, Drewinko B, Freireich EJ: Use of a 4'-(9-acridinylamino) methanesulfon-m-anisidide (AMSA), cytosine-arabinoside (Ara-C), vincristine, prednisone, combination (AMSA-DAP) in poor risk patients in acute leukemia. Proc Am Soc Clin Oncol (abstract) 22:479, 1981.

47. Cysyk RL, Shoemaker D, Adamson RH: The pharmacologic disposition of 4-(9-acridinylamino) methanesulfon-m-anisidide in mice and rats. Drug Metab Dispos 5:579–590, 1977.

48. Przybylski M, Adamson RH, Mean JAR et al.: Field desorption mass spectrometric identification of the conjugation products of m-AMSA (NSC-141549) with endogenous thiols *in vitro* and in rat bile. Proc Am Assoc Cancer Res 20:287, 1979.

49. Malspeis L, Padmanahban S, Bhat HB et al.: Proton magnetic resonance identification of the principle biliary metabolite of m-AMSA (NSC-249992). Proc Am Assoc Cancer Res 21:308, 1980.

50. Shoemaker D, Gormley P, Monks A et al.: Microsomal metabolism of m-AMSA (NSC-249992). Proc Am Assoc Cancer Res 21:306, 1980.

51. Staubus A, Neidhart J, Young D, Malspeis L: Pharmacokinetics of m-AMSA (NSC-249992) in humans. Proc Am Assoc Cancer Res (abstract) 21:1981, 1980.

52. Hall SW, Benjamin RS, Legha SS et al.: Clinical pharmacokinetics of the new antitumor agent AMSA. Proc Am Assoc Cancer Res (abstract) 20:175, 1979.

53. Hall SW, Friedman J, Legha SS et al.: Human pharmacokinetics of a new acridine derivative, 4'-(9-acidinylamino) methanosulfon-m-anisidide (NSC 249992). Cancer Res, 43:3422–3426, 1983.

54. Gormley PE, Cysyk R: A fluorescence assay for 4'-(9-acridinylamino)methanesulfon-m-anisidide, a new antitumor agent. Anal Biochem 96:504–507, 1979.

55. Burger RM, Peisach J, Horwitz SB: Mechanisms of bleomycin action: in vitro studies. Life Sci 28:715–727, 1981.

56. Yagoda A, Murkherji B, Young C, Etcubanas E, Lamonte C, Smith JR, Tan CTC, Karkoff IH: Bleomycin, an antitumor antibiotic. Clinical experience in 274 patients. Ann Intern Med 77:861–870, 1972.

57. Haas CD, Coltman CA Jr, Gottlieb JA, Hart A, Luce JK, Talley RW, Samal B, Wilson HE, Hoogstrateen B: Phase II evaluation of bleomycin. A Southwest Oncology Group Study. Cancer 38:8–12, 1976.

58. Bonadonna G, Delena M, Monfardini S, Bartoli C, Bajetta E, Beretta G, Fossati-Bellani G: Clinical trials with bleomycin in lymphomas and in solid tumors. Eur J Cancer 8:205–215, 1972.

59. Exelby PR: Testis cancer in children. Semin Oncol 6:116–120, 1979.

60. Yee GC, Crom WR, Lee FH, Smyth RD, Evans WE: Bleomycin disposition in children with cancer. Clin Pharmacol Ther 33:668–673, 1983.

61. Broughton A, Strong JE: Radioimmunoassay of bleomycin. Cancer Res, 36:1418–1421, 1976.

62. Yee GC, Crom WR, Champion JE, et al.: Cisplatin-induced changes in bleomycin elimination. Cancer Treat Rep 67:587–589, 1983.

63. Krakoff IH, Cvitkovic E, Curie V, Yeh S, Lamonte C: Clinical pharmacologic and therapeutic studies of bleomycin given by continuous infusion. Cancer 40:2027–2037, 1977.

64. Alberts DS, Chen HSG, Liu R, Himmelstein KJ, Mayersohn M, Perrier D, Gross J, Moon T, Broughton A, Salmon SE: Bleomycin pharmacokinetics in man. I. Intravenous administration. Cancer Chemother. Pharmacol 1:177–181, 1978.

65. Broughton A, Strong JE, Holoye PY, Bedrossian CWM: Clinical pharmacology of bleomycin following intravenous infusion as determined by radioimmunoassay. Cancer 40:2772–2778, 1977.

66. Green AA, Hayes FA, Pratt CB et al.: In: Cis-platin – Current Status and New Developments. Prestayko AW, Crooke ST, Carter SK (eds). Academic Press, New York, 1980.

67. Ochs JJ, Freeman AI, Douglass HO Jr et al.: Cis-Dichlorodiammineplatimum (II) in advanced osteogenic sarcoma. Cancer Treat Rep 63:239–245, 1978.

68. LeRoy AF, Lutz RJ, Dedrick RL et al.: Pharmacokinetic study of cis-dichlorodiammineplatium (II) (DDP) in the beagle dog: thermodynamic and kinetic behavior of DDP in a biologic milieu. Cancer Treat Rep 63:59–71, 1979.

69. Casper ES, Kelsen DP, Alcock WW et al.: Platinum concentrations in bile and plasma following rapid and 6-hour infusions of cis-dichlorodiammineplatinum (II). Cancer Treat Rep, 63:2023–2025, 1979.

70. Vermorken JB, van der Vijgh WJF, Pinedo HM: Pharmacokinetic evidence for an enterohepatic circulation in a patient treated with cis-dichlorodiammineplatinum (II). Res Commun Chem Pathol Pharmacol, 28:319–328, 1980.

71. DeSimone PA, Yancey RS, Coupal JJ et al.: Effect of a forced duresis on the distribution and excretion (via urine and bile) of 195m Platinum When given as 196m platinum cis-dichlorodiammineplatinum (II). Cancer Treat Rep 63:951–960, 1979.

72. Crom WR, Evans WE, Pratt CB et al.: Cisplatin disposition in children and adolsecents with cancer. Cancer Chemother Pharmacol, 6:95–99, 1981.

73. Gullo JJ, Litterst CL, Maguire PJ et al.: Pharmacokinetics and protein binding of cis-dichlorodiammineplatinum(II) administered as a one hour or as a twenty hour indusion. Cancer Chemother. Pharmacol 5:21–26, 1980.

74. Long DF, Repta AJ: Cisplatin: Chemistry, distribution and biotransformation. Biopharmaceutics Drug Dispos 2:1–16, 1981.

75. Litterst CL, Gram TE, Dedrick RL et al.: Distribution and disposition of platinum following intravenous administration of cis-dichlorodrammineplatinum (II) (NSC 119875) to dogs. Cancer Res 36:2340–2344, 1976.

76. DeConti RC, Toftness BR, Lange RC, Creasy WA: Clinical and pharmacological studies with cis-diamminedichloroplatinum (II). Cancer Res 33:1310–1315, 1973.

77. Gormley PE, Bull JM, LeRoy AF, Cysyk R: Kinetics of cisdichlorodiammineplatinum. Clin Pharmacol Ther 25:351–357, 1979.

78. Repta AJ, Long DF: In: Cisplatin – Current Status and New Developments. Prestayko AW, Crroke ST, Carter SK (eds). Academic Press, New York 285–304, 1980.

79. Prestayko AW, D'Aoust JC, Issel BJ, Crooke ST: Cisplatin (cis-diamminedichloroplatinum II). Cancer Treat Rev 6:17–39, 1979.

80. Frick GA, Ballentine R, Driever CW, Kramer WG: Renal excretion kinetics of high-dose cis-dichlorodiammineplatinum (II) administered with hydration and mannitol diuresis. Cancer Treat Rep 63:13–16,

81. Belt RJ, Himmelstein KJ, Patton TF et al.: Pharmacokinetics of non-protein-bound platinum species following administration of cis-dichlorodiammineplatinum(II). Cancer Treat Rep 63:1515–1521, 1979.

82. Himmelstein KJ, Patton TF, Belt RJ et al.: Clinical kinetics of intact cisplatinum and some related species. Clin Pharmacol Ther 29:658–664, 1981.

83. Patton TF, Himmelstein JK, Belt R et al.: Plasma levels and urinary excretion of filterable platinum species following bolus injection and IV infusion of cis-dichlorodiammineplatinum (II) in man. Cancer Treat Rep 62:1359–1362, 1978.

84. LeRoy AF, Wehling M, Gormley P et al.: Quantitative changes in cis-dichlorodiammineplatinum (II) speciation in excreted urine with times after IV infusion in man: Methods of analysis, preliminary studies, and clinical results. Cancer Treat Rep 64:123–132, 1980.

85. Chang Y, Sternson LA, Repta AJ: Development of a specific analytical method for cis-dichlorodiammineplatinan UM-(II) in plasma. Anal Lett. 11:339–459, 1978.

86. Sladek NE, Priest J, Doeden D et al.: Plasma half-life and urinary excretion of cyclophosphamide in children. Cancer Treat Rep 64:1061, 1980.

87. Mellett LB, El Darrer SM, Rall DP, Adamson RH: Metabolism of cyclophosphamide $C^{14}$ by various murine species. Arch Int Pharmacodyn Ther 177:60, 1969.

88. Friedman OM, Boger E: Colorimetric estimation of nitrogen mustards in aqueous media,hydrolytic behavior of bis(2-chloroethyl)amino, nor-HN2. Anal Cham 33:906, 1961.

89. Fenselau C, Kan MN, Rao SS et al.: Identification of aldophosphamide as a metabolite of cyclophosphamide in vitro and in vivo in humans. Cancer Res 37:2538, 1977.

90. Jardine I, Fenselau C, Appler M et al.: Quantitation by gas chromatography-chemical ionization mass specttometry of cyclophosphamide, phosphoramide mustard and nor-nitrogen mustard on the plasma and urine of patients receiving cyclophosphamide therapy. Cancer Res, 38:408, 1978.

91. Juma FD, Rogers HJ, Trounce JR: The pharmacokinetics of cyclophosphamide, phosphoramide mustard and nor-nitrogen mustard studied by gas chromatography in petients receiving cyclophosphamide therapy. Br J Clin Pharmacol 10:327, 1980.

92. Pantarotto C, Bossi A, Belvedere G et al.: Quantitative GLC determination of Cyclophosphamide and isophosphamide in biological specimens. J Pharm Sci 63:1554, 1974.

93. Juma FD, Rogers HJ, Trounce JR: Pharmacokineics of cyclophosphamide and alkylating activity in man after intravenous and oral administration. Br J Clin Pharmacol 8:209, 1979.

94. Bagley CM jr, Bostick FW, DeVita VT Jr: Clinical pharmacology of cyclophosphamide. Cancer Res 33:226, 1973.

95. Cohen JL, Jao JY, Jusko WJ: Pharmacokinetics of cyclophosphamide in man. Br J Pharmacol 43:677, 1971.

96. Duncan JH, Colvin MO, Fenselau C: Mass Spectrometric study of the distribution of cyclophosphamide in humans. Toxicol Appl Pharmacol 24:317, 1973.

97. Talha MR, Rogers HJ, Trounce JR: Distribution and pharmacokinetics of cyclophosphamide in the rat. Br J Cancer 41:140, 1980.

98. Edwards G, Calvert RT, Crowther D, Bramwell V, Scarffe H: Repeated investigations of cyclophosphamide disposition in myeloma patients receiving intermittent chemotherapy. Br J Clin Pharmacol 10:281, 1980.

99. Mouridsen HT, Jacobsen E: Pharmacokinetics of cyclophosphamide in renal failure. Acta Pharmacol Toxicol 409, 1975.

100. Grochow LB, Colvin M: Clinical pharmacokinetics of cyclophosphamide. Clin Pharmacokinet 4:380, 1979.

101. Connors TA: Alkylating drugs, nitrosurea, dialkyltriazenes. In: Cancer Chemotherapy. Pinedo HM (ed). Elsevier/North Holland, New York, 22–55, 1979.

102. Brock N, Stekar J, Pohl J, Niemeyer U, Scheffler G3 Acrolein, the causative factor of urotoxic side-effects of cyclophosphamide, ifosfamide, trofasfamide and sufosfamide. Arzneim Forsch 29:659, 1979.

103. Scheef W et al.: Controlled clinical studies in an antidote against the urotoxicity of oxazaphosphorines: preliminary results. Cancer Treat Rep 63:501, 1979.

104. Levy L, Harris Rb: Effect of N-acetylcysteine on some aspects of cyclophosphamide-induced toxicity and immunosuppression. Biochem Pharmacol 26:1015–1020, 1977.

105. Gerzon K: Dimeric catharanthus alkaloids. In: Anticancer Agents Based on Natural Products Model. Cassady JM, Douros JD (eds). Academic Press, New York 271-317, 1980.

106. Jackson DV, Bender RA: Clinical pharmacology of the vinca alkaloids, epipodophyllotoxins and maytansine. In: Clinical Pharmacology of Anti-Neoplastic Drugs. Pinedo HM (ed). Elsevier/North Holland, Biomedical Press, Amsterdam 277-293, 1978.

107. Nelson RL, Dyke RW, Root MA: Comparative pharmacokinetics of vincristine and vinblastine in patients with cancer. Cancer Treat Rev 7 (Suppl 1):17–24, 1980.

108. Holland JF, Glidewell O: Chemotherapy of acute lymphocytic leukemia of childhood. Cancer 30:1480, 1972.

109. Handbook on drugs of choice. Med Lett, 1977.

110. James DH Jr, George P: Vincristine in children with malignant solid tumors. J Pediatr 64:534–541, 1964.

111. Windmiller J, Berry DH, Haddy TB: Vincristine sulfate in the treatment of neuroblastoma in children. Am J Dis Child 111:75–78, 1966.

112. Sutow WW, Berry DH, Haddy TB, Sullivan MP, Watkins WL, Windmiller J: Vincristine sulfate therapy in children with metastatic soft tissue sarcoma. Pediatrics 38:465–472, 1966.

113. Bohannon RA, Miller DG, Diamond HD: Vincristine in the treatment of lymphomas and leukemia. Cancer Res 23:613–621, 1963.

114. Starling KA, Donaldson MH, Haggard ME: Therapy of histiocytosis X with vincristine, vinblastine and cyclophosphamide. The Southwest Cancer Chemotherapy Study Group. Am J Dis Child 123:105–110, 1972.

115. Einhorn LH, Donahue J: Cis-diamminedichloroplatinum, vinblastine, and bleomycin combination chemotherapy in disseminated testicular cancer. Ann Intern Med 87:293–298, 1977.

116. Gralla RJ, Tan CT, Young CW: Vindesine. A review of phase-II trials. Cancer Chemother Pharmacol 2(4):271–274, 1979.

117. Mathe G, Pico JL, Schwarzenberg L, Riband D, Musset M, Jasmin CL, DeLuca L: Phase II clinical trial with vindesine for remission induction in acute leukemia, blastic crisis of chronic myeloid leukemia, lymphosarcoma, and Hodgkin's disease: absence of cross-resistance with vincristine. Cancer Treat Rep 62:805–809, 1978.

118. Krivit W, Chilcote R, Pyesmany A, Anderson J, Hammond D: An initial report of a phase-III trial comparison vindesine and vincristine for acute lymphocytic leukemia of childhoud. Cancer Chemother. Pharmacol 2:267–270, 1979.

119. Hill BT, Whelan RDH: Comparative effects of vincristine and vindesine on cell cycle kinetics in vitro. Cancer Treat Rev 7(Suppl 1):5–15, 1980.

120. Valdivieso M: Phase I and II studies of vindesine. Cancer Treat Rev 7(Suppl 1):31–37, 1980.

121. Tan C: Current Chemotherapy. In: Proc 10th Int Congress of Chemotherapy, Vol 2. Zurich, September 1977.

122. Bender RA, Castle MC, Margileth DA, Oliverio VT: The pharmacokinetics of [³H]-vincristine in man. Clin Pharmacol Ther 22:430–435, 1977.

123. Creasey WA, Scott AI, Wei CC, Kutcher J, Schwartz A, March JC: Pharmacological studies with vinblastine in the dog. Cancer Res 35:1116–1120, 1975.

124. Pratt WB, Rudden RW (eds): The Anticancer Drugs. Oxford University Press, New York 227, 1979.

125. Nelson RL, Dyke RW, Root MA: Comparative pharmacokinetics of the vinca alkaloids in man. Clin Pharmacol Ther 21:112, 1977.

126. Jackson DV Jr, Castle MC, Bender RA: Biliary excretion of vincristine. Clin Pharmacol Ther 24:101–107, 1978.

127. Woods WG, O'Leary M, Nesbit ME: Life-threatening neuropathy and hepatotoxicity in infants during induction therapy for acute lymphoblastic leukemia. J Pediatr 98:642–645, 1981.

128. Owellen RJ, Hartke CA, Hains FO: Pharmacokinetics and metabolism of vinblastine in humans. Cancer Res, 37:2597–2602, 1977.

129. Castle MC, Mead JAR: Investigation of the metabolic fate of tritiated vincristine in the rat by high-pressure liquid chromotogrphy. Biochem Pharmacol 27:37–44, 1978.

130. Kelly MG, Hartwell JL: Biological effects and chemical composition f podophyllin: review. J Natl Cancer Inst, 14:967, 1954.

131. Brewer CF, Loike JD, Horwitz SB, Sternlicht H, Gensler WJ: Conformational analysis of podophyllotoxin and its congeners. Structure-activity relationship in microtubule assembly. J Med Chem 22:215–221, 1979.

132. Grieder A, Maurer R, Stahelin H: Effect of an epipodophyllotoxin derivative (VP-16–231) on macromolecular synthesis and mitosis in mastocytoma cells in vitro. Cancer Res 34:1788–1793, 1974.

133. Misra NC, Roberts DW: Inhibition by 4'-demethyl-epipodophyllotoxin 9-(4,6-O-2-thenylidene-beta-D-glucopyranoside) of human lymphoblast cultures in G2 phase of the cell cycle. Cancer Res 35:99–105, 1975.

134. Rivera G, Avery T, Pratt C: 4'-demethylepipodophyllotoxin 9-(4,6-O-2-thenylidene-beta-D-glucopyranoside) (NSC-122819; VM-26) and 4'-demethylepipodphyllotoxin 9-(4,6-O-ethylidene-beta-D-glucopyranoside) (NSC-14150; VP-16–213) in childhood cancer: preliminary observations. Cancer Chemother. Rep 59:743–749, 1975.

135. Bleyer WA, Krivit W, Chard RL Jr, Hammond D: Phase II study of VM-26 in acute leukemia, neuroblastoma and other refractory childhood malgnancies: a report from the Children's Cancer Study Group. Cancer Treat Rep 63:977–981, 1979.

136. Rivera G, Green A, Hayes A: Epipodophyllotoxin VM-26 in the treatment of childhood neuroblastoma. Cancer Treat Rep 61:1243–1248, 1977.

137. Rozencweig M, Von Hoff DD, Henney JE et al: VM-26 and VP-16–213: a comparative analysis. Cancer 40:334–342, 1977.

138. Seiler RW: Combination chemotherapy with VM-26 and CCNU in primary malignant brain tumors of children. Helv Pediatr Acta 35:51–56, 1980.

139. Sklansky BD, Mann-Kaplan RS, Reynolds AF Jr et al.: Proceedings: 4'-demethyl-epipodophyllotoxin-beta-D-thenylideneglucoside (PTG) in the treatment of malignant intracranial neoplasms. Cancer 33:460–467, 1974.

140. Issell BF, Crooke ST: Etoposide (VP-16–213). Cancer Treat Rev, 6:107, 1979.

141. Muggia FM, Selawry OS, Hansen HH: Clinical studies with a new Podophylloxin derivative, epipodophyllotoxin, 4'-demethyl-9-(4,6-O-2-thenylidene-D-glucopyranoside) (NSC-122819). Cancer Chemother Rep 55:575–581, 1971.

142. Venditti JM: Treatment schedule dependency of experimentally active antileukemic (L1210) drugs. Cancer Chemother. Rep 2(part 3):35–59, 1971.

143. Dombernowsky P, Nissen NI: Schedule dependency of the antileukemic activity of the podophyllotoxin-derivative VP-16–213 (NSC-141540) in L1210 leukemia. Acta Path Microbiol Scand 81:715–724, 1973.

144. D'Incalci M, Farina P, Fosoli M et al.: VP-16 plasma levels after IV and two methods of oral administration to choriocarcinoma patients. Proc Am Soc Clin Oncol 22:357, 1981.

145. Evans WE, Sinkule JA, Crom WR et al.: Pharmacokinetics of teniposide (VM-26) and etoposide (VP-16–213) in children with cancer. Cancer Chemother. Pharmacol 7:147–150, 1982.

146. Snodgrass W, Walker L, Tubergen D et al.: Kinetics of VP-16 epipodophyllotoxin in children with cancer. Proc Am Assoc Cancer Res 21:333, 1980.

147. Strife RJ, Jardine I, Colvin M: Analysis of the anticancer drugs etoposide (VP-16–213) and teniposide (VM-26) by high-performance liquid chromatography with fluorescence detection. J Chromatogr 224:168–174, 1981.

148. Allen LM, Creaven PJ: Comparison of the human pharmacokinetics of VM-26 and VP-16, two antineoplastic epipodophyllotoxin glucopyranoside derivatives. Eur J Cancer 11:697, 1975.

149. Sinkule JA, Stewart CF, Crom WR et al-: Teniposide (VM-26) disposition in children with leukemia. Cancer Res 44:1235–1237.

68

150. Evans WE, Sinkule JA, Rivera G, Dow L et al.: Clinical pharmacology of VM-26 (NSC-122819) and VP-16 (NSC-141540) in children with cancer. Proc Am Assoc Cancer Res 22:174, 1981.

151. Allen LM, Marcks C, Xreaven PJ: 4'-demethyl-epipodophyllic acid-9-(4,6-O-ethylidene-β-D-glucopyranoside), the major urinary metabolite of VP-16-213 in man. Proc am Assoc. Cancer Res 17:6, 1976.

152. D'Incalci M, Farina P, Sessa R, Conter P et al.: Mario Negri Institute, Milan, Italy, personal communications, 1981.

153. Hande KR, Wedlund PJ, Noon RM et al.: Pharmacokinetics of high-dose etoposide (VP-16-213) administered to cancer patients. Cancer Res 44:379–382, 1984.

154. Arbuck SG, Douglass HO, Goodwin P, Nava H, Clark J, Crom WR, Evans WE: Pharmacokinetics of etoposide (VP) in patients with normal and abnormal liver function. Proc Am Soc Clin Oncol 4:40, 1985.

155. Frei EIII, Bickers JN, Hewlett JS et al.: Dose schedule and antitumor studies of arakinosyl cytosine (NSC-63878). Cancer Res 29:1325–1332.

156. Pommier Y, Pochat L, Marie JP et al.: High-dose cytarabine in acute luekemia: toxicity and pharmacokinetics. Cancer Treat Rep 67:371–373, 1983.

157. Briethaupt H, Pralle H, Eckhardt T et al.: Clinical results and pharmacokinetics of high-dose cytosine arabinoside (HD ARA-C). Cancer 50:1248–1257, 1982.

158. Ho DHW, Frei EIII: Clinical pharmacology of 1-beta-d-arabinofuranosyl cytosine. Clin Pharmacol Ther 12:944–954, 1971.

159. Van Prooijen HC, Vierwinden G, Wessels J et al.: Cytosine arabinoside binding to human plasma proteins. Arch. Int Pharmacodyn. Ther 229:199–205, 1977.

160. Sinkule JA, Mauer EC, Ochs JJ, Rivera G, Evans WE: Pharmacokinetics of high-dose cytosine arabinoside (Ara-C) in children with refractory leukemia. Proc Amer Assoc Cancer Res 23:128, 1982.

161. Band PR, Holland JF, Bernand J et al.: Treatment of central nervous system leukemia with intrathecal cytosine arabinoside. Cancer 32:744–748, 1973.

162. Momparler RL: Kinetic and template studies with 1-D-arabinofurano-sylcytosine 5'triphosphate and mammalian deoxyribonucleic acid polymerase. Mol Pharmacol 8:362–370, 1972.

163. Momparler RL: Effect of cytosine arabinoside 5'triphosphate on mammalian DNA polymerase. Biochem Biophys Res Commun 34:464–471, 1969.

164. Coleman CN, Stoller RG, Drake JC et al.: Deoxycytidine kinease: properties of the enzyme from human leukemia granulocytes. Blood 46:791–803, 1975.

165. Creasey WA: In: Antineoplastic and Immunosuppressive Agents. Sartorelli AC, Johns DG (eds). Springer-Verlag, New York, 232–256, 1975.

166. Stoller RG, Coleman CN, Chang P et al.: Inb: Comparative Leukemia Research. Clemmesen J, Yohn DS (eds). Karger, Basel 531–533, 1976.

167. Wan SH, Huffman DH, Azarnoff DL et al.: Pharmacokinetics of 1-beta-D-arabinofuranosylcytosine in humans. Cancer Res, 34:392–397, 1974.

168. Finklestein JZ, Scher J, Karon M: Pharmacologic studies of tritiated cytosine arabinoside (NSC-63878) in children. Cancer Chemother Rep 54:35–39, 1970.

169. Chou TC, Arlin Z, Clarkson B et al.: Metabolism of 1-beta-D-arabinofuranosylcytosine in human leukemic cells. Cancer Res 37:3561–3570, 1977.

170. Ochs J, Sinkule J, Danks MK et al.: Continuous infusion high-dose cytosine arabinoside in refractory childhood leukemia. J Clin Oncol 2:1092–1097, 1984.

171. Rustum YMJ, Preisler HD: Correlation between leukemic cell retention of 1-beta-D-arabinofuranosycytosine 5'triphosphate and response to therapy. Cancer Res 39:42–49, 1979.

172. Elion GB, Hitchings AH, Van der Werff H: Antagonists of nucleic acid derivatives; purines. J Biol Chem 192:505–518, 1951.

173. Burchenal JH, Murphy ML, Ellison RR et al.: Clinical evaluation of new antimetabolite, 6-mercaptopurine, in treatment of leukemia an allied diseases. Blood 8:965–999, 1953.

174. Calabresi P, Parks RE Jr: Antiproliferative agents and drugs used for immunosuppression. In: The Pharmacological Basis of Therapeutics. Goodman & Gilman (eds). Macmillan, New York, 1256, 1980.

175. Ding TL, Benet LZ: Comparative bioavailability and pharmacokinetic studies of azathioprine and 6-mercaptopurine in the Rhesus monkey. Drug Metab Disp 7:373–377, 1979.

176. Loo TL, Luce JK, Sullivan MP, Frei EIII: Clinical pharmacologic observations on 6-mercaptopurine and 6-methylthiopurine ribonucleoside. Clin Pharmacol. Ther 9:180–194, 1968.

177. Zimm S, Collins JM, Riccardi R, O'Neill D, Narang PK, Chabner B, Poplack DG: Variable bioavailability of oral mercaptopurine. Is maintenance chemotherapy in acute lymphoblastic leukemia being optimally delivered? NEJM 308:1005–1009, 1983.

178. Coffey JJ, White CA, Lesk AB et al.: Effect of allopurinol on the pharmacokinetics of 6-mercaptopurine (NSC-755) in cancer patients. Cancer Res 32:1283–1289, 1972.

179. Therlikkis L, Ortega E, Solomon R, Day JL: Pharmacokinetics of mercaptopurine. J Pharm Sci 66:1454–1457, 1977.

180. Grindey GB: Clinical pharmacology of the 6-thiopurines. Cancer Treat Rev 6(Suppl):19–25, 1979.

181. Elion GB: Symposium of immunosuppressive drugs. Biochemistry and pharmacology of purine analogues. Fed Proc 26:898–904, 1967.

182. Vogler WR, Bain JA, Huguley CM Jr et al.: Metabolic and therapeutic effects of allopurinol in patients with leukemia and gout. Am J Med 40:548–559, 1966.

183. Goldin A, Vendetti JM, Humphreys SR et al.: Quantitative comparison of antileukemic effectiveness of 2 folic acid antagonist in mice. J Natl Cancer Inst 15:1657, 1955.

184. Haskell CM: In: Cancer Treatment. Haskell CM (ed). W.B. Saunders, Philadelphia, 79, 1980.

185. Valerino DM, Johns DG, Zaharko DS, Oliverio VT: Studies of the metabolism of methotrexate by intestinal flora. I. identification and study of biological properties of the metabolite 4-amino-4-deoxy-$N^{10}$-methylpteroic acid. Biochem Pharmacol 21:821–831, 1972.

186. Smith DK, Omura GA, Ostroy F: Clinical pharmacology of intermediate-dose oral methotrexate. Cancer Chemother Pharmacol 4:117–120, 1980.

187. Henderson ES, Adamson RH, Olicerio VT: The metabolic fate of tritiated methotrexate. II. Absorption and excretion in man. Cancer Res 25:1018–1024, 1965.

188. Wan SH, Huffman DH, Azarnoff DL et al.: Pharmacokinetics of 1-beta-D-arabinofuranosylcytosine in humans. Cancer Res 34:392–397, 1974.

189. Balis FM, Savitch JL, Bleyer WA: Pharmacokinetics or oral methotrexate in children. Cancer Res 43:2342–2345, 1983.

190. Cohen MH, Creaven PJ, Fossieck BE et al.: Effect of oral prophylactic broad spectrum nonabsorbable antibiotics on the gastrointestinal absorption of nutrients and methotrexate in small cell bronchogenic carcinoma patients. Cancer 38:1556, 1976.

191. Pinkerton CR, Welsham SG, Dempsey SI et al.: Absorption of methotrexate under standardized conditions in children with acute lymphoblastic leukemia. Br J Cancer 42:613–615, 1980.

192. Schornagel JH, Van Engelen ME, De Vos D: Bioavailability of methotrexate tablets. Pharmaceutisch Weekblad [Sci] Ed 4:89–90, 1982.

193. Stuart JF, Calman KC, Watters J et al.: Bioavailability of methotrexate: implications for clinical use. Cancer Chemother Pharmacol 3:239–241.

194. Harvey VJ, Slevin ML, Wollard RC et al.: The bioavailability of oral intermediate-dose methotrexate. Effect of dose subdivision, formulation and timing in the chemotherapy cycle. Cancer Chemother Pharmacol 13:91–94, 1984.

195. Christophidis N., Vajda FJ, Lucas I et al.: Comparison of intravenous and oral high-dose methotrexate in treatment of solid tumors. Br Med J 1:298–300, 1979.
196. Freeman-Narrod M, Gerstly BJ, Engstrom PF, Bornskin RS: Comparison of serum concentrations of methotrexate after various routes of administration. Cancer 36:1619, 1975.
197. Leme PR, Creaven PJ, Allen LM, Berman M: Kinetic model for the disposition and metabolism of moderate and high-dose methotrexate (NSC-740) in man. Cancer Chemother Rep 59:811, 1975.
198. Pratt CB, Howrath C, Ransom JL et al.: High-dose methotrexate used along and in combination for measurable primary or metastatic ostersarcoma. Cancer Treat Rep 64:11, 1980.
199. Zaharko DS, Dedrick RL, Bischoff KB et al.: Methotrexate tissue distribution: prediction by a mathematical model. J Natl Cancer Inst 46:775, 1971.
200. Bischoff KB, Dedrick RL, Zaharko DS, Longsheth JA: Methotrexate pharmacokinetics. J Pharm Sci 60:1128, 1971.
201. Evans WE, Pratt CB: Effect of pleural effusion on high-dose methotrexate kinetics. Clin Pharmacol Ther 23:68, 1978.
202. Evans WE: In: Applied Pharmacokinetics – Principles of Therapeutic Drug Monitoring. Evans WE, Schentag JJ, Jusko WJ (eds). Applied Therapeutics 518, 1980.
203. Evans WE, Hutson PR, Stewart CF et al.: Methotrexate cerebrospinal fluid and serum concentrations after intermediate-dose methotrexate infusion. Clin Pharmacol Ther 33:301–307, 1983.
204. Jacobs SA, Stoller RG, Chabner BA, Johns DG: 7-hydroxymethotrexate as a urinary metabolite in human subjects and rhesus monkeys receiving high-dose methotrexate. J Clin Invest 57:534, 1976.
205. Johns DG, Loo TL: Metabolite of 4-amino-4-deoxy-$N^{10}$-methylpteroylglutamic acid (methotrexate). J Pharm Sci 56:356, 1967.
206. Wang YM, Howell SK, Smith RG et al.: Effect of metabolism on pharmacokinetics and toxicity of high dose methotrexate (HD-MTX) therapy in children. Proc Am Soc Clin Oncol 20:334, 1979.
207. Baugh CM, Krumdieck CL, Nair MG: Polygammaglutamyl metabolites of methotrexate. Biochem Biophys Res Commun 52:27–34, 1973.
208. Brown JP, Davidson GE, Weir DC, Scott JM: Specificity of folate-y-L-glutamate ligase in rate liver and kidney. Biosynthesis of Poly-y-L-glutamates of unreduced methotrexate and the effect of methotrexate on folate polyglutamate biosynthesis. Int J Biochem 5:727–733, 1974.
209. Jacobs SA, Adamson RH, Chabner BA et al.: Stoichiometric inhibition of mammalian dihydrofolate reductase by the gamma-glutamyl metabolite of methotrexate, 4-amino-4-dexoy-N-10-methylpteroylglutamyl-y-glutamate. Biochem Biophys Res Commun 63:692–698.
210. Whitehead VM, Perrault MM, Stelcner S: Tissue-specific synthesis of methotrexate polyglutamates in the rat. Cancer Res 35:2985–2990, 1975.
211. Hoffbrand AV, Tripp E, lavoie A: Synthesis of folate polyglutamates in human cells. Clin Sci Mol Med 50:61–68.
212. Whitehead VM, Perrault MM, Stelcner S: Tissue-specific synthesis of methotrexate polyglutamates in the rat. In: Chemistry and Biology of Pteridines. Pfleiderer W (ed). Walterde Gryter, Berlin 475–483, 1975.
213. Jacobs SA, Derr CJ, Johns DG: Accumulation of methotrexate diglutamate in human liver during methotrexate therapy. Biochem Pharmacol 26:2310–2313, 1977.
214. Whitehead VM: Synthesis of methotrexate polyglutamates in L1210 murine leukemia cells. Cancer Res 37:408–412, 1977.

215. Rosenblatt DS, Whitehead VM, Dupont MM et al.: Synthesis of methotrexate polyglutamates in cultured human cells. Mol Pharmacol 14:210–214, 1978.

216. Rosenblatt DS, Whitehead VM, Vera N et al.: Prolonged inhibition of DNA synthesis associated with the accumulation of methotrexate polyglutamates by cultured human cells. Mol Pharmacol 14:1143–1147, 1978.

217. Whitehead VM, Rosenblatt DS: Decreased synthesis of methotrexate polyglutamates in mutant-hamster cells and in folinic acidtreated human-fibroblasts. In: Chemistry and Biology of Pteridines. Kisliuk RL, Brown GM (eds). Elsevier/North Holland, New York 689–694, 1979.

218. Galivan J: Transport and metabolism of methotrexate in normal and resistant cultured rat hepatoma cells. Cander Res 39:735–743, 1979.

219. Gewirtz DA, White JC, Randolph JK et al.: Formation of methotrexate polyglutamates in rat hepatocytes. Cancer Res 39:2914–2918, 1979.

220. Witte A, Whitehead VM, Rosenblatt DS et al.: Synthesis of methotrexate polyglutamates by bone marrow cells from patients with leukemia and lymphoma. Dev Pharmacol Ther, 1:40–46, 1980.

221. McGuire JJ, Bertino JR: Enzymatic synthesis and function of folylpoly-glutamates. Mol Cellular Biochem (Spec No Pt 1 38:19–48, 1981.

222. Galivan J: Evidence for the cytotoxic activity of polyglutamate derivatives of methotrexate. Mol Pharmacol 17:105–110, 1980.

223. Schilsky RL, Bailey BD, Chabner BA: Methotrexate polyglutamate synthesis by cultured human breast cancer cells. Proc Natl Acad Sci USA 77:2919–2922, 1980.

224. Fabre G, Matherly LH, Fabre I, Cano J-P, Goldman ID: Interactions between 7-hydroxymethotrexate and methotrexate at the cellular level in the Ehrlich ascites tumor in vitro. Cancer Res 44:970–975, 1984.

225. Huffman DH, Wan SH, Azarnoff DL, Hoogstraten B: Pharmacokinetics of methotrexate. Clin Pharmacol Ther 14:572–579, 1973.

226. Evans WE, Tsiatis A, Crom WR, Brodeur G, Coburn T, Pratt CB: Pharmacokinetics of sustained serum methotrexate concentrations secondary to gastrointestinal obstruction. J Pharm Sci 70:1194–1198, 1981.

227. Shen DD, Azarnoff DL: Clinical pharmacokinetics of methotrexate. Clin Pharmacokinet 3:1–13, 1978.

228. Ziegler DG, Henderson ES, Hahn MA, Oliverio VT: The effect of organic acids on renal clearance of methotrexate in man. Clin Pharmacol Ther 10:849–857, 1969.

229. Evans WE, Stewart CF, Hutson PR, Cairnes DA, Bowman WP, Yee GC, Crom WR: Disposition of intermediate-dose methotrexate in children with acute lymphocytic leukemia. Drug Intell Clin Pharm 16:839–842, 1982.

230. Wang YM, Sutow WW, Romsdahl MM, Perez C: Age-related pharmacokinetics of high-dose methotrexate in patients with osteosarcoma. Cancer Treat Rep 63:405–410, 1979.

231. Evans WE, Crom WR, Stewart CF et al.: Methotrexate systemic clearance influences probability of relapse in children with standard-risk acute lymphocytic leukaemia. Lancet 1:359–362, 1984.

232. Look AT, Melvin SL, Williams DL et al.: Aneuploidy and percentage of S-phase cells determined by flow cytometry correlate with cell phenotype in childhood acute leukemia. Blood 60:959–967, 1982.

233. Evans WE, Abromowitch M, Look AT, Williams D, Crom WR: Variability – drug clearance can influence risk of relapse in children with acute lymphocytic leukemia (ALL). Clin Pharmacol Ther 37:194, 1985.

# Pharmacologic reasons for treatment failure

# 4. Drug resistance in medical and pediatric oncology

KENNETH H. COWAN

## Introduction

Significant progress has been achieved in the treatment of cancer and leukemia over the past two decades. Through the use of combination chemotherapy and combined modality therapy, complete remissions can now be achieved in the vast majority of patients with acute lymphocytic leukemia (ALL), Hodgkin's and non-Hodgkin's lymphoma, testicular cancer, Ewing's sarcoma, and osteogenic sarcoma. Even in the more common adult malignancies such as breast cancer, small cell lung cancer, and ovarian cancer, combination chemotherapy regimens are capable of of achieving meaningful clinical remissions in a high proportion of patients. Unfortunately many of these patients will eventually relapse. While durable second and even third remissions are frequently achieved in some diseases such as ALL [1], relapses in most cancers are associated with the development of drug resistance and salvage therapy is relatively ineffective. Indeed, one of the important problems in clinical oncology is the identification of the mechanisms involved in the development of clinical drug resistance so that effective second line therapies may be more rationally designed.

Drug resistant tumors have been empirically divided into two distinct clinical entities based on the relative response to initial therapy. Tumors which are unresponsive to primary chemotherapy regimens are considered to have inherent resistance. Included in this group are tumors such as colon cancer, non-small cell lung cancer, and malignant melanoma. In contrast, resistance that develops in malignancies that were initially responsive to chemotherapy are considered to have acquired a drug resistant phenotype during therapy. Although, entirely arbitrary this subdivision is useful in order to emphasize that the mechanisms associated with the lack of effective clinical response under these two clinical circumstances may be different and may, therefore, require different therapeutic approaches.

## Pharmacologic factors in drug resistance

As will be described below tumor cells can develop resistance to cytotoxic drugs at the cellular level through a variety of different mechanisms. However, it is important to bear in mind that there are also many pharmacologic factors which may influence the clinical outcome. Thus, as shown in Table 1, there are a variety of host factors which may influence the concentration of drug to which otherwise drug sensitive tumor cells are exposed. For example, there is significant interindividual variation in the bioavailability of certain drugs including phenylalanine mustard [2], hexylmethylmelamine [3], and mercaptopurine [4] following the oral administration of these agents. In the case of mercaptopurine, Zimm *et al.* [4] observed over a six-fold variation in the peak plasma level of this drug following oral administration to patients with acute lymphoblastic leukemia. In addition, there may be important differences among patients in the rate of drug metabolism or elimination. Furthermore, tumors which develop in sanctuary sites such as the CNS or testes are more refractory to systemic therapy presumably as a result of the poor penetration of most chemotherapeutic agents into these areas. Patients who have been exposed to extensive prior therapy, either radiation therapy or chemotherapy, may have excessive toxicity and be unable to tolerate even conventional doses of salvage chemotherapy. Moreover, large tumor masses may be refractory to chemotherapy for a variety of reasons including limited diffusion of drug into large masses, the availability of increased concentrations of salvage nucleosides, the presence of central areas of relative tissue hypoxia, and the presence of a higher fraction of less vulnerable non-cycling cells in these masses. Each of the factors shown in Table 1 can limit the exposure of tumor cells to otherwise effective concentrations of cytotoxic agents and may be at least in part responsible for drug resistance.

*Table 1.* Pharmacologic factors involved in relative "drug resistance" (ineffective drug concentrations at site of tumor).

1. Variations in drug bioavailability
2. Variations in drug metabolism
3. Variations in drug elimination
4. Presence of tumor in inaccessible sanctuary sites
5. Excessive host toxicity
6. Limited drug diffusion
7. Differences in cell kinetics
8. Variation in salvage factors

## Genetic mechanisms of drug resistance

As alluded to earlier, studies in drug resistant tumor cell lines have identified many different mechanisms associated with the development of resistance to antineoplastic agents. A few basic principles must be kept in mind when one is evaluating these mechanisms. First, for any given drug several different cellular mechanisms may result in the development of resistance to that agent. At low levels of drug resistance, these mechanisms are usually present as isolated defects, while at higher levels of drug resistance, which is commonly the case in *in vitro* studies, multiple mechanisms may be acting

*Table 2.* Mechanisms of drug resistance.

| | |
|---|---|
| Alterations in drug uptake (carrier mediated) | MTX <br> Melphelan <br> Methchlorethamine |
| Alterations in intracellular drug accumulation | Doxorubicin <br> Vinca Alkaloids <br> Actinomycin D |
| Decreased drug activation | Cytosine Arabinoside <br> 5-Fluorouracil <br> 6-Mercaptopurine <br> 6-Thioguanine <br> Methotrexate |
| Increased metabolic inactivation | 6-Mercaptopurine <br> 6-Thioguanine <br> Cytosine Arabinoside <br> Alkylators <br> Cisplatin |
| Alterations in target proteins | MTX <br> Steroid Hormones <br> Vinca Alkaloids <br> FUDR |
| Alterations in cellular metabolism | Cytosine Arabinosine <br> 5-Fluorouracil <br> Methotrexate <br> 6-Mercaptopurine |
| Alterations in cofactor levels | 6-Thioguanine <br> FUDR |
| Alterations in cellular repair mechanisms | Alkylators <br> Nitrosoureas |
| Increased levels of target proteins | MTX <br> Phosphonoacetyl-L-Aspartate <br> FUDR <br> Deoxycoformycin |

METHOTREXATE POLYGLUTAMATES

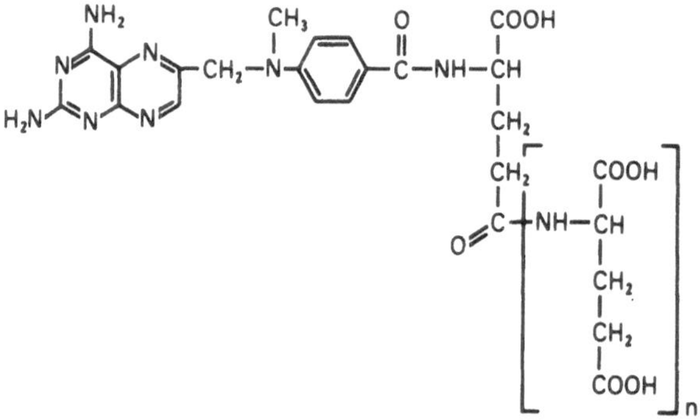


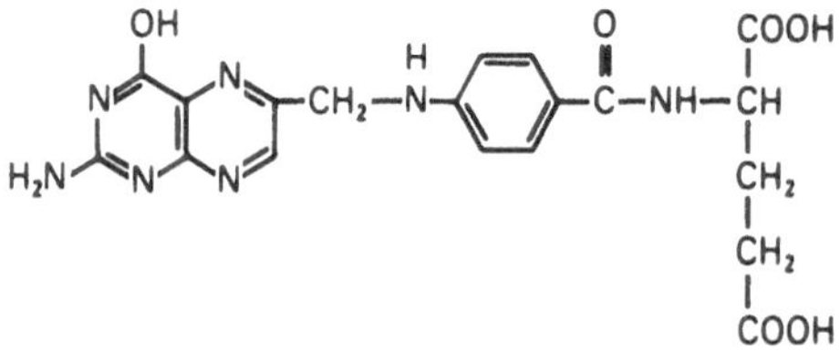


FOLIC ACID

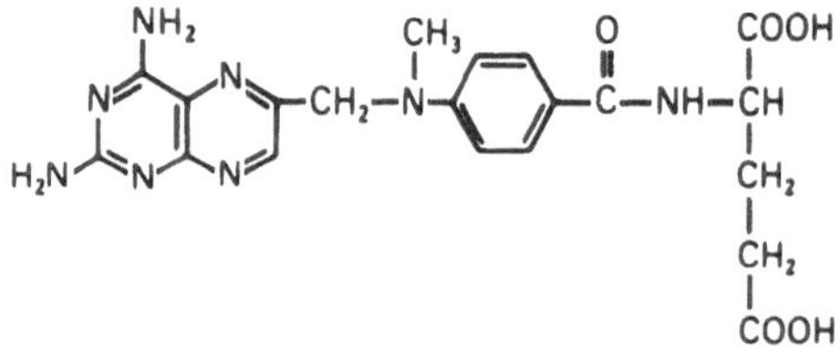


METHOTREXATE

*Figure 1.* Structure of methotrexate, folic acid, and methotrexate polyglutamates.

in any given cell. Secondly, some mechanisms are quite specific and result in resistance to a specific drug or class of drugs. In this case the cell may still be sensitive to other classes of cytotoxic drugs. For example, cells resistant to methotrexate may be cross resistant to other antifolates such as aminopterin, but are generally sensitive to anthracyclines [5]. In contrast, cells which have been selected for resistance to vinca alkaloids or anthracyclines frequently develop a high degree of cross resistance to other structurally dissimilar agents. This latter class of drug resistance has been referred to as pleiotropic or multi-drug resistance.

Some of the mechanisms associated with the development of drug resistance are shown in Table 2. Drug transport into cells has been identified as a mechanism of resistance to methotrexate, nitrogen mustard, and phenylalanine mustard. In these cells the defects apparently involve specific carrier mediated drug transport systems. The phenotype of multidrug or pleiotropic drug resistance is also frequently associated with decreased intracellular accumulation of drug. Although the precise mechanism involved in the development of pleiotropic drug resistance is not known it appears to frequently involve an increase in drug efflux.

Many antineoplastic drugs are actually inactive pro-drugs which need to be metabolically converted to their active species in order to exert their cytoxic effects. This is particularly true of antimetabolites including cytosine arabinoside, thiopurines, and fluorouracil. Resistance to these agents frequently involves defects in cellular activating enzymes. Recent work in our own laboratory has identified another example, in which decreased metabolism of methotrexate to methotrexate polyglutamate forms is associated with resistance in a human breast cancer cell line [6]. Although studies by a number a of laboratories have shown that in most cells methotrexate is converted to a series of derivatives formed by the variable addition of from 1 to 4 glutamyl residues to the native structure (see Figure 1), the isolation of a cell line which was defective in this conversion was the first demonstration that altered cellular metabolism could be associated with methotrexate resistance [6]. Other studies by Curt et al. [7] on cell lines obtained from patients with small cell lung cancer suggest that this may be a common mechanism of clinical resistance to methotrexate.

Other mechanisms involved in the development of drug resistance include the increased metabolism of cytotoxic drugs to inactive metabolites. This has been demonstrated to result in resistance to mercaptopurines and cytosine arabinoside. In both instances resistant cells contain increased levels of drug metabolizing enzymes. Increased drug inactivation can also result from the increased concentrations of scavenger substances such as metallothionein and glutathione. Cells containing increased amounts of these sulphydryl rich peptides have been shown to be resistant to alkylating agents as well as cisplatinum [8–10].

Alterations in specific target proteins can also result in drug resistance. The best example in this class are MTX resistant cells which contain alterations in the DHFR enzyme [11]. In one example, a single amino acid substition in this enzyme can apparently produce an enzyme which has a markedly reduced binding affinity for methotrexate [12]. Other examples in this class include vinca alkaloid resistant cells containing altered tubulin [13], steroid hormone resistant cells containing altered receptors [14], and fluorodeoxyuridine resistant cells which contain an altered thymidylate synthase enzyme [15].

Changes in various metabolic pathways can also lead to insensitivity to various drugs. For example cells containing expanded CTP pools are resistant to cytosine arabinoside and flourouracil [16, 17]. Alterations in the extracellular concentrations of salvage nucleosides can effect the toxicity of certain drugs including methotrexate and thiopurines [18, 19], while intra-cellular concentrations of various cofactors can modulate the cytotoxicity of certain drugs. For example, the intracellular pools of PRPP can effect thio-purine [20] as well as fluorouracil conversion to their active intermediates, while the intracellular pool of reduced folates can effect the toxicity of fluoropyrimidines by limiting the inhibition of thymidylate synthase [21].

Another mechanism associated with the development of drug resistance is the increased ability to repair damage done by these agents. Thus, cells resistant to alkylating agents or to cis platinum may have an increased abil-ity to correct the damage done to DNA by these drugs. This phenotype appears to involve changes in the enzyme activities involved in the repair of damaged DNA [22].

One of the most common mechanisms associated with the development of *in vitro* resistance to agents which are potent enzyme inhibitors, such as methotrexate, is the development of increased levels of their respective tar-get enzymes in the resistant cells. This mechanism is of particular interest because of the finding that the increased levels of enzymes in these cells resulted from the amplification of the gene sequences which codes for these proteins [23].

## Gene amplification and drug resistance

The first report of increased levels of DHFR in MTX resistant cells appeared almost 25 years ago [24]. At that time it was proposed that there was an increase in the regulation of DHFR gene expression in the resistant cell lines which resulted in the increased enzyme levels. However studies by Biedler and Spengler [25] opened the door for new interpretations regarding the mechanism involved in the development of this phenotypic change. These workers demonstrated that methotrexate resistant cells contained dis-tinct cytogenetic abnormalities in the form of large elongated marker chro-mosomes which stained homogenously grey on chromosomal banding stu-dies and hence were called HSRs (homogeneously staining regions). These abnormalities have subsequently been identified in many other animal and human MTX resistant cell lines (Figure 2). Although the finding of these elongated marker chromosomes suggested the presence of excess or ampli-fied DNA sequences, the precise significance of this cytogenetic abnormality remained unclear until Alt *et al.* [22] demonstrated that methotrexate resis-tant cells containing increased levels of DHFR enzyme also contained amplified DNA sequences coding for this enzyme. This was the first demon-stration that amplification of a specific gene could occur in somatic cells in order to alter the overall level of its expression. Further studies subsequently

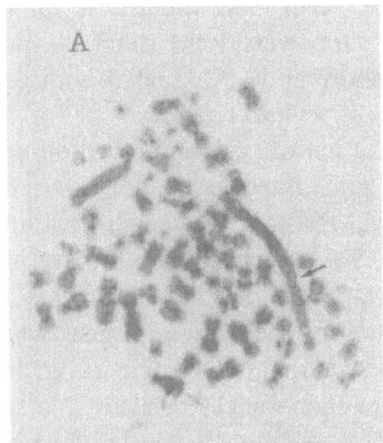 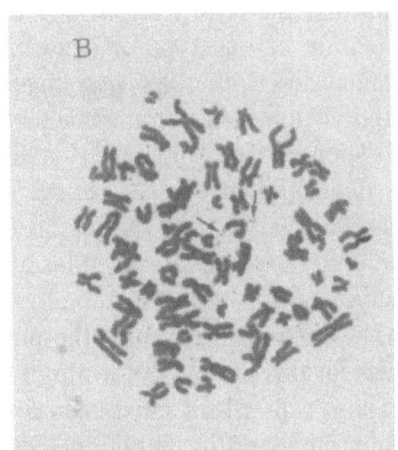

*Figure 2.* (A) Metaphase spread of a methotrexate resistant human breast cancer cell line [26] containing increased levels of dihydrofolate reductase enzyme and amplified dihydrofolate reductase genes. The arrow indicates an HSR which is present in the resistant cell line and not in the parental drug sensitive cell line. (B) Metaphase analysis of 249P small cell lung cancer cell line [39]. The arrows indicate numerous double minute chromosomes.

demonstrated by *in situ* hybridization that the amplified DHFR genes were indeed located within the HSRs presumably as tandem repetitive elements [27].

Gene-amplified methotrexate-resistant cells were subsequently found to be either stably or unstably resistant during subsequent passages in nonselective (drug-free) media. Stably resistant cell lines maintained high levels of drug resistance, high levels of DHFR enzyme, and amplified DHFR gene sequences for prolonged periods of time (greater than a year). In contrast, unstably resistant cell lines readily lose their amplified DNA sequences and revert to a drug sensitive phenotype with lower DHFR enzyme levels. Although unstably resistant cells do not contain HSRs, they instead frequently contain a variable number of small extrachromosomal structures called double minutes (DMs) (Figure 2). These structures have also been shown to have amplified DHFR gene sequences [28]. Since DMs lack centromeres, they segregate unequally into replicating daughter cells. This results in their loss from cell populations once the selective pressure to maintain the amplified DNA sequences is removed.

During the early stages of the development of gene amplification, most cell lines are found to be unstably resistant, a finding which suggests that during the initial stages the amplified DNA is present in an extrachromosomal form. It is only during subsequent selection for higher levels of resistance that the amplified sequences can be seen in the form of HSRs or DMs. The observation that certain cell lines tend to form one type of cytogenetic structure (and hence develop a stably or unstably inherited phenotype) suggests that there are certain cell properties which may predispose for the formation of one type of cytogenetic structure versus the other. A more detailed description of the cytogenetic abnormalities associated with gene amplification can be found in several recent reviews [29-32].

It soon became apparent that the association of gene amplification with the development of drug resistance was not limited to methotrexate. For example, Wahl et al. [33] demonstrated that resistance to the enzyme inhibitor PALA (phosphonoacetyl-1-aspartate) was associated with the overproduction of the multifunctional protein containing the target enzyme for PALA (CAD protein) and the amplification of the gene sequences which codes for this protein. Shown in Table 3, is a partial list of some of the drug resistant cells which have been found to contain increased levels of a specific protein and/or amplified gene sequences. Thus, cells selected for resistance to the toxic effects of the heavy metal cadmium have been shown to contain increased levels of metallothionein, a sulfur rich protein which can bind heavy metals and apparently protect cells from toxicity. As noted earlier, cells containing increased levels of metallothionein are collaterally resistant to cis platinum [10] as well as chlorambucil [9] presumably through the increased binding of these drugs or various metabolites to this scavenger protein. Other examples in which drug resistance is associated with the development of increased proteins and/or amplified genes sequences include deoxycoformycin (adenosine deaminase), flourodeoxyuridine (thymidylate synthetase), and pyrazofurin (UMP synthetase).

Gene amplification apparently also plays a role in the development of pleiotropic resistance. As noted earlier, cells which are selected for resis-

*Table 3.* Gene amplification and drug resistance.

| Selection | Protein overproduced | Gene amplification demonstrated |
|---|---|---|
| MTX | DihydrofolateReductase | + |
| PALA | CAD Protein | + |
| FUDR | Thymidylate Synthetase | + |
| Deoxycoformycin | Adenosine Deaminase | + |
| Hydroxyurea | Ribonucleotide Reductase | |
| Dimethylfluoroornithine | Ornithine Decarboxylase | + |
| Cadmium | Metallothionein | + |
| Vinca Alkaloids | 17OK Glycoprotein | |
| Actinomycin D | 15OK Glycoprotein | |
| | 19K Protein | |
| Compactin | Hydroxymethylglutaryl-CoA Reductase | + |
| Methionine Sulfoximine | Glutamine Synthetase | + |
| Pyrazofurin Azauridine | UMP Synthetase | + |

tance to a single agent frequently will develop cross resistance to a wide variety of structurally dissimilar agents. This is particularly noted in cells which are selected for resistance to vinca alkaloids or to antitumor antibiotics. Thus cells selected for resistance to vincristine or vinblastine are not only cross resistant to other alkaloids but are also cross resistant to adriamycin and other antibiotics including actinomycin D and mitomycin. Although the mechanism of pleiotropic resistance is not known, increased levels of specific membrane proteins have been frequently noted in this class of cells. For example Ling and coworkers [34] have found an increase in a 170 k dalton glycopeptide, which they have referred to as P-glycoprotein, in pleiotropic resistant chinese hamster cells. Other high molecular weight membrane proteins have been found in drug resistant cells isolated by Biedler and coworkers [35] as well as by Beck and coworkers [36], while Fine *et al.* [37] have shown that pleiotropic resistant cell lines contain increased levels of certain phosphorylated membrane proteins. Recently, amplified gene sequences have been cloned from one of these cell lines [38]. If this gene sequence is amplified in other drug resitant cells, it will provide an important insight into the mechanism involved in the development of pleiotropic drug resistance as well as a unique probe for the screening for clinical drug resistance.

### Gene amplification and clinical drug resistance

Although the studies listed in Table 3 clearly demonstrate that gene amplification is a common mechanism in the development of drug resistance *in vitro*, it has now been established that similar mechanisms are associated with the development of clinical drug resistance. Curt *et al.* [39] studied a tumor cell line established from a patient with small cell lung cancer who had developed progressive disease after treatment with methotrexate. This cell line (249P) was shown to be resistant to MTX *in vitro* and had elevated levels of DHFR enzyme and amplified DHFR genes relative to other drug sensitive tumor cell lines. Moreover, the drug resistant cells had numerous double minute chromosomes which suggested that it would have an unstably inherited resistant phenotype (see Figure 2B). Indeed during passage in culture in drug free medium for 6 months this tumor cell line lost its DM chromosomes and amplified DHFR gene sequences and became progressively more sensitive to methotrexate. Studies by other investigators have confirmed that DHFR gene amplification does occur clinically [40–42]. Whether this is a common mechanism involved in the development of clinical resistance to methotrexate and whether gene amplification is involved in the development of clinical resistance to other agents remains to be determined.

In this regard, it is of interest to note recent studies by Bell *et al.* [42] in which an antibody against a membrane protein found amplified in a pleiotropic drug resistant chinese hamster ovary cell line was used to screen cells obtained from patients with ovarian cancer. These workers found an increase in a cross reactive protein in two patients previously treated with chemotherapy, suggesting that the overproduction of this protein may play a role in clinical drug resistance. However, these results are quite preliminary and future prospective studies are needed in order to determine whether the level of expression of this protein is indeed involved in the development of drug resistance in some patients.

## Conclusions

It is obvious from reviewing the studies on drug resistance that cells can develop resistance to cytotoxic agents through a variety of mechanisms. In order to develop pharmacological approaches to the clinical problem of drug resistance it is first necessary to identify which of these mechanisms are involved in the development of drug resistance *in vivo*. Given this information it may be then possible to develop treatments which either bypass the mechanism of resistance, or it may be possible to actually exploit a particular mechanism employed by cells since these changes may in fact render the resistant cells colaterally more sensitive to specific salvage therapies [43]. Future progress in the management of malignant diseases is dependent upon finding non-cross resistant therapies which will be effective when resistance to primary regimens is established. Thus, identifying the biochemical and genetic mechanisms involved in the development of acquired and inherent clinical drug resistance is one of the most important problems facing clinical oncologists today.

## References

1. Simone JV, Cassady JR, Filler RM, Cancers of Childhood: In: Cancer: Principles and Practice of Oncology. DeVita VT Jr, Hellman S, Rosenberg SA (eds). J.B. Lippincott, Philadelphia 125–1316, 1982.
2. Alberts DS, Chang SY, Chen H-SG et al.: Comparative pharmacokinetics of chlorambucil and melphalan in man. Recent Results in Canc Res 74:124–130, 1980.
3. D'Incalcci M, Bolis G, Mangioni C et al.: Variable absorption of hexamethylmelamine in man. Cancer Treat Rep 62:2117–2119, 1978.
4. Zimm S, Collins JM, Ricarrdi R, O'Neill D, Narang PK, Chabner B, Poplack DG: Variable bioavailability of oral mercaptopurine: Is maintenance chemotherapy in acute lymphoblastic leukemia being optimally delivered. N Eng J Med 308:1005–1009, 1983.
5. Hill BT, Price LA, Goldie JH: The value of adriamycin in overcoming resistance to methotrexate in tissue culture. Eur J Cancer 12:541–549, 1976.

6. Cowan KH, Jolivet J: A novel mechanism of resistance to methotrexate in human breast cancer cells: lack of methotrexate polyglutamate formation. J Biol Chem 259:10793–10800, 1984.

7. Curt GA, Carney DN, Jolivet J et al.: Defective methotrexate polyglutamation: a mechanism of in vivo resistance in human small cell lung cancer. Proc Am Assoc Clin Res 24:283, 1983.

8. Suzukake K, Vistica BP, Vistica DT: Dechlorination of 1-phenylalanine mustard by sensitive and resistant tumor cells and its relationship to intracellular glutathione content. Biochem Pharmacol 32:165–167, 1983.

9. Endresen L, Bakka A, Rugstad HE: Increased resistance to chlorambucil in cultured cells with a high concentration of cytoplasmic metallothionein. Cancer Res 43:2918–2926, 1983.

10. Bakka A, Endresen L, Johnson ABS et al.: Resistance against cis-dichloro-diaminoplatinum in cultured cells with a high content of metallothionein. Toxicol Appl Pharmacol 61:215–226, 1981.

11. Flintoff WF, Essani K: Methotrexate-resistant Chinese hamster ovary cells contain a dihydrofolate reductase with an altered affinity for methotrexate. Biochem 19:4321–4432, 1980.

12. Simonsen CC, Levinson AD: Isolation and expression of an altered mouse dihydrofolate reductase cDNA. Proc Natl Acad Sci USA 80:2495–2499, 1983.

13. Ling V, Aubin JE, Chase A et al.: Mutants of Chinese hamster ovary (CHO) cells with altered colcemid binding affinity. Cell 18:423–430, 1979.

14. Nawata H, Bronzert D, Lippman ME: Isolation and characterization of tamoxifen-resistant cell line derived from MCF-7 human breast cancer cells. J Biol Chem 256:5016–5021, 1983.

15. Heidelberger C, Kaldor G, Mukherjee KL et al.: Studies on fluorinated pyrimidines. XI. In Vitro studies on tumor resistance. Cancer Res 20:903–909, 1960.

16. Aronow B, Watts T, Lassetter J, Washtien WJ, Ullman B: Biochemical phenotype of 5-fluorouracil-resistant murine T lymphoblasts with genetically altered CTP synthetase activity. J Biol Chem 259:9033–9043, 1984.

17. Desaint Vincent BR, Butten G: Studies on 1-beta-D-arabinofuranosylcytosine-resistant mutants of Chinese hamster fibroblasts. III. Joint resistance to arabinofuranosylcytosine and to thymidine-a semidominant manifestation of deoxycytidine triphosphate pool expansion. Somat Cell Genet 5:67–82, 1979.

18. Howell SB, Mansfield SJ, Taetle R: Thymidine and hypoxanthine requirements of normal and malignant human cells for protection against methotrexate cytotoxicity. Cancer Res 41:945–951, 1981.

19. Browman GP, Csullog GW: Modification of in vivo methotrexate antitumor effect in L1210 leukemia by induced impairment of purine salvage. Biochem Pharmacol 30:869–871, 1981.

20. Kimiko I, Sartorelli AC: Altered 5-phosphoribosyl-pyrophosphate amido-transferase activity in 6-thioguanine resistant HL 60 promyelocytic leukemia cells. Cancer Res 44:3679–3685, 1984.

21. Houghton JA, Maroda SJ, Phillips JO et al.: Biochemical determinants of responsiveness to 5-fluorouracil and its derivatives in xenografts of human colorectal adenocarcinomas in mice. Cancer Res 42:144–149, 1982.

22. Parsons PG, Smellie SG, Manson LE et al.: Properties of human melanoma cells resistant to 5-(3', 3'-dimethyl-1-triazeno)imidazole-4-carboxamido and other methylating agents. Cancer Res 42:1454–1461, 1982.

23. Alt FW, Kellem RE, Bertino JR, Schimke RT: Selective Amplification of dihydrofolate reductase genes in methotrexate resistant variants of cultured murine cells J Biol Chem 253:1357–1370. 1978.

24. Fischer GA: Increased levels of folic reductase as a mechanism of resistance to amethopterin in leukemia cells. Biochem Pharmacol 7:75-77, 1961.
25. Biedler JL, Spengler BA: Metaphase chromosome anomaly: Association with drug resistance and cell specific products. Science 191:185-187, 1976.
26. Cowan KH, Goldsmith ME, Levine RM, Aitken SC, Douglass E, Clendeninn N, Nienhuis AW, Lippman ME: Possible rearrangment of amplified dihydrofolate reductase gene in a methotrexate resistant estrogen sensitive human breast cancer cell line. J Biol Chem 257:15079-15086, 1982.
27. Dolnick BJ, Berenson RJ, Bertino JR, Kaufman RJ, Numberg JH, Schimke RT: Correlation of dihydrofolate reductase elevation and gene amplification in a homogeneously staining region in L51784 cells. J Cell Biol 83:394-402, 1979.
28. Brown PC, Beverly SM, Schimke RT: Relationship of amplified dihydrofolate reductase genes to double minute chromosomes in unstably resistant cell lines. Mol Cell Biol 1:1077-1083, 1981.
29. Schimke RT: Gene amplification, drug resistance, and cancer. Cancer Res 44:1735-1742, 1984.
30. Biedler JL, Myers MB, Spengler BA: Homogeneously staining regions and double minute chromosomes, prevalent cytogenetic abnormalities of human neuroblastoma cells. Adv Cell Neurobiol 4:267-307, 1983.
31. Cowell JK: Double minutes and homogeneously staining regions: gene amplification in mammalian cells. Ann Rev Genet 16:21-59, 1982.
32. Stark GR, Wahl GM: Gene amplification. Ann Rev Biochem 53:447-491, 1984.
33. Wahl GM, Pudgett RA, Stark GR: Gene amplification causes overproduction of the first three enzymes of UMP synthesis in N-(phosphonoacetyl)-L-aspartate resistant hamster cells. J Biol Chem 254:8679-8689, 1979.
34. Juliano RL, Ling V: a surface glycoprotein modulating drug permeability in Chinese hamster ovary cells mutants. Biochem Biophys Acta 455:152-162, 1976.
35. Peterson PHF, Myers MB, Spengler BA, Biedler JL: Alteration of plasma membrane glycopeptides and gangliosides of Chinese hamster cells accompanying development of resistance to daunorubicin and vincristine. Cancer Res 43:222-228, 1983.
36. Beck WT, Mueller TJ, Tanzer LR: Altered surface membrane glycoproteins in vinca alkaloid resistant human leukemia lymphoblasts. Cancer Res 39:2070-2076, 1979.
37. Fine RL, Patel J, Allegra CJ, Curt GA, Cowan KH, Ozols RF, Lippman ME, McDevitt R, Chabner BA: Increased phosphorylation of a 20,000 M.W. protein in pleiotriopic drug-resistant MCF-7 human breast cancer cell lines. Proc Am Assoc Canc Res, 1985.
38. Roninson IB, Abelson HJ, Housman DE, Howell N, Varshavsky A: Amplification of specific DNA sequences correlates with multi-drug resistance in Chinese hamster cells. Nature 309:626-688, 1984.
39. Curt GA, Carney DM, Cowan KH, Jolivet J, Balley BD, Drake JC, Kao-Shan CW, Minna JD, Chabner BA: Unstable methotrexate resistance in human small cell carcinoma associated with double minute chromosomes. N Engl J Med 308:199-202, 1983.
40. Trent JM, Buick RM, Olson S, Horns RC, Schimke RT: Cytologic support for gene amplification in methotrexate-resistant cells obtained from a patient with ovarian adenocarcinoma. J Clin Oncol 2:8-15, 1984.
41. Horns RC, Dower WJ, Schimke RT: Gene amplification in a leukemic patient treated with methotrexate. J Clin Oncol 2:1-7, 1984.
42. Cardman MD, Schornagel JH, Rivest RS, Srimatkandada S, Portlock CS, Duffey T, Bertino JR: Resistance to methotrexate due to gene amplification in a patient with acute leukemia. J Clin Oncol 2:16-20, 1984.
43. Bell DR, Gerlach JH, Kartner N, Buick Rn, Ling V: Detection of P-glycoprotein in ovarian cancer: a molecular marker associated with multidrug resistance. J Clin Oncol 3:311-315, 1985.

44. Ozols RF, Cowan KC: New Aspects of clinical Drug Resistance: the role of gene amplification and the reversal of resistance in drug refractory cancer. In: Important Advances in Oncology 1986. Devita VT Jr, Hellman S, Rosenberg SA (eds). J.B. Lippincott, Philadelphia, 1986.

# 5. Genetic reasons for pharmacologic treatment failure: gene amplification

GIUSEPPE TORELLI

## Introduction

In 1983 in her Nobel Lecture delivered in Stockholm under the title 'The significance of responses of the genome to challenge' Dr B. McClintock stated: "There are 'shocks' that a genome must face repeatedly, and for which it is prepared to respond in a programmed manner. Examples are the 'heat shock' responses in eukaryotic organisms and the 'SOS' responses in bacteria. Each of these initiates a highly programmed sequence of events within the cell that serves to cushion the effects of the shock. But there are also responses of genomes to unanticipated challenges that are not so precisely programmed. The genome is unprepared for these shocks. Nevertheless they are sensed, and the genome responds in a discernible but initially unforseen manner" [1]. For our purposes we may consider for a moment that antineoplastic chemotherapy is a kind of 'unanticipated challenge' that the human genome is able to manage successfully, more frequently than we expect or, in this case, than we hope. The result of the genome response is the acquired resistance of cancer cells to one or several cytotoxic drugs, that is a well established phenomenon at the experimental level and is a very likely reason for many clinical treatment failures.

It is possible to speculate that a genome may acquire drug resistance in several different ways, implying different types of changes at the genome level (mutations, rearrangements, amplifications, etc.) leading to the same or different resistance phenotypes (altered drug affinity, altered drug transport, etc.). We might postulate, for example, that a mutation of a target gene may make a protein less susceptible to a chemotherapeutic agent, or a mutation in the genetic elements controlling the expression of a gene may make a drug ineffective by permitting it to surround, for example, a metabolic block. Other mutations may affect genes able to influence the transmembrane transport of a drug, or the amplification of a gene may make a cell resistant by amplifying a target product. This is obviously only a partial list of the possible mechanisms. Some of these are already under strict experimental scrutiny, while others may only be envisaged at the present moment. Not only is it possible that different genomic changes may determine the same kind of resistance phenotype, but also that the same kind of genomic change, as we will see later, may produce different resistance phenotypes. In spite of the possible existence of several different genetic mechanisms underlying mammalian cell resistance to drugs, until now gene amplification is by far the best known.

### Genetic systems of drug resistance in mammalian cells

Today the genetic systems of clinical relevance involving mammalian cells resistant to cytotoxic drugs are the following two:
1. Cells resistant to methotrexate by overproduction of dihydrofolate reductase [2];
2. Cells cross-resistant to colchicine, Vinca alkaloids, puromycin, adriamycin, actinomycin D and other drugs by reduced cellular uptake [3].

In both cases the genetic mechanism involved is gene amplification, a phenomenon known to occur only occasionally in the development of higher animals, when the organism must face extraordinarily high transcriptional requirements. The classic examples are the amplification of ribosomal RNA genes in Xenopus oocytes [4] and that of chorion genes in Drosophila eggs [5].

Methotrexate (MTX) is a potent inhibitor of the enzyme dihydrofolate reductase (DHFR) and methotrexate resistance may result from three different mechanisms: (1) altered MTX transport; (2) altered affinity of DHFR for MTX; and (3) overproduction of DHFR. A possible fourth mechanism, diminished formation of methotrexate polyglutamates, was recently proposed. The possible role of thymidilate synthetase activity, which makes cells less susceptible to MTX when thymidilate synthesis is low is unclear [6].

In 1978 Schimke and coworkers [7] reported that the overproduction of DHFR (the third resistance mechanism) is the result of a dose related amplification of the DHFR genes in cultured mammalian cells. The same author [8] has indicated the following general properties of MTX resistance by DHFR gene amplification:
1. Cells with up to 1,000 DHFR genes are obtained by stepwise selection, gradually increasing the MTX in the medium. This behaviour suggests that amplification probably occurs in small increments;
2. Drug resistance is the result of an increase in DHFR messenger RNA and final overproduction of the target enzyme;
3. The amplified genes, and the resultant drug resistance, can be stable for hundreds of cell doublings, declining slowly over a period of 6 to 12

months, or unstable, disappearing after two weeks, or about twenty cell doublings;

4. Unstably amplified genes are associated with those extrachromosomal elements known as double minutes (DM). DM do not contain centromeres, and thus are unequally distributed in daughter cells. They may be lost easily through micronucleation. The stably amplified genes are located on chromosomal homogeneously staining regions (HSR) sometimes, but not always, present on one of the two homologous chromosomes normally carrying the nonamplified gene [9];

5. Generally the cells emerging from a first period of selection have unstably amplified genes, while if the selective pressure is maintained for some time the resulting populations have stably amplified genes.

Acquired MTX resistance is certainly the best known example of gene amplification in somatic cells, but, since the first report, the amplification of a number of genes has been reported, always induced using a specific enzyme inhibitor to obtain resistant cell variants. Already established is the amplification of the genes coding for CAD, UMP synthetase, metallothionine, thymidylate synthetase, adenosine deaminase, glutamine synthetase, ribonucleotide reductase, hydroxymethylglutaryl CoA reductase, hypoxanthine-guanine phosphoribosyltransferase, ornithine decarboxylase and asparagine synthetase (for review see [8, 10]). It is now clear that, in cultured cells, using an enzyme inhibitor binding tightly to a protein, it is possible to produce amplification of the gene corresponding to that protein.

More interesting from our point of view is the type of multi-drug resistance that can be obtained by selecting different mammalian cell lines (human included) for resistance to a single cytocidal drug, such as colchicine [11], Vinca alkaloids [12] or other compounds. Cells obtained by this procedure are resistant because of a decrease in the cellular uptake of the selecting drug [13] and the same mechanism is the basis of the resistance of the same cells to other drugs [11] structurally and functionally unrelated, such as actinomycin D, puromycin and adriamycin. The decreased membrane permeability is associated with the presence in the membrane of a glycoprotein, called P-glycoprotein (m.w. about 170,000), previously undetectable in the same cells [14–16]. The observation of the presence of double minutes or homogeneously staining regions in some of these multi-drug resistant cell lines suggested that a gene amplification phenomenon underlies the acquired resistance. On this assumption Varshavsky and coworkers [17] were able to isolate from these cell lines DNA fragments amplified in common in multi-drug resistant cells. So it seems highly probable that, in this case as well, gene amplification is the genetic basis of a resistance phenotype, different from that involved in MTX resistance, but yet one which may lead to treatment failure.

## Occurrence and mechanisms of gene amplification

Because gene amplification seems to play an important role in acquired drug resistance, we must pay some attention to certain details of the process that have possible relevance to the clinical problems of drug resistance.

We do not know if amplification has been observed only in tumor cells or in cells adapted to growth in culture. Gene amplification may certainly occur in the absence of selection pressure, as demonstrated in experiments with fluorescein conjugated MTX [18], although selective pressure increases the frequency of the phenomenon. In addition, we know that the resistance of a cell population does not necessarily involve the selection of a preexisting mutant, but may be in fact induced by the treatment. Moreover, a number of experiments suggest that any agents (tumor promotors, UV, etc.) that affect DNA structure or synthesis greatly increase the frequency of the amplification phenomena. This holds for chemotherapeutic agents like hydroxyurea, as well [19].

The amplified DNA is made by several copies of a DNA segment comprising the active gene and some flanking sequences (the so-called 'amplification unit'). Surprisingly enough, the length of this unit is different in different cell lines and its chromosomal location is not necessarily near the site of the original nonamplified gene. Furthermore the amplified segment undergoes variable rearrangement phenomena at the recombination site. Thus far no sequence specificity for these recombination sites has been observed [8]. It is reasonable to think that this variability is keeping with what Dr McClintock defined as 'responses of genomes to unanticipated challenges that are not so precisely programmed'. However this variability may maintain the amplified genes under the influence of naturally occurring control elements, as shown in human breast cancer cells, where the amplified genes are still susceptible to hormone induction [20].

The mechanism by which gene amplification occurs at the DNA level is still poorly understood. Three general mechanisms can be hypothesized (for review see [8]):

1. The uptake of DNA segments from dead cells with subsequent integration in the genome of the recipient cells, in a way similar to that of transfection experiments;
2. Unequal crossing over events which may determine gene amplification, for example, by unequal sister chromatid exchange. On the basis of this model the generation of multiple copies of one gene requires a high number of mitoses. Moreover, the amplified genes should be located, at least in principle, on chromosomes. This mechanism was proposed first for ribosomal DNA amplification in Drosophilia [21], and cannot be excluded in mammalian cells;

3. Gene amplification by disproportionate replication, a mechanism requiring that the same DNA segment may be replicated more than one time in a single cell cycle. This contrasts with the idea that there is a single initiation of replication of DNA in each S phase. We might imagine a segment of DNA in which more than one replication cycle took place, forming free strands of DNA (the so-called 'onion skin' replication model) [22]. It is now possible to suggest the recombination of the loose ends of these segments leading to the formation of circular extrachromosomal structures or to chromosomally localized sequences, when the recombination event takes place into the chromosomal backbone.

In the protozoa Leishmania tropica, which can acquire MTX resistance by gene amplification, a mechanism involving the formation of circular DNA structures and then chromosomal arrays has been demonstrated [23]. The large majority of authors favor this last mechanism as that most likely involved in generation of gene amplification. There are circumstantial evidences in favor of this mechanism, mainly from the observation that if we block the DNA synthesis of synchronized cells after the first two hours of the S phase, and then remove the blocking agent (hydroxyurea) allowing the cells to resume DNA synthesis, almost all the DNA synthesized prior to the block is now re-replicated. Most of the re-replicated DNA is rapidly lost, but a portion is retained on the genome as a result of rearrangement-recombination events [24]. Also supporting this mechanism are reports of the existence of extrachromosomal circular DNA sequences in cultured cells [25, 26] as well as the observation that a particular 'inter Alu' sequence is present as extrachromosomal circular DNA in different copy numbers in different intact human tissues [27].

This last observation introduces a fundamental question: is gene amplification relevant to drug resistance phenomena so frequently observed in human cancers? The only answer is that in fact there are reports of DHFR gene amplification associated with MTX resistance in human cancer cells derived from two leukemia cases [28, 29], from one small cell carcinoma of the lung [30] and from one ovarian adenocarcinoma [31]. Considering the possible relevance of this type of data one would expect a lot more information about this subject, nevertheless the overall data available argue strongly in favor of the occurrence of this phenomenon *in vivo*. If this is true, cancer chemotherapy must be administered in a way which minimizes the possibility of the emergence of amplification phenomena [10]. So, for example, the doses of the drugs used should be cytocidal, because sublethal doses may produce transient inhibition of DNA synthesis resulting in over-replication of DNA sequences. Similarly, in theory, chemotherapeutic agents damaging DNA, such as alkylating agents, should be avoided, if possible, in the treatment of fast growing cellular populations, because this kind of agent greatly enhances the overreplication of cells in S phase. To encourage the loss of amplified genes in cells with acquired unstable resistance, the various chemotherapy regimens theoretically should not be used for prolonged periods of time, because we know that this type of resistance tends to become stable under prolonged selective pressure. Possibly relevant to this issue is the observation that noncytotoxic concentrations of hydroxyurea are able to greatly accelerate *in vitro* the loss of unstably amplified DHFR genes [32].

Finally, it is of interest that recent studies suggest that gene amplification phenomena may be increasingly involved in the process of carcinogenesis, through mechanisms similar to those described above [33, 34]. Thus, we must keep this recent clue to the pathogenesis of human cancer in mind not only to adapt our treatment schedules, but also to define, if possible, new strategies in cancer therapy.

## References

1. McClintock B: The significance of responses of the genome to challenge. Science 226:792–801, 1984.
2. Schimke RT (ed): Gene Amplification. Cold Spring Harbor Laboratory, New York, 1982.
3. Ling V: Genetic basis of drug resistance in mammalian cells. In: Drug and hormone resistance in neoplasia, Vol. 1. Bruchovsky N, Goldie JH (eds). CRC Press, Boca Raton 1-19, 1982.
4. Brown DD, David IB: Specific gene amplification in ocytes. Science 160:272–280, 1980.
5. Spradling AC, Mahowald AP: Amplification of genes for chorion proteins during oogenesis in Drosopila melanogaster. Proc Nat Acad Sci USA 77:1096–2002, 1980.
6. Jolivet J, Cowan KH, Curt GA, Clendeninn NJ, Chabner BA: The pharmacology and clinical use of methotrexate. N Eng J Med 309:1094–1104, 1983.
7. Schimke RT, Alt FW, Kellems RE, Kaufman RJ, Bertino JR: Amplification of dihydrofolate reductase genes in methotrexate-resistant cultured mouse cells. Cold Spring Harbor Symp Quant Biol 42:649–657, 1978.
8. Schimke RT: Gene amplification in cultured animal cells. Cell 37:705–713, 1984.
9. Cowell JK: Double minutes and homogeneously staining regions: Gene amplification in mammalian cells. Ann Rev Genet 16:21–59, 1982.
10. Schimke RT: Gene amplification, drug resistance and cancer. Cancer Res 44:1735–1742, 1984.
11. Bech-Hansen NT, Till JI, Ling V: Pleiotropic phenotype of colchicine-resistant CHO cells: cross-resistance and collateral sensitivity. J Cell Physiol 88:23–32, 1976.
12. Beck WT, Mueller TJ, Tanzen LR: Altered surface membrane glycoproteins in Vinca alkaloid-resistant human leukemic lymphoblasts. Cancer Res 39:2070–2076, 1979.
13. Ling V, Thompson LH: Reduced permeability in CHO cells as a mechanism of resistance to colchicine. J Cell Physiol 83:103–116, 1974.
14. Kartner N, Shales M, Riordan JR, Ling V: Daunorubicin resitant Chinese hamster ovary cells ecpressing multi-drug resistance and cell surface P-glycoprotein. Cancer Res 43:4413–4419, 1983.
15. Biedler JL, Peterson RHF: In: Molecular actions and targets for cancer chemotherapeutic agents. Sartorelli AC, Lazo JS, Bertino JR (eds). Academic Press, Inc., New York 1981.

16. Garman D, Center MS: Alterations in cell surface membranes in Chinese hamster lung cells resistant to adriamycin. Biochem Biophys Res Commun 105:157–163, 1982.

17. Roninson IB, Abelson HT, Housman DE, Howell N, Varshavsky A: Amplification of specific DNA sequences correlates with multi-drug resistance in Chinese hamster cells. Nature 309:626–628, 1984.

18. Johnston RN, Beverley SM, Schimke RT: Rapid spontaneous dihydrofolate reductase gene amplification shown by fluorescence activated cell sorting. Proc Nat Acad Sci USA 80:3711–3715, 1983.

19. Brown PC, Tisty TD, Schimke RT: Enhancement of methotrexate resistance and dihydrofolate reductase gene amplification by treatment of mouse 3T6 cells with hydroxyurea. Mol Cell Biol 3:1097–1107, 1982.

20. Cowan KH, Goldsmith ME, Levine RM, Aitken SC, Douglass E, Clendeninn N, Nienhuis AW, Lippman ME: Dihydrofolate reductase gene amplification and possible rearrangement in estrogen-responsive methotrexate-resistant human breast cancer cells. J Biol Chem 257:15079–15086, 1982.

21. Tartof KD: Unequal mitotic sister chromatid exchange as the mechanism of ribosomal RNA gene magnification. Proc Nat Acad Sci USA 71:1272–1276, 1974.

22. Botchan MW, Topp W, Sambrook J: Studies on SV40 excision from cellular chromosomes. Cold Spring Harbor Symp Quant Biol 43:709–719, 1979.

23. Beverley SM, Coderre JA, Santi DV, Schimke RTE Unstable DNA amplifications in methotrexate resistant Leishmania consist of extrachromosomal circles which relocalize during stabilization. Cell 38:431–439, 1984.

24. Mariani BD, Schimke RT: Gene amplification in a single cell cycle in Chinese hamster ovary cells. J Biol Chem 259:1901–1910, 1984.

25. Smith CA, Vinograd J: Small polydisperse circular DNA of HeLa cells. J Mol Biol 69:163–168, 1972.

26. Stanfield SW, Helinsky DR: Cloning and characterization of small circular DNA from Chinese Hamster ovary cells. Mol Cell Biol 4:173–180, 1984.

27. Calabretta B, Robberson DL, Barrera-Saldana HA, Lambrou TP, Saunders GF: Genome instability in a region of human DNA enriched in Alu repeat sequences. Nature 296:219–225, 1982.

28. Cadman MD, Shomagel JH, Rivest RS, Srimatkandada S, Portlock CS, Duffy T, Bertino JR: Resistance to methotrexate due to gene amplification in a patient with acute leukemia. J Clin Oncol 2:16–20, 1984.

29. Horns RC, Dower WJ, Schimke RT: Gene amplification in a leukemic patient treated with methotrexate. J Clin Oncol 2:1–7, 1984.

30. Curt GA, Carney DM, Cowan KH, Jolivet J, Bailey BD, Drake J, Kao-Shan CW, Minna JD, Chabner BA: Unstable methotrexate resistance in human small-cell carcinoma associated with double minute chromosomes. N Eng J Med 308:199–202, 1983.

31. Trent JM, Buick RM, Olson S, Horns RC, Schimke RT: Cytologic support for gene amplification in methotrexate resistant cells obtained from a patient with ovarian adenocarcinoma. J Clin Oncol 2:8–15, 1984.

32. Snapka RM, Varshavsky A: Loss of unstably amplified dihydrofolate reductase genes from mouse cells is greatly accelerated by hydroxyurea. Proc Nat Acad Sci USA 80:7533–7537, 1983.

33. Marx JL: Oncogenes amplified in cancer cells. Science 223:40–41, 1984.

34. Arrighi FE: Gene amplification in human tumor cells. In: 13th Int. Cancer Congr., Part C: Biology of cancer (2). ARLis New York 259–268, 1983.

# 6. New approaches to overcome drug resistance

VASSILIOS AVRAMIS, ROBERT BIENER and
JOHN HOLCENBERG

The development of acquired resistance to antitumor agents is a major impediment to the cure of pediatric cancers and leukemias. The causes of drug resistance include: (1) defective drug transport, (2) defective drug metabolism to active species, (3) altered intracellular pools of nucleotides, (4) increased drug inactivation, (5) altered DNA repair, (6) gene amplification and (7) altered target proteins [1–3]. These mechanisms may be due to enhanced expression of specific genes as seen in cells that have amplification of dihyrofolate dehydrogenase (DHFR), adenosine deaminase, ribonucleotide reductase, and possibly pleotropic drug resistance, a condition where cells are resistant to anthracyclines, vinca alkaloids and dactinomycin [4–6]. Alternatively, resistant cells may have altered genes or reduced expression of the genes that code for transport proteins, drug receptors and enzymes that activate certain antitumor agents. In most cases of drug resistance, we do not know the mechanisms for this altered gene expression.

Several approaches are now available to counteract drug resistance. Certain drugs have been found to have increased effect on tumor cells resistant to specific agents. This is called *collateral sensitivity*. Recently, biochemical studies of resistant cell lines have led to rational approaches to the design of new agents that can exploit metabolic changes in the resistant cells [7]. By use of alternating non-cross-resistant chemotherapy, one may be able to maintain a population of tumor cells with sensitivity to both therapies [8, 9].

Another approach is to directly alter the expression of the genes associated with the drug resistance by the design of agents that target to specific sequences of DNA or RNA, by the design of drugs that interact with the gene products causing drug resistance, or by pharmacologically producing changes in the methylation patterns of DNA. This chapter will summarize current research in collateral sensitivity and these other approaches concentrating on modification of DNA methylation which shows promise in counteracting resistance to cytosine arabinoside (ara-C).

## Collateral Sensitivity

One of the earliest examples of collateral sensitivity was the empirical observation that L1210 leukemic cells resistant to 6-MP have increased sensitivity to methotrexate [10]. Wallerstein *et al.* [9] have shown that resistance to each of these drugs can be delayed in mice bearing L1210 leukemia by alternating courses of methotrexate plus hypoxanthine and 6-MP plus folic acid. A similar collateral sensitivity may explain the prolonged effectiveness of 6-MP and methotrexate in the maintenance phase of therapy for acute lymphocytic leukemia.

Shabel and co-workers [11] have shown that L1210 and P388 mouse leukemia cells resistant to ara-C are frequently much more sensitive to inhibitors of *de novo* pyrimidine biosynthesis. For example, PALA, acivicin, pyrazofurin, and dihydro-5-azacytidine produced $3-5$ $\log_{10}$ greater cell kill in the resistant than the sensitive lines. Other examples include increased effect of methotrexate in adriamycin resistant CHO cells [12] and increased vinca alkaloid activity in cis-platinum resistant Ehrlich ascites cells [13].

Recently Cheng and Brockman [7] have reviewed research designed to rationally exploit collateral sensitivity. Promising approaches include:

1. use of lipophilic antifols in cells lacking a transport system for methotrexate and reduced folates;
2. increased conversion of 2′-fluoro-2′-deoxy-5-iodo-1-β-D-arabino-furanosylcytosine to an active uracil compound in cells with high activity of deoxycytidine deaminase, an enzyme that degrades ara-C;
3. Increased sensitivity to inhibitors of *de novo* synthesis in cells lacking salvage pathways for purines and pyrimidines;
4. increased sensitivity of human KB cells with overexpression of ribonucleotide reductase to thioguanine which is converted by this enzyme to its deoxynucleotide;
5. design of drug analogues that exploit differences in drug binding affinity to altered targed enzymes.

## Targeting to Specific DNA or RNA Sequences

This specific approach to drug resistance is now possible because of the vast increase in our knowledge of cellular and molecular biology in the last few years. DNA and RNA sequences are now known for enzymes like dihydrofolate dehydrogenase and adenosine deaminase that are overexpressed in some drug resistant lines [4, 14, 15]. If exposed coding sequences of DNA or messenger RNA for these enzymes are paired, matched or blocked by appropriate complementary sequences of artificial analogues, their expression should be greatly decreased, thereby restoring drug sensitivity. The analogue must have the following characteristics [16]:

1. absolute specificity for the base sequence of the targeted DNA or RNA;
2. high binding affinity for the targeted sequence;
3. ability to penetrate the cell with ease;
4. stability within the cell

The first two characteristics require that the selected target be a unique sequence for the gene. Hybridization experiments have shown that 15 to 20 bases are needed for unique complementary binding. The last two characteristics make unmodified oligonucleotides unsuitable as they have highly charged phosphate groups and are readily degraded-

Several approaches are currently being explored. Weintraub and co-workers [17] have introduced specific DNA sequences into cells that produce an antisense message. This antisense RNA binds to messenger RNA and decreases expression of the specific gene product. Activity of the important salvage enzyme, thymidine kinase, has been greatly reduced by this approach. An efficient method to introduce this antisense DNA selectively into resistant cells has not been developed.

Certain polymeric drugs like netropsin selectively bind to the minor groove of the B configuration of DNA duplexes with a strong preference for regions containing stretches of dA · dT base pairs [18]. Dickerson et al. [19] have shown that this selectivity is due to specific hydrophobic and steric interactions. By altering the polymer length and the heterocyclic residues in the polymer, they are designing drugs that can bind along the minor groove to specific known gene sequences. Such binding may interfere with interconversions of DNA configurations and transcription of these sequences.

Ts'o and co-workers [16, 20] have pioneered the synthesis and biologic evaluation of oligonucleotide derivatives which contain either esters of the phosphate backbone or substitution of the phosphates with methylphosphonates. The latter compounds appear to be more stable in vivo. They are transported passively into mammalian cells, are degraded very slowly within cells, and bind with a higher degree of stability to polynucleotide sequences than natural oligonucleotides. Specific sequences of any length can be synthesized and purified by modifications of the standard chemical methods of gene synthesis. Work is just beginning to see if these oligonucleotide derivatives can reverse drug resistance.

## Targeting to Specific Gene Products

Now that the structure and function of many of the enzymes and proteins involved in drug resistance have been characterized, antitumor agents can be designed to interact specifically with these targets. For example, Cheng and co-workers [7], have reported that the viral DNA polymerase in phosphonoformate-resistant, herpes simplex virus-infected KOS cells is more sensitive to aphidicolin, a drug that binds to this enzyme. Similarly, acyclovir and other recent antiviral drugs selectively inhibit viral derived enzymes of nucleic acid synthesis [21]. This approach should be applicable to some drug resistant cell lines.

Another example is pharmacologic reduction of glutathione levels in tumor cells resistant to alkylating agents because of increased content of this detoxifying agent [22, 23]. Finally, several groups have attempted to reverse the pleotropic drug resistance to antitumor antibiotics and alkaloids that is due to decreased drug accumulation and retention. The resistance is associated with a high molecular weight glycoprotein that appears in these resistant cells. Recently, calcium channel blockers or calmodulin inhibitors have been shown to reverse resistance to some of these drugs [24].

## Alteration in Methylation Patterns in DNA

The degree and pattern of 5-methylation of deoxycytosine bases in DNA appear to have a major role in mammalian gene regulation [25, 26]. Hypermethylation is associated with decreased gene expression. After incorporation into DNA, azacytidine and related 5-substituted cytidine derivatives prevent the formation of 5-methyl-cytosine by inactivating DNA methylase. Once a cytosine residue is demethylated, further strands formed during cell division will retain the demethylated pattern since the methylase only methylates the complementary strand of Me-C · G pairs. Thus, the methylation pattern is retained for at least several cell divisions even if the azacytidine derivative is no longer present [25]. Treatment of cells with azacytidine and its derivatives have caused differentiation of tumor cells; reactivation of inactive X-linked genes for HGPRTase, glucose 6-phosphate dehydrogenase and phosphoglucokinase in hybrid cells; restoration of glucocorticoid sensitivity and activation of latent genes and viruses [25].

Ara-C is one of the most active drugs in the treatment of acute myelogenous leukemia in man. Acquired resistance can be due to many factors, but the most important is the lack of deoxycytidine kinase (dCk), the enzyme responsible for the phosphorylation of ara-C to ara-CMP, which is then phosphorylated further by pyrimidine nucleoside monophosphate kinase to form ara-CDP and by nucleoside diphosphate kinase to form ara-CTP, the active metabolite of ara-C. Avramis *et al.* [27] have been investigating whether one form of resistance to ara-C is due to hypermethylation of the gene that codes for dCk and whether this gene can be reactivated by azacytidine analogues.

EXPERIMENTAL PROTOCOL

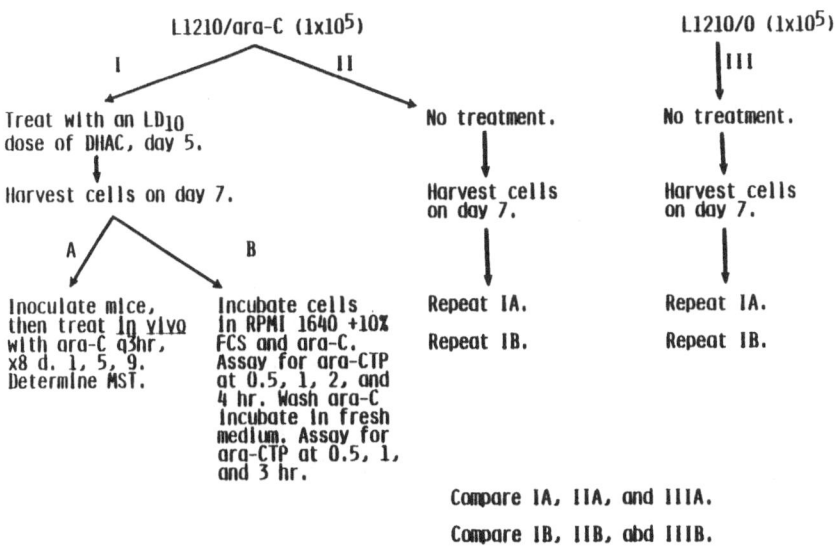

*Figure 1.* Diagram of experimental protocol.

5-Azacytidine (5-Aza-C), a nitrogen bioisostere of cytidine, is an antimetabolite with antineoplastic, mitogenic and leukopenic activity. 5-Aza-C is thought to exert its pharmacologic effects through an interference with nucleic acid metabolism [28]. Dihydro-5-Azacytidine (DHAC) is a hydrolytically stable analog of 5-Aza-C with potent anti-leukemic activity against experimental leukemias, and like 5-Aza-C and 5-Aza-dCyt causes hypomethylation of the DNA of cells [29]. DHAC is more efficacious against the ara-C resistant murine luekemia line L1210/ara-C than the parent L1210/0 and is cross-resistant to a 5-Aza-C resistant line, L1210/aza-C [11, 30]. The L1210/ara-C line is resistant to ara-C because it lacks dCk. In these studies we investigated whether DHAC treatment could induce expression of dCk activity in L1210/ara-C cells and restore their sensitivity to ara-C treatment.

*Experimental Reversal of Tumor Resistance in L1210/ara-C Cells*

One $\times 10^5$ L1210/ara-C or L1210/0 cells were inoculated into DBA/2 mice on day 0. On day 5 post-inoculation, at which point approximately $10^8$ cells were in the peritoneal cavity of the mouse, four mice bearing L1210/ara-C and one mouse bearing L1210/0 were treated i.p. with an $LD_{10}$ single dose of DHAC (I) (Figure 1). Four mice with L1210/ara-C (II) and four mice with L1210/0 (III) were not treated (Figure 1).

On day 7 when approximately four to five cell replications had occurred, the surviving cells from DHAC treatment and the untreated animals were harvested, pooled per group, counted and sized. A fraction fo these cells (IA, IIA and IIIA) was used to inoculate healthy BD2F$_1$ mice ($1 \times 10^5$ cells per mouse of each tumor line). The mice were then treated *in vivo* with ara-C 15 mg/kg, q3h $\times$ 8 on days 1, 5 and 9 post-inoculation (LD$_{10}$). Table 1 presents the median survival time (MST) and increase in life span (ILS) for these groups. The mean $\pm$SD for ILS was $22.3 \pm 8.8\%$ for the groups of mice that were inoculated with $1 \times 10^5$ L1210/ara-C cells, pretreated with an LD$_{10}$ dose of DHAC 48 h earlier and treated with ara-C when compared to either L1210/ara-C not pretreated with DHAC or L1210/0 not treated with ara-C. Our positive control groups that were inoculated with L1210/0 and treated with ara-C had a much higher % ILS of 75%.

No increase in % ILS was obtained when L1210/ara-C cells were pretreated with a single LD$_{10}$ dose of 5-Aza-dCyd 48 h earlier, inoculated into healthy BD2F$_1$ mice and treated with ara-C. Additional treatment schedules will be tested to determine whehter DHAC, which is much more stable in aqueous solutions than either 5-Aza-C or 5-Aza-dCyd, is more efficient in converting a tumor line resistant to ara-C into a partially sensitive one.

*Table 1.* Antitumor effect of ara-C against L1210 and L1210/ara-C pretreated with DHAC tumor lines. Tumor cells ($1 \times 10^5$) were implanted i.p. on Day 0; treatment regimen: ara-C 15 mg/kg q3h $\times$ 8 on days 1, 5 and 9, i.p.

| # | Tumor line | Treatment | # of mice | Toxic deaths[a] | MST, days[b] | Mean/range, days | % Ils |
|---|------------|-----------|-----------|------------------|--------------|------------------|-------|
| 1 | L1210/0 | saline | 18 | — | 8 | 7.70/7–9 | — |
| 2 | L1210/ara-C | saline | 16 | — | 8 | 7.89/7–8 | — |
| 3 | L1210/ara-C +DHAC | saline | 16 | — | 8 | 8.00/7–9 | — |
| 4 | L1210/0 | ara-C | 18 | 1 | 14 | 13.89/13–17 | 75.0 |
| 5 | L1210/ara-C | ara-C | 16 | — | 8 | 7.80/7–8 | — |
| 6 | L1210/ara-C +DHAC | ara-C | 10 | 2 | 11 | 12.40/10–12 | 29.4 |
| 7 | L1210/ara-C +DHAC | ara-C | 10 | 1 | 9 | 10.00/8–18 | 12.5 |
| 8 | L1210/ara-C +DHAC | ara-C | 10 | — | 10 | 10.60/9–13 | 25.0 |
| 9 | Average 6, 7 and 8 | | | | | | $22.3 \pm 8.8$[c] |

[a] Toxic deaths = deaths by day 6 post-inoculation.
[b] MST = median survival time.
[c] Mean, $\pm$S.D., n = 3.

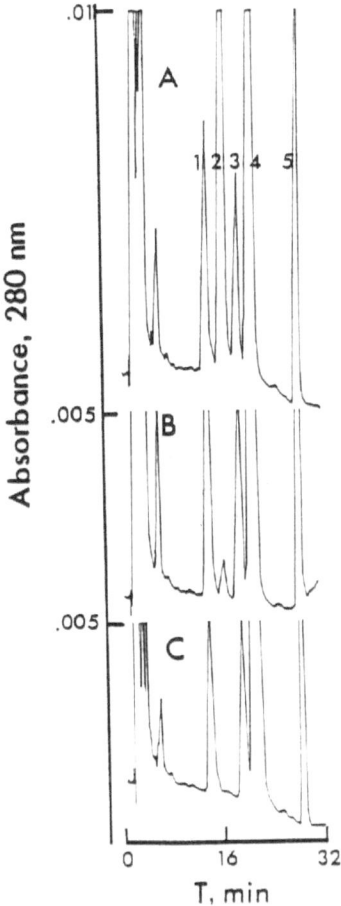

*Figure 2.* HPLC separation of L1210/0 and L1210/ara-C cellular nucleotides. (A) Chromatogram of nucleotides from $1 \times 10^7$ L1210/0 cells treated with 1 mM ara-C for a h at 37°. The sequence of the numbered peaks is: CTP (1), ara-CTP (2), UTP (3), ATP (4), and GTP (5). (B) chromatogram of nucleotides from $1 \times 10^7$ L1210/ara-C cells pretreated with DHAC and then treated with 1 mM ara-C for 1 h at 37°C. (C) Chromatogram of nucleotides from $1 \times 10^7$ L1210/ara-C cells. Full-Scale absorbance, 0-01 AU.

The remaining cells from groups IB, IIB and IIIB were split into three portions for each tumor line. The cells were washed and $5 \times 10^6$ cell/ml of RPMI 1640 + 10% fetal calf serum were incubated with 1 mM of ara-C 37°C in 5% $CO_2$/humidified air incubators. After 0.5, 1, 2, and 4 h, aliquots were removed from the incubation flasks, washed of exogenous ara-C and extracted twice with 0.4 N perchloric acid (PCA) as described previously [31, 32]. Neutralized soluble acid extracts were assayed for nucleoside triphosphates (NTP's) and ara-CTP by high pressure liquid chromatography.

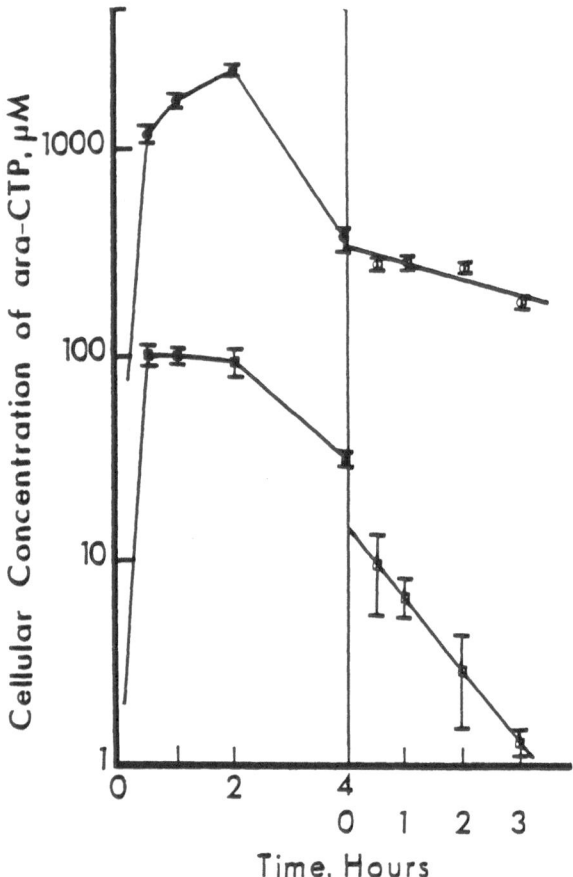

*Figure 3.* Accumulation and elimination kinetics of intracellular concentrations of ara CTP in L1210/0 (●) and L1210/ara-C (□) pretreated with DHAC after *in vitro* incubation with 1 mM ara-C at 37°. At 4 h the cells were washed twice and incubated in ara-C-free medium to determine the degradation kinetics of ara-CTP. The $t_{1/2}$, el of ara-CTP in L1210/0 and L1210/ara-C (+DHAC) cells is 3.60 and 0.86 h, respectively (bars, S.D., n = 3).

At 4 h, the remaining cells in the incubation flasks were washed twice of exogenous ara-C and incubated in fresh growth medium. At 0.5, 1, 2, and 3 h, aliquots of the cells were removed, washed and extracted with PCA. The neutralized acid extracts were assayed for NTP's and ara-CTP by HPLC. In a similarly designed experiment, the fractions IB, IIB and IIIB were incubated *in vitro* with various concentrations of ara-C for 1 h. The cells were extracted with PCA and the neutralized soluble acid extracts were assayed for ara-CTP by HPLC.

The NTP's in the acid extracts of these cells and the ara-CTP concentrations are depicted in Figures 2 and 3. L1210/0 cells (IIIB) accumulated over 2000 µM ara-CTP within 2 h, a highly toxic concentration of ara-CTP. As a result the cells started lysing between 2 and 4 h. L1210/ara-C cells (IIB) that were not pretreated with DHAC did not form any detectable ara-CTP (Fig-

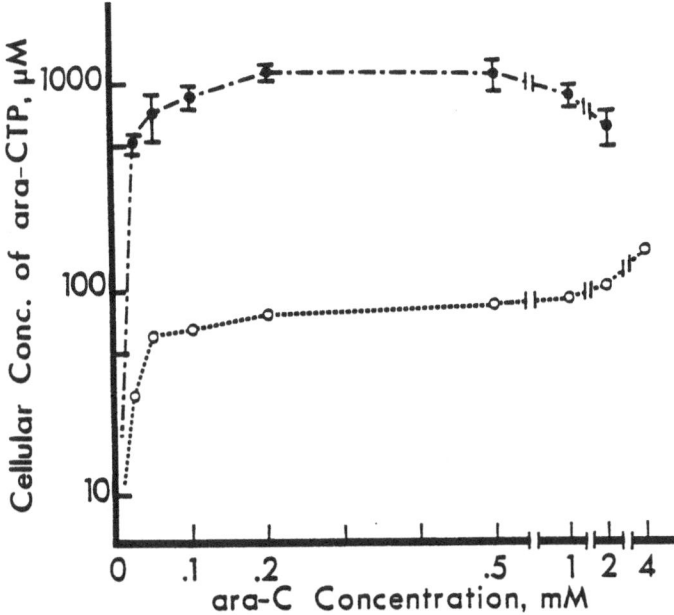

*Figure 4.* Intracellular concentrations of ara-CTP in L1210/0 (●) and L1210/ara-C (○) pre-treated with DHAC cells after *in vitro* incubations with various concentrations of ara-C for 1 h at 37°C (bars, S.D., n = 3).

ure 2C), whereas the L1210/ara-C pretreated with DHAC 48 h earlier were able to form ara-CTP up to 100 µM (Figure 2B). This concentration was approximately 1/20 the intracellular concentration of control (L1210/0) cells.

In the *in vitro* experiment, the intracellular concentration of ara-CTP in L1210/ara-C + DHAC was only 1/15 to 1/20 of that in the L1210/0 leukemia cells after incubations with 1 µM ara-C over 1 to 2 h. After washing the cells and incubating in drug-free medium, the half-life of elimination ($t_{1/2}$, el.) of ara-CTP in the L1210/0 cells was 3.6 h (n = 3), while the $t_{1/2}$, el. of ara-CTP in the L1210/ara-C pretreated with DHAC was 0.86 h (n = 3). Thus, the hydrolytic activity of ara-CTP is four times higher in the ara-C resistant tumor line than the L1210/0 cells (Figure 3). When L1210/0 cells were pretreated *in vivo* 48 h earlier with a single $LD_{10}$ dose of DHAC, the $t_{1/2}$, el. of ara-CTP was 4.8 h, indicating that DHAC pretreatment does not enhance degradation of ara-CTP.

In a similarly prepared experiment, the IB, IIB and IIIB cells were incubated for 1 h with various ara-C concentrations of 0, 25, 50, 100, 200, 500, 1000, 2000 and 4000 µM. Once again, the L1210/ara-C cells pretreated with DHAC (IB) formed ara-CTP (Figure 4). These intracellular concentrations reached a plateau at 50 µM ara-C, possibly indicating saturation of the kinase responsible for phosphorylating ara-C. A plateau was also observed in the L1210/0 (IIB) cells after 200 μM of ara-C, but at about 15 times the intracellular level of the IB cells (Figure 4). The L1210/ara-C (IIB) cells without pretreatment formed no detectable ara-CTP.

*Therapeutic Efficacy of Ara-C and DHAC*

The tumor titration studies of L1210/0, L1210/ara-C and L1210/ara-C pretreated with DHAC resulted in similar duplication times and identical median survival times for all serial inocula but the last one ($1 \times 10^7$ cells/mouse). The cell doubling times were 11.0, 9.0, 12.5 h for L1210/0, L1210/ara-C and L1210/ara-C pretreated with DHAC, respectively. These values are in excellent agreement with values from L1210/0 in larger numbers of mice [33]. These results indicate that the three tumor lines had similar growth rates and that the L1210/ara-C cells surviving DHAC pretreatment had not lost their tumorigenic activity.

DHAC was tested alone against L1210/0 and L1210/ara-C. Groups of $BD2F_1$ mice (eight mice each) were inoculated with $1 \times 10^5$ L1210/0 and treated with either the $LD_{10}$ single dose (two groups) or the $LD_{10}$ qd $\times$ 5 dose (two groups). Four groups of $BD2F_1$ mice were inoculated with $1 \times 10^5$ L1210/ara-C and treated with DHAC. There was no statistical difference between the single dose *vs.* multiple dose of DHAC against either tumor line after accounting for the number of treatment days in the multiple dose regimen. Nevertheless, the multiple DHAC regimen was more effective against L1210/ara-C than against L1210/0 (P<0.002), whereas the single dose regimen was not (P>0.2).

*Enhancement of Expression of Deoxycytidine Kinase in the Human Cell Lines CCRF/CEM/0 and CCRF/CEM/dCk− by DHAC*

Human lymphoid cells cultured *in vitro* were tested for intracellular ara-CTP formation and accumulation after incubations with 1 mM ara-C for 1 h. The experimental cell lines were pretreated with 0.1 mM DHAC for 24 h, a dose that decreased growth by 50%. The surviving fraction of the cells were cultured for three more days in fresh medium and then treated with ara-C. After pretreatment with DHAC, a cell line with decreased dCk activity, CEM/dCk−, showed 1.3- to 1.8-fold greater ara-CTP accumulation than untreated CEM/dCk− cells. Two subclones of CEM/dCk− have been isolated in our laboratory. These cell lines accumulated cellular ara-CTP concentrations approximately 53% and 11% of control (CEM/O) after 1 h incubation with ara-C and 20% and 5% after 4 h incubation. Both subclones of CEM/dCk− showed enhanced cellular ara-CTP accumulation

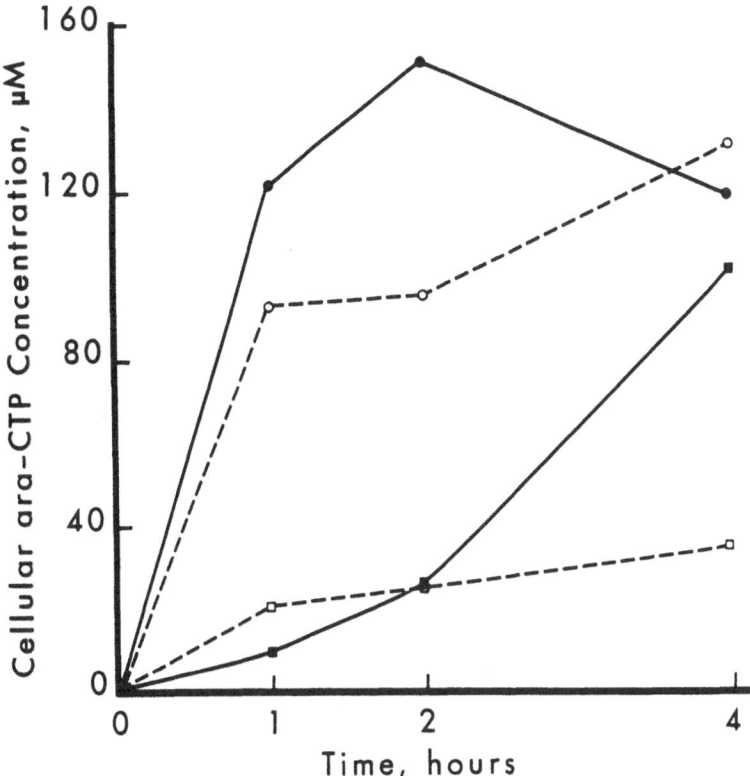

*Figure 5.* Accumulation of cellular ara-CTP concentrations in two subclones of CEM/dCk⁻ with
(●, ○) and without (■, □) DHAC pretreatment, after *in vitro* incubation with (³H)ara-C. The
PCA-soluble extract from these cells was assayed on HPLC.

after DHAC pretreatment (Figure 5). CEM/0 cells showed a small but not
significant cellular ara-CTP concentration after DHAC pretreatment. Further studies are in progress with CEM/dCk− clones that are unable to accumulate any ara-CTP.

Certain questions remain unanswered by these studies. First, it is unknown whether all the L1210/ara-C cells that were pretreated with DHAC
express a small copy number of dCk, a few cells express an adequate number, or even fewer cells express as much as the sensitive cells L1210/0. This
question will be addressed by evaluation of dCk activity in single origin cells
cloned in soft agar. If only a small proportion of the cells express dCk,
experiments will be directed to increase the proportion by repeated treatments or other agents that select for the revertants. The second and most
important question is whether this phenomenon of partial reversal of tumor
drug resistance is a transient effect and if so, what is its duration. Finally, we
must establish whether the degree of hypomethylation after *in vivo* treatment with DHAC correlates with the degree of expression of dCk activity. A

selective media has been developed to clone dCk revertants so that their enzyme activity and methylation pattern can be analyzed.

## In Vivo *Human Studies of Reversal of Tumor Drug Resistance*

Even though these animals and cell culture experiments show a limited reversion to ara-C sensitivity, the collateral sensitivity of ara-C and 5-Aza-C makes the following treatment sequence worth investigating: ara-C, 5-Aza-C and then ara-C again. Ara-C will kill the sensitive tumor cells. The surviving resistant cells may be collaterally more sensitive to 5-Aza-C compounds. As we have demonstrated, a portion of cells surviving therapy with 5-Aza-C or its derivatives may have regained sensitivity to ara-C. A second treatment with ara-C would kill these revertants. We are now testing this approach.

Three pediatric patients with acute lymphocytic leukemia who had multiple bone marrow relapses and who had not responded to a high dose ara-C (HDara-C) regimen, were treated with a continuous infusion of 150 mg/m$^2$ of 5-aza-C. Bone marrow and peripheral blood specimens were obtained. The blast cells were separated, isolated, and their cell number and cell size determined. A portion of the cells were tested for dCk activity by measuring ara-CTP accumulation after 1 h incubation with 1 mM ara-C at 37 °C. Another fraction of the leukemic cells were tested for DNA synthetic capacity (DSC) by thymidine incorporation after 1 h incubation with 1 mM ara-C. These patients received another course of HDara-C 1 to 9 days after the 5-aza-C treatment. During this study, sequential heparinized blood samples were obtained, and the circulating blasts were isolated and extracted for nucleotides and ara-CTP.

Control leukemic cells from patient #1 formed similar cellular ara-CTP concentrations in peripheral blast cells (PBC) after 1 h incubations with 0.2 or 1 mM ara-C (Figure 6). Three days after the patient finished the 5-day 5-Aza-C regimen, the PBCs accumulated >1000 µM ara-CTP, a 3.6-fold increase over control. Nine days after the end of 5-Aza-C treatment, the PBCs accumulated >700 µM ara-CTP, 2.2-fold higher than control, but 30% lower than at 3 days post 5-Aza-C. At the same time the BM blasts accumulated >570 µM ara-CTP. The DSC was approximately 20% of control before and 3 days after 5-Aza-C. By day 9 post treatment, the DSC had increased to 58% and 34% of the PBCs and BM controls, respectively.

The 5-Aza-C treatment did not decrease the blast count. The patient received the second high dose ara-C regimen on day 9. Five hours after the first dose of ara-C, the PBCs contained >1250 µM peak ara-CTP concentrations. The $t_{1/2}$, el. of ara-CTP in the PBC was 13.5 h. These values produce an area under the curve for cellular ara-CTP greater than any value seen in

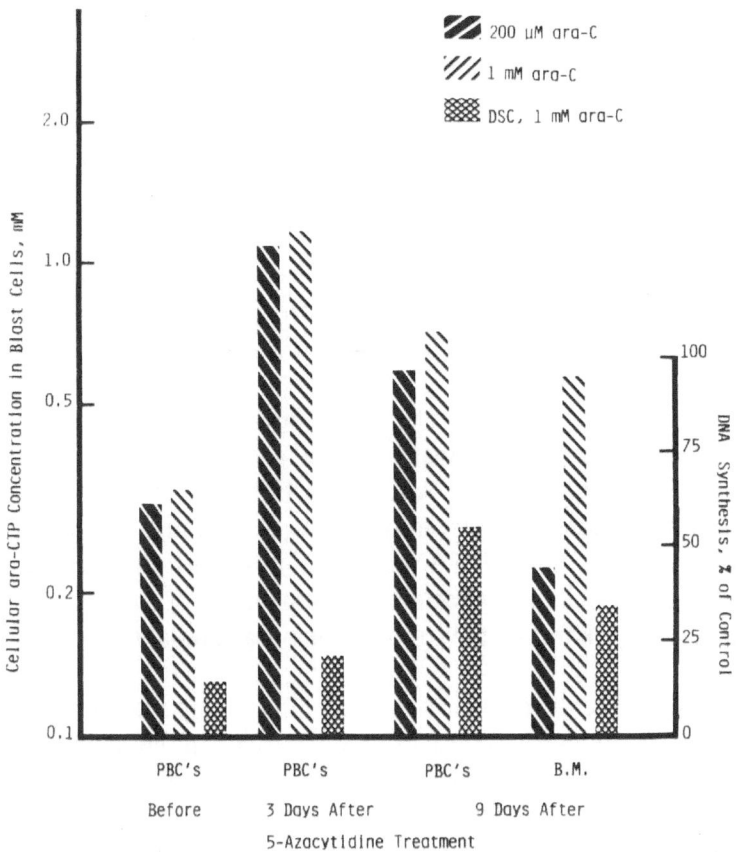

*Figure 6.* Cellular ara-CTP concentrations in peripheral (PBC) and bone marrow blast cells (BM) from patient #1 after 1 h incubations with ara-C. The tests were conducted before, 3 days after and 9 days after 5-Aza-C treatment *in vivo*.

our HDara-C study. Previous studies have shown that the $t_{1/2}$ and AUC correlate with antileukemic effect of HDara-C [24, 34–36]. No DSC studies were performed in this patient after the second HDara-C regimen due to specimen limitations. This patient had clearing of peripheral lymphoblasts but he died of sepsis 8 days after the HDara-C treatment.

The blast cells of patient #2 showed slightly more accumulation of ara-CTP cellular concentrations in both peripheral and BM blasts after the 5-Aza-C treatment (Table 2). The DSC of the peripheral blast cells was 52% and 25% of their respective controls, before and 4 days after the 5-Aza-C treatment. However, the DSC of the BM blast cells was 85% of their control. The lymphoblast count rose from 13,000 to 40,000/mm$^3$ during the 5-Aza-C treatment. This patient received HDara-C 5 days after the 5-Aza-C infusion. The blast count fell to zero 4 days after the start of this infusion. The biochemical and pharmacological parameters, such as cellular ara-CTP concentrations (peak and through), the $t_{1/2}$, el. of ara-CTP from blasts and the DSC, were similar for the HDara-C administered before and 5 days after 5-Aza-C. Preliminary studies show that the 5-Aza-C treatment greatly decreased the percentage of 5-methyl-cytosine bases in this DNA. He died of infection 17 days after the HDara-C treatment. There was no evidence of leukemia at post-mortem examination.

Blast cells from a third patient were studied. The cellular ara-CTP concentration increased slightly after 5-Aza-C treatment. This was associated with a decrease in DSC after incubations with 1 mM ara-C. This patient had a blast count of over $300,000/\text{mm}^3$. He showed no clinical response to the 5-Aza-C and died 22 h after the start of HDara-C treatments.

These clinical studies suggest that enhanced antileukemic and toxic effects are seen with the sequence of 5-Aza-C and HDara-C. Additional patients will be treated to confirm these results and to investigate whether these effects correlate with altered DNA methylation patterns. We will attempt to decrease the infectious complications by adjustment of the HD-ara-C dosage and by use of laminar flow rooms plus oral non-absorbable antibiotics.

Other forms of drug resistance may be affected by alteration in DNA methylation. We are currently attempting to reactivate HGPRTase in various cell lines lacking this activity. In this system, an increase in gene expression could occur on the active X chromosome in male tumor cells and in either the active or inactivated X chromosome in female tumor cells [20]. This strategy to change DNA methylation will also be tested in tumor cells resitant to other drugs that require metabolic activation, transport proteins or specific binding proteins.

Table 2. Biochemical and pharmacological parameters in circulating blast cells of patient #2 after *in vivo* HDara-C administered before and 5 days post 5-Aza-C.

| Treatment | Ara-CTP µM | | Ara-CTP $t_{1/2}$, el. (hours) | DSC % of Control | | $t_{1/2}$, el. of blasts (hours) |
|---|---|---|---|---|---|---|
| | Peak (3 h) | Trough (12 h) | | Nadir | 12 Hours | |
| HDara-C first regimen | 460.0 | 120.0 | 4.93 | 4.34% | 18.7% | 7.1 |
| HDara-C second regimen | 398.8 | 106.4 | 5.20 | 2.72% | 22.2% | 10.2 |

# Conclusion

Our new understanding of the targets of antitumor agents and the molecular biology of gene expression have lead to promising approaches to counteract acquired drug resistance in cancer cells. Further investigations should lead to clinical applications of drug combinations that delay the emergence of resistance, exploit the biochemical changes that have allowed resistance, and directly alter the gene expression causing the resistance.

# References

1. Curt GA, Clendeninn NJ, Chabner BA: Cancer Treat Rep 68:87–99, 1984.
2. Lane M: Fed Proc 38:103–107, 1979.
3. Bertino JR: Med Pediat Oncol 5:105–114, 1978.
4. Schimke RT, Beverley S, Brown P et al.: Drug resistance and gene amplification in euka-ryotic cells. In: Mechanisms of Drug Action. Singh T, Monsour T, Ondarza R (eds). Acad Press New York, 107–117, 1983.
5. Conter V, Beck WT: Cancer Treat Rep 68:831–839, 1984.
6. Roninson IB, Abelson HT, Housman DE, Howell N, Varshavsky A: Nature 309:626–628, 1984.
7. Cheng Y-C, Brockman RW: Mechanisms of drug resistance and collateral sensitivity: bases for development of chemotherapeutic agents. In: Development of Target-Oriented Anti-cancer Drugs. Chang Y-C, Goz B, Minkoff M (eds). Prog Cancer Res Ther 28. Raven Press, New York, 107–117, 1983.
8. Wallerstein H, Slater LM, Eng B, Calman N: Cancer Res 32:2235–2240, 1972.
9. Goldie JH, Coldman AJ, Gudauskas GA: Cancer Treat Rep 66:439–449, 1982.
10. Schmid FA, Hutchinson DJ: Cancer Res 32:808–812, 1972.
11. Schabel FM Jr, Skipper HE, Trader MW, Brockman RW, Laster WR Jr, Corbett TH, Gris-wold DP Jr: Med Ped Onc (Suppl) 1:125–148, 1982.
12. Herman TS, Cress AE, Gerner EW: Cancer Res 39:1937–1942, 1979.
13. Seeber S, Osieka R, Schmidt CG, Achterrath W, Cooke ST: Cancer Res 42:4719–4725, 1982.
14. Horns RC, Dower WJ, Schimke RT: J Clin Oncol 2:2–7, 1984.
15. Hunt SW, Hoffee PA: J Biol Chem 258:13185–13192, 1983.
16. Ts'o POP, Miller PS, Greene JJ: Nucleic acid analogs with targeted delibery as chemother-apeutic agents. In: Development of Target-Oriented Antivancer Drugs. Chang YC, Goz B, Minkoff M (eds). Prog Cancer Res Ther 28. Raven Press, 189–206, 1983.
17. Izant JG, Weintraub H: Cell 36:1007–1015, 1984.
18. Marky LA, Curry J, Breslaver KJ: Netropsin binding to poly d(AT) . poly d(AT) and to poly dA . poly dT: A comparative thermodynamic study. IN: Molecular Basis of Cancer, Part B. Rein R (ed). A. Liss, New York, 155–173, 1985.
19. Kopka ML, Yoon C, Goodsell S, Pjurs P, Dickerson RE: Proc Natl Acad Sci USA 82:1376–1380, 1985.
20. Miller PS, Agris CH, Murakami A, Reddy PM, Spitz SA, Ts'o POP: Nucleid Acid Res 11:6225–6242, 1983.
21. Dolin R: Science 227:1296–1303, 1985.
22. Arrick BS, Nathan CF: Cancer Res 44:4224–4232, 1984.
23. Somfai-Relle S, Suzukake K, Vistica B, Vistica DT: Biochem Pharmacol 33:485–490, 1984.

24. Beck WT: Cellular Pharmacology of vinca alkaloids resistance and its circumvention. In: Adv Enz Reg, Vol. 22. Weber G (ed). Perfamon Press, New York, 207–227, 1984.

25. Jones PA: Gene activation by 5-azacytidine. In: DNA Methylation-Biochemistry and Biological Significance. Razin A, Cedar H, Riggs AD (eds). Springer-Verlag, 165–187, 1984.

26. Riggs AD: X Inactivation, DNA Methylation and differentiation revisited. In: DNA Methylation-Biochemistry and biological Significance. Razin A, Cedar H, Riggs AD (eds). Springer-Verlag, 269–278, 1984.

27. Avramis VI, Holcenberg JS: Proc Am Assoc Cancer Res 25:333, 1984.

28. Vesely J, Cihak A: Pharmac Ther A 2:813–840, 1978.

29. Jones PA, Taylor SM: Cell 20:85–93, 1980.

30. Schabel FM Jr, Skipper HE, Trader MW, Laster WR Jr, Griswold DP Jr, Corbett TH: Cancer Treat Rep 67:905–922, 1983.

31. Plunkett W, Chubb S, Alexander L, Montgomery JA: Cancer Res 40:2349–2355, 1980.

32. Plunkett W, Hug V, Keating MJ, Chubb S: Cancer Res 40:588–591, 1980.

33. Schabel FM Jr, Griswold DP, Laster WR Jr, Corbett TH, Lloyd HH: Pharmacol Ther A 1:411–435, 1977.

34. Avramis VI, Holcenberg JS: Biochemical pharmacology of high dose cytosine arabinoside (HDara-C). In: Childhood leukemia. Submitted to Cancer Res.

35. Avramis VI, Biener R, Ettinger LJ, Holcenberg JS, Finkelstein JZ, Laug W, Williams K Shore N, Siegel SE: Proc Am Assoc Clin Oncology, 1985 (in press).

36. Plunkett W, Iacoboni S, Danhauser L, Estey E, Walters R, keating M, McCredie K, Freireich EJ: Proc Am Assoc Cancer Res 25:166, 1984.

# Methods of drug delivery

# 7. New methods of administering old drugs: IV infusion of mercaptopurine

SOLOMON ZIMM and DAVID G. POPLACK

## Introduction

In order to maximize an anti-neoplastic agent's activity it is essential to consider the drug's pharmacokinetics. The importance of route and schedule of administration has been well exemplified by the experience with cytosine arabinoside and doxorubicin [1, 2]. We have been interested in the pharmacology of mercaptopurine (MP), particularly its clinical pharmacokinetics and have examined several of its characteristics [3–7]. In this chapter we will review our initial clinical pharmacologic studies as well as our recently completed phase I and pharmacologic study of MP administered as a prolonged iv infusion, a study that was prompted by our earlier observations.

## Background

MP is an analog of the naturally occurring purine base, hypoxanthine. It was synthesized in 1952 [8] and as such is one of the oldest anti-cancer agents in current use. Clear anti-leukemic activity was demonstrated for MP in initial and follow-up clinical trials [9, 10]. MP was administered orally on a daily basis in low doses in these studies. Based on these clinical trials MP came to have an established place in acute lymphoblastic leukemia (ALL) maintenance chemotherapy regimens, and this continues to constitute the drug's primary clinical use [11]. Daily oral administration of MP in relatively low doses (50–75 mg/sq m) is the conventional schedule of administration in these remission maintenance regimens.

Despite the use of oral MP in ALL therapy for over 20 years, little was known about the drug's clinical pharmacology. This was due to the lack of analytical methodology with sufficient sensitivity and specificity to measure the low levels of MP found in biological fluids and clearly separate it from its major plasma metabolite, thiouric acid (TU). In one earlier study in which radiolabeled MP was administered to several patients, total radioactivity was measured in plasma following oral and iv administration [12]. Analysis of the data from this study suggested that oral MP had a bioavailability of approximately 50%. The major problem with this study, however, was that levels of MP were determined from measurements of total radioactivity in plasma. This is not accurate for highly metabolized compounds, like MP. In these situations one is measuring not only the parent compound but also the various metabolites formed. This could lead to the conclusion that a drug's bioavailability is good, when in fact, it may be quite poor due to a substantial amount of first-pass metabolism.

## Initial Studies

In order to study the clinical pharmacology of MP in patients with leukemia, it was first necessary to develop a sensitive and specific assay for MP in biologic fluids. This was accomplished by developing a reverse phase high pressure liquid chromatography (HPLC) assay that clearly separated MP from its major plasma metabolite, TU. The lower limit of assay sensitivity for MP quantitation was 10 ng/ml [13].

In our initial study we examined the pharmacokinetics of MP following oral and iv administration to children with ALL in remission [3]. A conventional dose of MP (75 mg/sq m) was administered on two separate occasions to the identical seven children by both the oral and iv routes. Plasma MP concentrations were measured over the following 6 h. The results are shown in Figure 1. The bioavailability of oral MP (defined as the fraction of orally administered drug that gains access to the systemic circulation as parent compound) was determined by dividing the area under the concentration-time curve (AUC) following oral dosing by the AUC following iv dosing. The bioavailability of oral MP was calculated to be 16%, far less than previously reported [12]. Intravenously administered MP had an elimination half-life of 0.9 h and a total body clearance of 719 ml/min/sq m.

Given the poor bioavailability of oral MP, we then asked the question: can predictable plasma concentrations of MP be achieved following uniform oral dosing? To answer this question we administered MP 75 mg/sq m by the oral route to fourteen children with ALL in remission. They were fasted for 12 h prior to study and all other medications were witheld for 24 h. Despite controlling for these factors, we could not achieve predictable plasma concentrations following administration of uniform doses of oral MP. As shown in Table 1, there was marked variability in peak plasma concentration, AUC, and time to peak concentration. The variable and low mean peak plasma MP levels (less than 1.0 µM) coupled with *in vitro* cytotoxicity

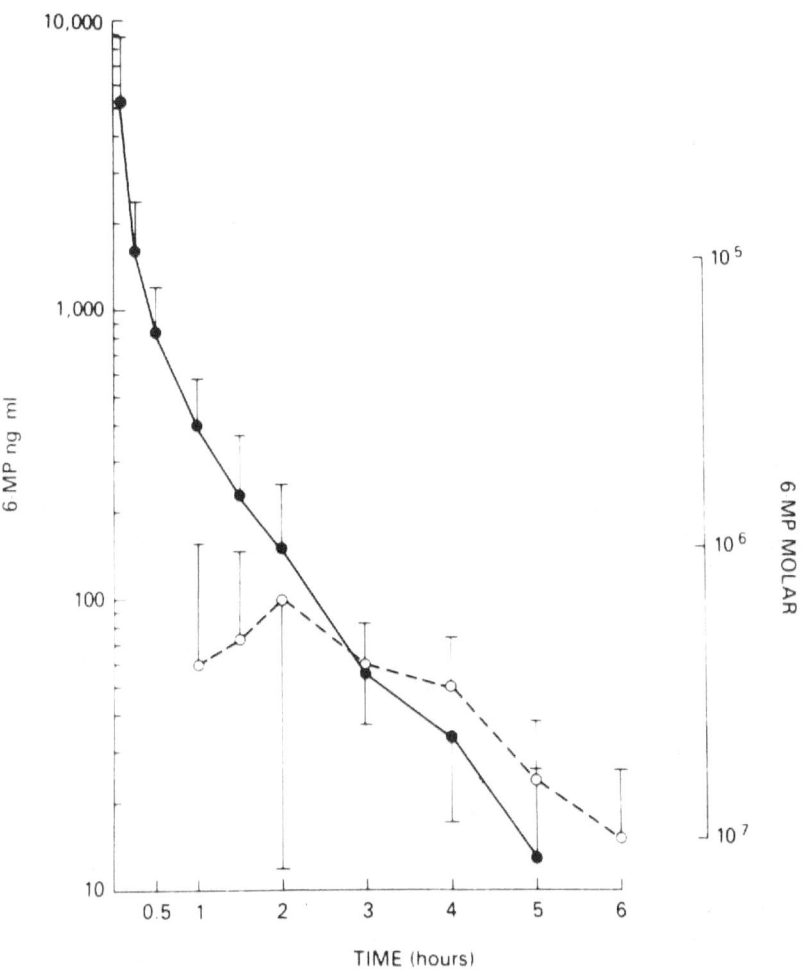

*Figure 1.* Plasma MP levels in seven patients following oral (○) and iv (●) administration of 75 mg/sq m. Mean +/− S.D. From Zimm et al. (3).

*Table 1.* Oral MP: pharmacokinetic values.

| Parameter | Value[a] |
|---|---|
| Peak plasma concentration (μM) | 0.9+/−0.5 |
| (range) | (0.3–1.8) |
| Time to peak (h) | 2.2+/−1.0 |
| (range) | (0.5–4.0) |
| AUC (μM-min) | 139+/−67 |
| (range) | (52–273) |

[a] Mean +/− standard deviation.

studies that have suggested that MP levels of 1–10 µM maintained for at least 12 h are required to achieve a substantial anti-neoplastic effect [7, 14] led us to ask if the current method of MP dosing for ALL remission maintenance is optimal. This study suggested that it was now appropriate to conduct clinical investigations of alternate dosing strategies that were more pharmacologically rational.

### Delivery of MP by Intravenous Infusion

The strategy we chose to investigate involved the administration of MP by prolonged intravenous infusion. We therefore initiated a pediatric phase I and clinical pharmacological study of MP administered as a prolonged intravenous infusion [6]. It was expected that this approach would result in less interpatient variability in plasma drug levels. In addition, MP's short half-life and the known cell-cycle dependence of the anti-metabolite class of agents suggested that administration of this compound by prolonged iv infusion would be more pharmacologically rational.

In this study MP was administered at an infusion rate of 50 mg/sq m/h (an infusion rate calculated to achieve steady state MP levels in plasma of approximately 5 µM) to all patients. The initial duration of infusion was 12 h. The dose rate was held constant throughout the study, while the duration of infusion was escalated in 12 h increments. Forty-four patients were entered on this study, and 38 were evaluable for response and toxicity. This study was conducted in a pediatric patient population with a median age of 10 yr. Nineteen patients had ALL. MP and its metabolites were measured in plasma, CSF, urine, and erythrocytes using a modified version of the previously published reverse phase HPLC assay as well as by anion exchange HPLC (for erythrocyte thiopurine levels) [15].

### Toxicities and Responses

The primary toxicities seen in this study were mucositis, myelosuppression, and hepatotoxicity. The dose-limiting toxicity was mucositis. None was observed with infusions of up to 24 h in length. However, infusions of 60 h in length were associated with frequent episodes of mucositis (6 of 13 cycles). Mucositis was judged acceptable with infusions of 48 h in duration (7 of 24 cycles). Based on these findings, it was recommended that phase II trials of iv MP infusions (at the same 50 mg/sq m/h dose rate) be initiated at infusion durations of 48 h.

No bone marrow toxicity was seen until infusions were administered for 48–60 h. At these durations transient depression of WBC, granulocyte, and

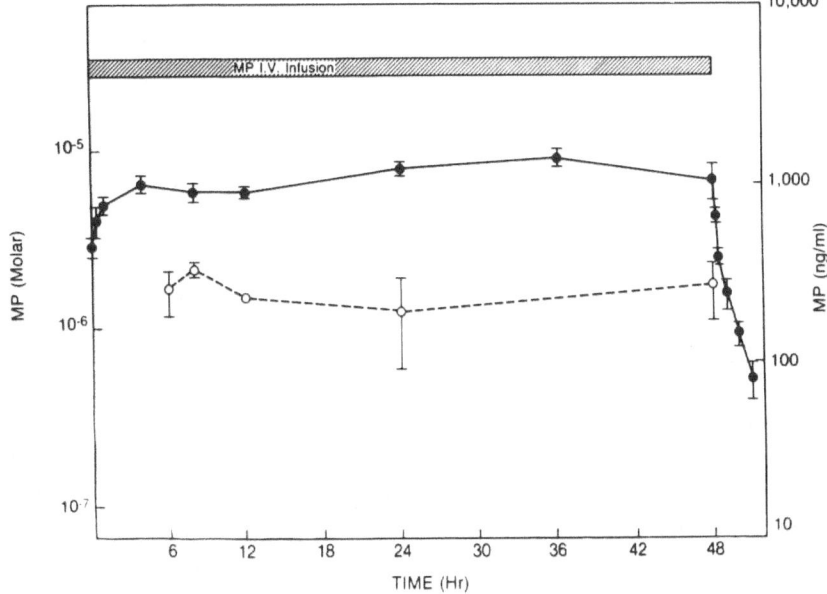

*Figure 2.* Plasma (●) and CSF (○) MP levels in 22 and 8 patients respectively during and following MP iv infusions at 50 mg/sq m/h. Mean +/− S.E. From Zimm et al. (3).

platelet counts were seen. Hepatotoxicity was also noted in this study. It was not dose-related and was manifested primarily as elevated transaminases, although hyperbilirubinemia was also observed. Hepatotoxicity was usually transient with liver chemistries returning to normal within 7–10 days. Nausea and vomiting in this study were mild. There was no renal or CNS toxicity.

Five responses were seen. One patient with a neuroblastoma had a partial response. Three patients with ALL had minor responses (all of whom had received prior oral MP), and one patient with an ependymoma also had a minor response.

## Pharmacology

The plasma pharmacokinetics of MP were determined in 22 patients and the CSF kinetics in 8 patients. As shown in Figure 2, steady-state plasma MP levels were in excess of 5 uM and CSF steady state levels approached 2 μM. Upon completion of the infusion MP levels in plasma declined rapidly and were less than 1 μM within 2 h post-infusion. The major pharmacokinetic valus for MP administered as a prolonged iv infusion are shown in Table 2. Intravenous administration of MP at this dose rate on this study was associated with good penetration of the central nervous system (CNS)

*Table 2.* MP iv infusion: pharmacokinetic values.

| Parameter | Values[a] |
|---|---|
| Css plasma (μM) | 6.9+/−0.4 |
| Css CSF (μM) | 1.7+/−0.3 |
| CSF/plasma ratio | 0.27+/−0.05 |
| Half-life (h) | 0.9+/−0.04 |
| Clearance (ml/min/sq m) | 864+/−49 |

[a] Mean +/− S.E.

with a CSF/plasma ratio of 0.27. In contrast, following administration of standard doses of oral MP to six patients, we were unable to detect the drug in CSF (<0.1 μM). The reported CSF/plasma ratio in our study is approximately ten-fold greater than that reported for methotrexate and similar to that reported with cytosine arabinoside when administered as a high dose infusion. This favorable penetration of the CNS suggests that MP may be of value in the treatment and perhaps the prevention of meningeal leukemia and other primary and metastatic CNS malignancies.

MP metabolites were measured in erythrocytes obtained from nine patients. Thioguanosine triphosphate was the major MP metabolite detected in erythrocytes. Of interest, despite the short half-life of MP in plasma (<1 h), the elimination half-life of erythrocyte thiopurines was quite long, 3.6 days.

### Interaction of MP and allopurinol

Patients treated with MP iv infusions who were receiving concurrent allopurinol did not have their dose of MP reduced. This policy was followed based on the results of our previous study [4]. In that study we administered the same dose of MP orally and subsequently as an iv bolus to five patients. They then received the same oral and iv doses of MP, but this time preceded by 24 h of oral allopurinol (300 mg/day). Allopurinol pretreatment resulted in a 500% increase in peak plasma MP concentration and AUC when MP was administered orally. In contrast, allopurinol pretreatment had no significant effect on the pharmacokinetics of intravenously administered MP. These results indicated that it is appropriate to reduce the dose of orally administered MP when given with allopurinol; there appears to be no pharmacokinetic justification for dose reduction of intravenously administered MP when co-administered with allopurinol. This differential effect of allopurinol on the pharmacokinetics of oral and iv MP is a result of inhibition of first pass metabolism. Xanthine oxidase, the primary catabolic

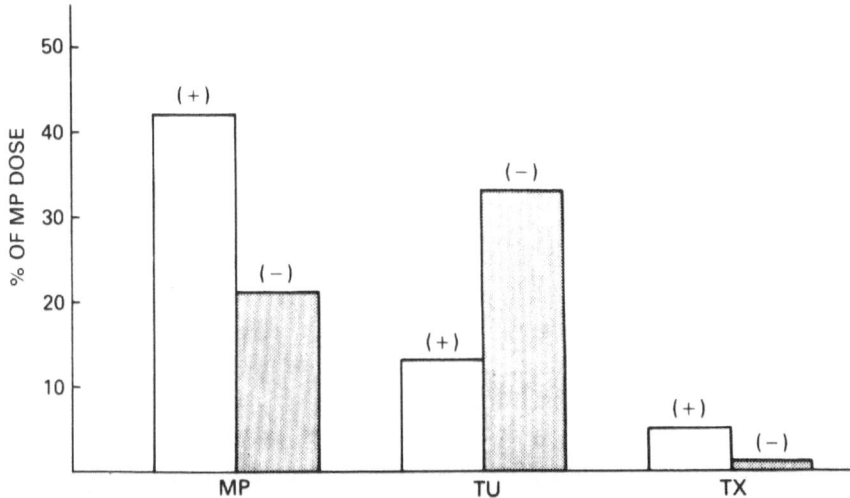

*Figure 3.* MP and metabolite urinary elimination expressed as a percentage of the administered dose of MP in patients receiving (+) or not receiving (−) allopurinol.

enzyme of MP, is mainly located in the gut mucosa and liver [16]. When administered orally, the entire dose of MP must traverse the two major sites of metabolism prior to gaining access to the systemic circulation. For a high extraction drug like MP whose clearance is flow-limited [17, 18], this results in very little drug reaching the systemic circulation as parent compound. When administered intravenously, however, only 25% of the drug reaches the liver during any one circulation, as this is the fraction of the cardiac output that supplies the liver. As a result, the effect of xanthine oxidase and its inhibition by allopurinol is markedly reduced.

Based on the above observations, none of the eight patients on the MP iv infusion study who were receiving allopurinol had their dose of MP reduced. Although the number of patients treated at any specific infusion duration was small, there was no evidence of increased MP-induced toxicity in the patients who received concurrent allopurinol. The pharmacokinetics of MP were studied in six patients who were receiving both allopurinol and MP. Steady-state MP plasma levels and total body clearance of MP were not significantly altered in the patients who received allopurinol compared to those who did not. The urinary metabolite elimination pattern, however, was significantly influenced by allopurinol treatment. As shown in Figure 3, the four patients on allopurinol excreted approximately half as much TU and thioxanthine and twice as much MP in their urine as did the six patients not receiving allopurinol. Whether the patients did or did not receive allopurinol, MP accounted for a substantial fraction of the administered dose appearing in the urine (42% with allopurinol, 21% without allopurinol). In contrast, following oral MP administration only 7% of the administered dose appears in the urine as MP.

## Summary and conclusions

We have identified several pharmacological disadvantages to the conventional (daily, low doses administered orally) method of MP administration, an approach in use for over 25 years. The bioavailability of oral MP was found to be poor, and it was not possible to achieve predictable plasma MP levels following uniform dosing. In addition, oral administration does not result in detectable MP levels in the CSF. In an attempt to circumvent these problems, we initiated a phase I trial in which MP was administered as a prolonged.

The results indicate that MP can be safely administered as a 48 h infusion at a dose rate of 50 mg/sq m/h. The dose-limiting toxicity was mucositis with myelosuppression (dose-related) and hepatotoxicity (not dose-related) also seen. The five responses seen, three in patients previously treated with oral MP, suggest that this dose and schedule of administration has clinical activity.

In addition, pharmacokinetic studies indicated that this approach was successful in achieving and maintaining steady-state plasma MP levels in excess of 5.0 μM and steady-state CSF MP levels greater than 1.0 μM with minimal interpatient variability, concentrations of MP that are cytotoxic to neoplastic cells *in vitro*. The ability to achieve high levels of MP in the CNS is an important attribute of this mode of MP administration and may have relevance for the treatment of neoplasms with a high frequency of spread to the CNS.

Based on these early, encouraging results we have initiated phase II trials of MP administered as a 48 h iv infusion at a dose-rate of 50 mg/sq m/h in both children and adults.

## References

1. Mellett LB: Considerations in design of optimal therapeutic schedules. In: Pharmacology and the Future of Man. Proc 5th Int Congr Pharmacology, Vol. 3. (Karger, Basel), 333–353, 1972.
2. Legha SS, Benjamin RS, MacKay B et al.: Reduction of doxorubicin cardiotoxicity by prolonged continuous intravenous infusion. Ann Int Med 96:133–139, 1982.
3. Zimm S, Collins JM, O'Neill D et al.: Variable bioavailability of oral mercaptopurine: Is maintenance chemotherapy in acute lymphoblastic leukemia being optimally delivered? N Engl J Med 308:1005–1009, 1983.
4. Zimm S, Collins JM, O'Neill D, Chabner BA, Poplack DG: Inhibition of first-pass metabolism in cancer chemotherapy: Interaction of 6-mercaptopurine and allopurinol. Clin Pharmacol Ther 34:810–817, 1983.

5. Zimm S, Grygiel JJ, Strong JM, Monks TJ, Poplack DG: Identification of 6-mercaptopurine riboside in patients receiving 6-mercaptopurine as a prolonged intravenous infusion. Biochem Pharm 33:4089–4092, 1984.

6. Zimm S, Ettinger L, Holcenberg J et al.: Mercaptopurine administered as a prolonged intravenous infusion: A phase I and clinical pharmacologic study. Cancer Res, 1985 (in Press).

7. Zimm S, Johnson GE, Chabner BA, Poplack DG: Cellular pharmacokinetics of mercaptopurine in human neoplastic cells and cell lines. Cancer Res (submitted for publication).

8. Elion GB, Burgi E, Hitchings GH: Studies on condensed pyrimidine systems IX. The synthesis of some 6-substituteed purines. J Am Chem Soc 74:411–414, 1952.

9. Burchenal JH, Murphy ML, Ellison RR et al.: Clinical evaluation of a new anti-metabolite, 6-mercaptopurine, in the treatment of acute leukemia and allied diseases. Blood 8:965–999, 1953.

10. Freireich EJ, Gehan E, Frei E III et al.: The effect of 6-mercaptopurine on the duration of steroid-induced remissions in acute leukemia: A model for evaluation of other potentially useful therapy. Blood 21:699–716, 1963.

11. Poplack DC: Acute lymphoblastic leukemia and less frequently occurring leukemias in the young. In: Cancer in the Young. Masson, New York, 405–460, 1982.

12. Loo TL, Luce JK, Sullivan MP, Frei E III: Clinical pharmacologic observations on 6-mercaptopurine and 6-methylthiopurine ribonucleoside. Clin Pharmacol Ther 9:180–194, 1967.

13. Narang PK, Yeager RL, Chatterji DC: Quantitation of 6-mercaptopurine in biologic fluids using high performance liquid chromatography: a selective and novel procedure. J Chromatog 230:373–380, 1982.

14. Tidd DM, Paterson ARP: A biochemical mechanism for the delayed cytotoxic reaction of 6-mercaptopurine. Cancer Res 34:738–746, 1974.

15. Lavi L, Holcenberg JS: A rapid and sensitive high performance liquid chromatographic assay for 6-mercaptopurine metabolites in red blood cells. Anal Biochem, 1985 (in press).

16. Huh K, Yamomoto I, Ghoda E, Iwata H: Tissue distribution and characteristics of xanthine oxidase and allopurinol oxidizing enzyme. Jpn J Pharmacol 26:719–724, 1976.

17. Perrier D, Gibaldi M: Clearance and biologic half-life as indices of intrinsic hepatic metabolism. J pharmacol Exp Ther 191:17–24, 1974.

18. Wilkinson GR, Shand DG: A physiological approach to hepatic drug clearance. Clin Pharmacol Ther 18:377–390, 1975.

19. Elion GB, Callahan S, Rundles RW et al.: Potentiation by inhibition of drug degradation: 6-substituted purines and xanthine oxidase. Biochem Pharmacol 12:85–93, 1963.

# 8. Regional therapy: an overview

JERRY M. COLLINS

## Abstract

Reginal drug delivery includes the intra-arterial route and a variety of intra-cavitary routes of administration. The principal goal of regional therapy is to *selectively* increase drug concentrations at the target (tumor) site without changing host tissue concentrations. The increase in concentration at the target site, relative to levels achievable via systemic drug delivery, is determined by the ratio of total body clearance for the drug to the local exchange rate with the systemic circulation. For most regional delivery situations, it is possible to calculate in advance the potential pharmacokinetic advantage. The ultimate usefulness of the pharmacokinetic advantage depends upon the steepness of the response-concentration curve. Arteries with low flow rates are more favorable sites than those with high flow. For any particular site, drugs with high total body clearance are more favorable than drugs with low rates of elimination from the body. The local exchange rate for intracavitary drug delivery tends to be much lower than for intra-arterial delivery; thus, drugs which are unattractive for the intra-arterial route may be reasonable candidates for intracavitary trials. Pharmacokinetic calculations can serve as guides for clinical trial design, within the limits of normal tissue sensitivity and the concentration-response curve.

## Introduction

Regional drug delivery is an area which is enjoying considerable interest in adult oncology. For pediatric oncologists, the therapeutic value of regional drug delivery has been clearly demonstrated through the use of intrathecal therapy for the prophylaxis and/or treatment of meningeal leukemia.

Regional therapy can be divided into the intra-arterial and intracavitary routes of administration. The principal areas of interest for intra-arterial therapy are liver metastases (usually from colon cancer), primary brain tumors, and sarcomas of the extremities. By far, the majority of clinical trials have involved liver infusions, but these trials are of little interest to a pediatric audience. On the other hand, the brain tumor work is more relevant, since this comprises the most common class of pediatric solid tumors. Intracavitary therapy has been applied to many areas in the body. Currently, there is much excitement about the use of intraperitoneal therapy for ovarian and colon cancers. Intravesical instillation has been shown to be efficacious in early stages of bladder cancer. Trials with intrapleural therapy are also occasionally reported. Generally, the diseases for which there is interest for intracavitary therapy are not common in childhood. However, the pharmacologic principles of intracavitary therapy are similar for most sites in the body; thus, intraperitoneal examples are appropriate. In addition, Dr Poplack's chapter will discuss intrathecal delivery.

Every anticancer drug has a narrow therapeutic index, i.e., the dose which must be given for efficacy is a dose which is close to the maximum tolerable concentration. The goal of regional therapy is to provide selective changes in concentrations: to increase tumor concentrations without raising the host tissue concentrations, and/or to decrease host tissue concentrations without lowering tumor concentrations.

In the evaluation of the potential advantage of regional drug delivery, the fundamental principle is that all of the advantage must result from the *first* time the drug reaches its target. After the drug leaves the target and reaches the systemic circulation, it behaves the same as if it were delivered intravenously.

As part of an overall evaluation of regional delivery techniques, pharmacokinetics can provide a quantiative perspective. Some drugs are attractive candidates for regional infusion while others are unattractive, and some sites of delivery are more favorable than others [1-6]. From a practical standpoint, one quick calculation can save years of clinical effort. Ideally, pharmacologic principles can help to allocate resources into high-probability areas.

## Increased local drug concentration

The advantage of regional administration should be assessed with reference to concentrations which are achievable by intravenous drug delivery. The increase in target concentrations for regional vs. intravenous delivery can be defined:

$$R_d = C_{target}(reg.)/C_{target}(i.v.) \tag{1}$$

Equation (1) is a general definition of the advantage of regional delivery which can be used to directly evaluate experimental results. The next step in

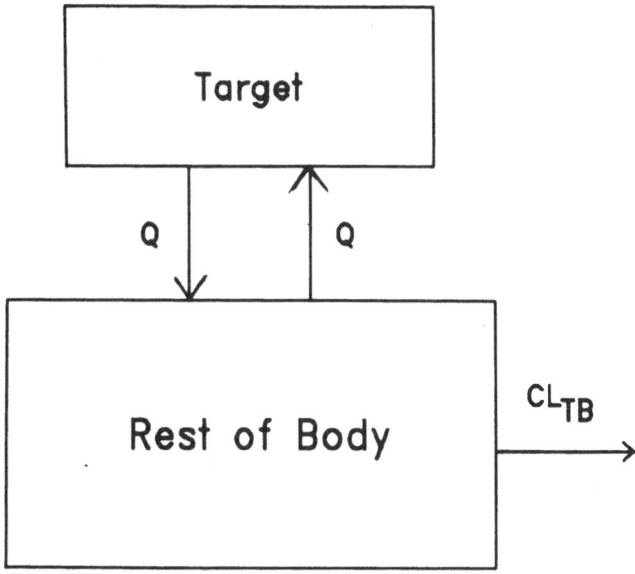

*Figure 1.* Schematic diagram for regional drug delivery without a first-pass effect.

this analysis is to use the results from pharmacokinetic modeling (described in detail elsewhere [4]) to calculate $R_d$ for various regional delivery situations.

A general analysis of regional delivery should include a section on presystemic clearance ('first-pass effect'). For the purposes of this chapter, we will only describe cases for which there is no first-pass effect, that is, in which the drug is *not* metabolized locally before it reaches the systemic circulation. Figure 1 is a schematic representation of this case. For the same dose given regionally and intravenously, $R_d$ is the ratio of target concentrations:

$$R_d = \frac{C_{target}(reg.)}{C_{target}(i.v.)} = 1 + \frac{CL_{TB}}{Q} \qquad (2)$$

$CL_{TB}$ is total body clearance of the drug, which can be found in the literature or determined from intravenous doses. $Q$ is the local exchange rate with the systemic circulation. The ratio of $CL_{TB}$ to $Q$ is the sole determinant of drug delivery advantage. This advantage can be calculated *before* doing an experiment or clinical study. Such calculations should influence the selection of drugs and delivery sites, based upon $CL_{TB}$, $Q$, and the steepness of the dose-response curve (discussed below).

As used in this presentation, the word 'concentration' denotes the steady-state drug level achieved during a constant infusion. If 'concentration' is interpreted as CxT, all formulas in this chapter are also valid for intermittent drug exposures. For both the bolus and the infusional cases, drug deliv-

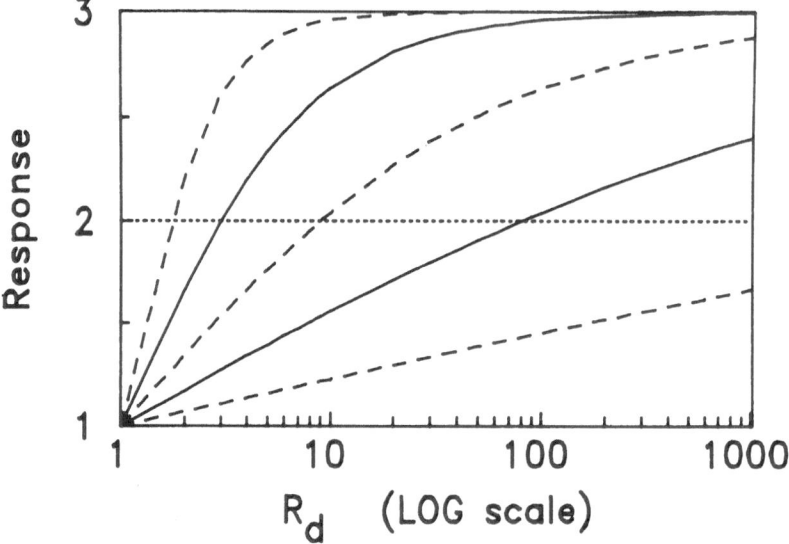

*Figure 2.* Relationship between pharmacodynamic advantage (increase in therapeutic effect) and pharmacokinetic advantage (increase in drug concentration at target site). From Collins [6].

ery ratios are limited to a description of total drug exposure. For anticancer drugs, time of exposure or threshold concentrations must often be considered in addition to total exposure.

## Pharmacologic response of tumor and normal host tissues

One of the conditions for Equation (2) is that the comparison between regional and intravenous routes is based upon equal doses. This implies that the limiting host tissue is *outside* the region to which drug is delivered (e.g., gastrointestinal toxicity is limiting for CNS delivery). If local toxicity is limiting, then regional administration of the same dose is not possible.

It must be emphasized that the measurement (or prediction) of $R_d$ is only the first step in the evaluation of the pharmacologic advantage of regional infusions. The second step is a consideration of the concentration-response curve. A large value of $R_d$ (e.g., 500) may appear to be more impressive than a small value (e.g., 3), but the therapeutic advantage depends upon the slope of the concentration-response curve.

Figure 2 illustrates the influence of the steepness of the concentration-response curve. The curves on the left half of the graph illustrate situations in which small changes in $R_d$ are expressed as large changes in target response. Moving towards the right half of the graph, very large changes in target drug concentration produce only small changes in target response.

One of the drugs with the most favorable pharmacokinetic properties for regional infusion is fluorodeoxyuridine (FUdR), yet the improvement in therapy for hepatic intraarterial vs. intravenous delivery can't be consistently demonstrated. One interpretation of the FUdR results is that the response vs. concentration curve for FUdR must be very shallow. Also, the local toxicity, chemical hepatitis, limits the full exploitation of the potential advantage of FUdR. Similarly, for essentially all drugs, neurotoxicity limits the intrathecal dose to less than the intravenous dose.

## Intra-arterial drug delivery

There seem to be two opposing philosophies regarding intra-arterial drug delivery: some think it's so technically complex that it's *never* worthwhile; others get carried away by the alluring concept that if you deliver a drug directly to the tumor, it *must* be better than intravenous delivery, regardless of the drug or the site.

The complexity of intra-arterial procedures has been a serious obstacle. Recently, the development of implantable pumps and other technical advances have made intra-arterial infusions more widely available. However, simply because intra-arterial therapy is more widely available does not mean that all clinical trials should be attempted. Intra-arterial infusion remains a dramatic intervention, and we should make sure that the chances for success warrant the risks and difficulties. Again, our focus is to use pharmacologic principles to guide trial design.

Arteries with low flow rates are the most favorable sites for intra-arterial drug delivery. However, most clinical experience is with organs with high flow, especially the liver, or moderate-flow vessels such as the carotid artery. Knowledge of flow rates can guide the decision to try or not to try intra-arterial delivery. Once the site has been fixed, selection of the drug to be used can be assisted by pharmacokinetics, specifically the total body clearance. It is essential that the drug have activity against the particular disease being treated, for it is unlikely that regional drug delivery will transform an inactive agent into a spectacular success. A more reasonable goal is to improve an established agent, perhaps to convert partial responses into complete responses.

Table 1 ranks selected anticancer drugs in order of total body clearance. The pharmacokinetic advantage, $R_d$, is calculated for a variety of exchange rates, Q. The last two columns correspond to arteries with low flow (Q = 100 ml/min) or high flow (Q = 1000 ml/min). Only drugs in the upper part of Table 1 have total body clearance values which can produce large $R_d$ values in high flow arteries. At lower arterial flow rates, drugs in the middle of Table 1 also become attractive. Drugs with very low clearance rates (bot-

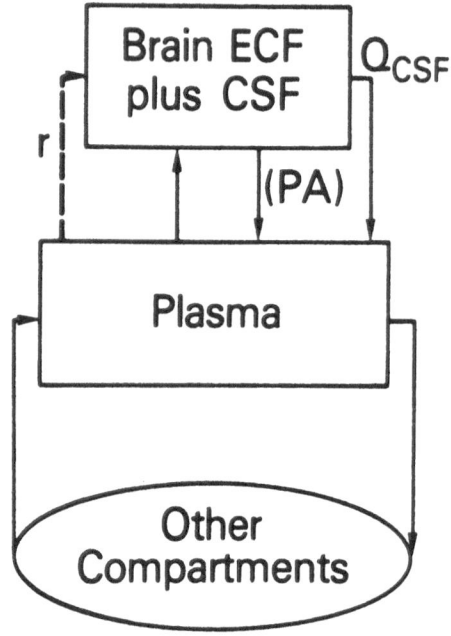

*Figure 3.* Compartmental model for intrathecal drug delivery. From Dedrick et al. [7].

*Table 1.* Regional drug delivery advantage, $R_d$ for some anticancer drugs. Based upon Equation (2).

| $CL_{TB}$ ml/min | Drug | $R_d$ Q = 10 ml/min | Q = 100 ml/min | Q = 1000 ml/min |
|---|---|---|---|---|
| 25000 | Fluorodeoxyuridine | 2501 | 251 | 26 |
| 5000 | Teroxirone | 501 | 51 | 6 |
| 4000 | Fluorouracil | 401 | 41 | 5 |
| 3000 | Cytosine arabinoside | 301 | 31 | 4 |
| 1000 | BCNU | 101 | 11 | 2 |
| 900 | Doxorubicin | 91 | 10 | 1.9 |
| 400 | Diaziquone | 41 | 5 | 1.4 |
| 400 | Cisplatin | 41 | 4 | 1.4 |
| 200 | Methotrexate | 21 | 3 | 1.2 |
| 120 | Carboplatin | 13 | 2.2 | 1.1 |
| 40 | Etoposide | 5 | 1.4 | 1.04 |
| — [a] | Cyclophosphamide | 1 | 1 | 1 |

[a] Drugs which must be activated at a side other than the arterial infusion site have *no* drug delivery advantage.

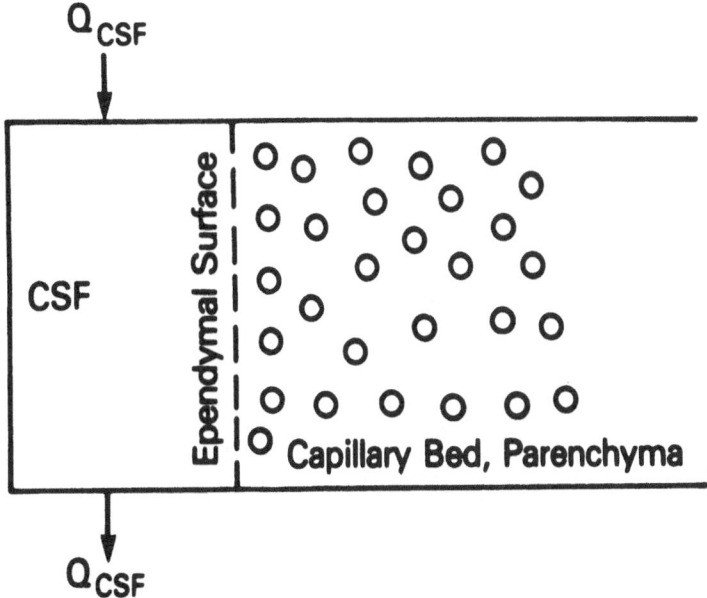

*Figure 4.* Distributed model for intrathecal drug delivery. From Collins [9].

tom third of Table 1) are never attractive for intra-arterial delivery. Drugs which must be activated by the liver (or any site outside of the infused region) should *never* be used intra-arterially.

## Intracavitary concepts

### Application to intrathecal therapy

Intrathecal therapy for meningeal leukemia is the most widely accepted indication for intracavitary therapy. Since this topic is covered by Dr Poplack in the next chapter, my remarks on the subject will be limited.

Dedrick and coworkers [7] described intrathecal MTX delivery with a compartmental model (Figure 3) which is very similar to the one shown in Figure 1 for regional delivery. Although the intrathecal route has had demonstrable success for treating meningeal disease, one must keep in mind that parenchymal brain tumors can't be successfully treated with this approach.

The concept of penetration depth (distributed model) has been effectively presented for intraventricular therapy by Blasberg and colleagues [8]. Conceptually, we realize that the closer a tumor cell is to CSF, the higher its exposure. But what are the quantitative dimensions: how close is 'close enough'? We can approach these quantitative aspects with mathematical

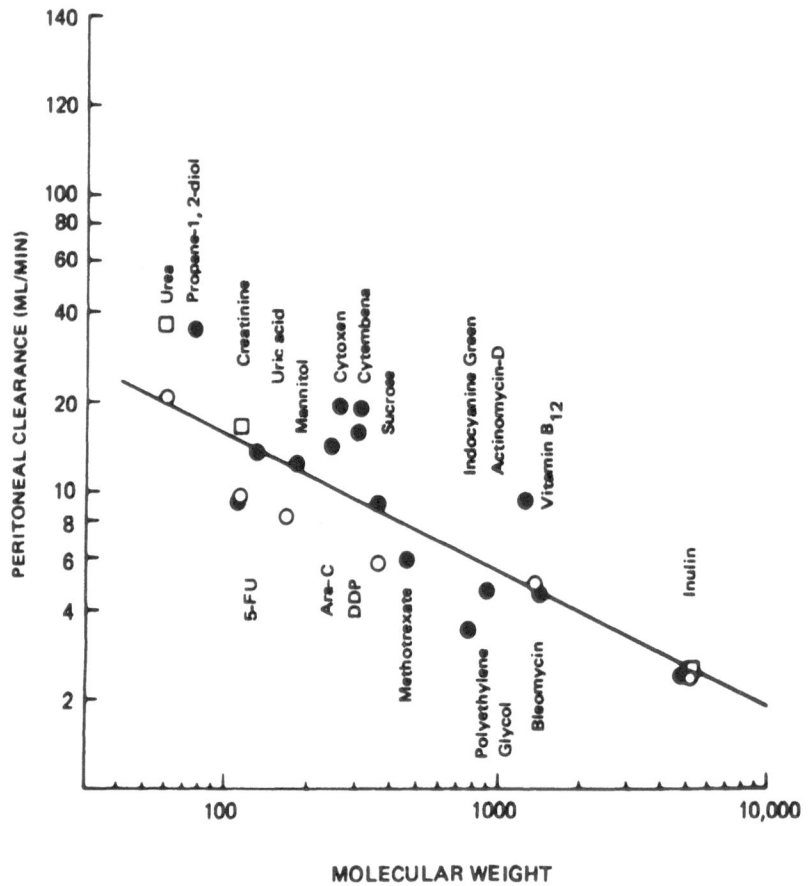

*Figure 5.* Relationship between PA and molecular weight for hydrophilic substances. From Myers and Collins [10].

modeling, but the type of model is rather different from the lumped compartmental approaches used to model regional drug delivery. As drug molecules diffuse across the meningeal surfaces and into parenchymal tissue, they cross capillaries and are washed away by blood. Thus, blood flow acts as a 'sink' for the drug. Drug concentration in the tissues adjacent to the meningeal surfaces depends upon the *distance* away from the meningeal surface as well as time. This type of model is shown in Figure 4.

*Intraperitoneal drug delivery*

In Figure 1 and Equation (2), the rate of exchange of drug between the local site and the rest of the body is denoted by the term 'Q'. For intra-arterial drug delivery, Q is easily described as arterial flow rate. For intracavitary drug delivery, Q is usually a permeability rate. Permeability depends strong-

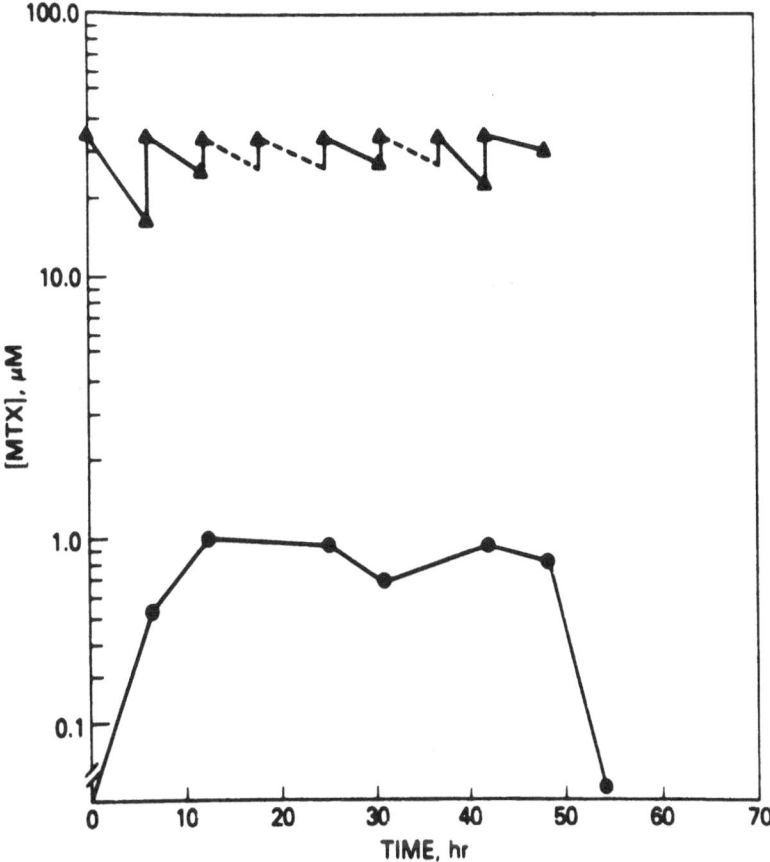

*Figure 6.* Concentrations of methotrexate are approximately 20-fold higher in peritoneal fluid than in plasma following intraperitoneal delivery. From Jones et al. 811].

ly upon the physico-chemical properties of the drug. For example, the permeability rate (PA) for intraperitoneal absorption has been shown to be inversely related to molecular weight for hydrophillic substances (Figure 5).

The success of Equation (2) in predicting and describing intraperitoneal drug delivery has been established [10–12]. The first drug which was tested clinically was methotrexate [11]. It was found that there was a 20-fold advantage for intraperitoneal delivery of this drug (Figure 6). It must be emphasized that the exchange rates for intracavitary drug delivery are usually far lower than for intra-arterial drug delivery. Thus, a drug such as methotrexate, which has already been shown to be a poor candidate for intra-arterial delivery, becomes attractive for intracavitary delivery in situations where Q is less than 20 ml/min.

As shown in Table 1, 5-fluorouracil has a very high rate of clearance from the body. When this favorable pharmacokinetic property is combined with

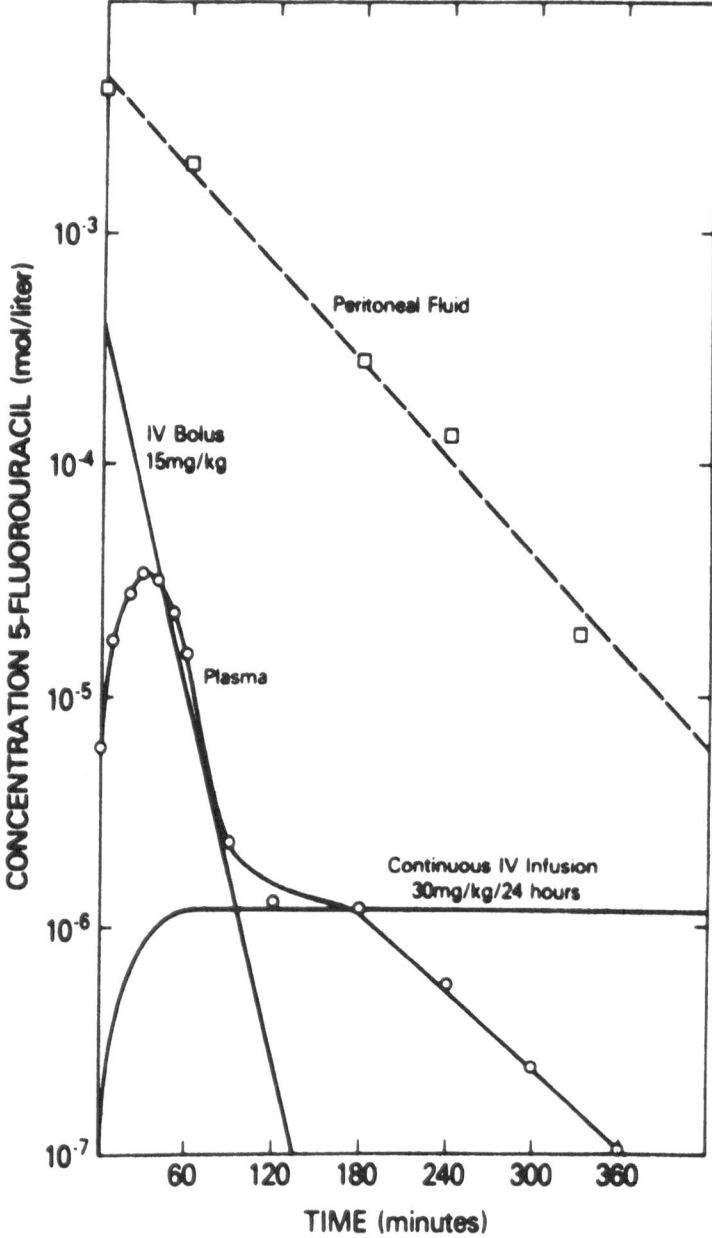

*Figure 7.* Concentrations of 5-fluorouracil are 300-fold greater in in peritoneal fluid than in plasma folowing intraperitoneal delivery. From Speyer et al. [12].

the relatively slow rate of absorption from the peritoneum, a large drug delivery advantage can be obtained [12]. As shown in Figure 7, $R_d$ values of 300 were demonstrated, consistent with Equation (2).

## Conclusion

Pharmacokinetics offers a powerful tool for the prediction of concentrations which are achievable by use of the regional route. These predictions can be used to guide clinical trial design. However, a complete pharmacologic evaluation of the potential advantage of regional delivery requires consideration of both the tumor response at higher concentrations and also the limits imposed by the chemosensitivity of normal host tissues.

## References

1. Eckman WW, Patlak CS, Fenstermacher JD: A critical evaluation of the principles governing the advantages of intra-arterial infusions. J Pharmacokinet Biopharm 2:257–285, 1974.
2. Chen HSG, Gross JF: Intra-arterial infusion of anticancer drugs theoretic aspects of drug delivery and review of responses. Cancer Treat Rep 64:31–40, 1980.
3. Collins JM, Dedrick RL: Pharmacokinetics of Anticancer Drugs. In: Pharmacologic Principles of Cancer Treatment. Chabner BA (ed). W.B. Saunders, Philadelphia, 77–99, 1982.
4. Collins JM: Pharmacologic rationale for regional drug delivery. J Clin Oncol 2:498–504, 1984.
5. Ensminger WD, Gyves JW: Regional cancer chemotherapy. Cancer Treat Rep 68:101–115, 1984.
6. Collins JM: Pharmacologic rationale for intra-arterial Therapy. In: Therapeutic strategies in Primary and Metastatic Liver Cancer. Herfarth C, Schlag P (eds). Springer Verlag, Heidelberg, Sept. 1984. (in press).
7. Dedrick RL, Zaharko DS, Bender RA, Bleyer WA, Lutz RJ: Pharmacokinetic considerations on resistance to anticancer drugs. Cancer Chemother Rep 59:795–804, 1975.
8. Blasberg R, Patlak CS, Fenstermacher JD: Intrathecal chemotherapy: Brain tissue profiles after ventriculocisternal perfusion. J Pharmacol EXP Ther 195:73–83, 1975.
9. Collins JM: Pharmacokinetics of intraventricular administration. J Neuro-Oncol 1:283–291, 1983.
10. Myers CE, Collins JM: Pharmacology of intraperitoneal chemotherapy. Cancer Invest 1:395–407, 1983.
11. Jones RB, Collins JM, Myers CE, Brooks AE, Hubbard SM, Balow JE, Brennan MF, Dedrick RL, DeVita VT: High-volume intraperitoneal chemotherapy with methotrexate in patients with cancer. Cancer Res 41:55–59, 1981.
12. Speyer JL, Collins JM, Dedrick RL, Brennan MF, Buckpitt AR, Londer H, DeVita VT, Myers CE: Phase I and pharmacological studies of intraperitoneal 5-fluorouracil. Cancer Res 40:567–572, 1980.

# 9. Pharmacologic approaches to the treatment of central nervous system malignancy

DAVID G. POPLACK and RICCARDO RICCARDI

## Introduction

The identification of effective chemotherapy for the treatment of central nervous system (CNS) malignancy poses a major challenge to the oncologist. Although anti-neoplastic chemotherapy has become a mainstay in the treatment of many malignancies which develop outside the CNS, surgery and radiotherapy are the primary modalities utilized to treat malignant tumors of the CNS. To a considerable degree this situation reflects the unique problem in the delivery of chemotherapeutic agents to the CNS. Despite the availability of a number of systemically active antitumor drugs many do not possess those pharmacologic properties which enable them to cross the 'blood-brain barrier' [1]. Thus the number of drugs which are suitable candidates for the treatment of primary (or metastatic) brain tumors is limited [2, 3].

The present chapter focuses upon the unique pharmacological problems encountered in attempting to treat CNS malignancy and reviews the different pharmacologic approaches currently in use. Recent developments in this field are discussed and perspectives for future directions are presented. Emphasis is placed on recent studies in a unique subhuman primate model.

## Factors Influencing Drug Delivery to the CNS

A number of factors influence the delivery of antineoplastic agents to the CNS. These include: (1) the blood-brain barrier, (2) the anatomic location of the tumor, (3) the physiocochemical characteristics of the drug, (4) the distribution of the drug, (5) the dose and schedule of drug administration and (6) the route of drug administration [4]. An appreciation of the role of these factors is central to an understanding of the problems associated with attempts to deliver antineoplastic therapy to the CNS.

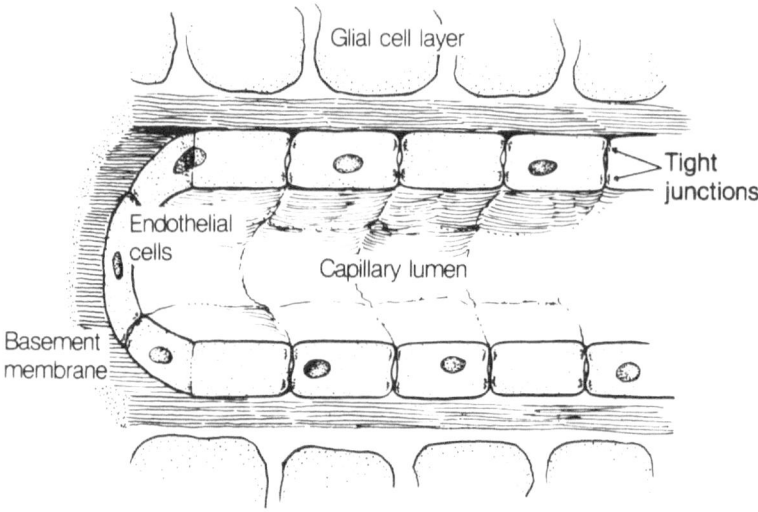

*Figure 1.* Cerebral capillary. Endothelial cells are connected by rings of tight junctions which restrict the movement of solutes between adjacent cells. Modified from Rapoport [6], with permission.

## The Blood-Brain Barrier

The 'blood-brain barrier', is the major obstacle to optimal delivery of systemically administered chemotherapeutic agents to the CNS. The barrier can be conceptualized as a physiological separation between the blood in the brain capillaries and the extracellular fluid of the brain. The anatomic basis of the barrier resides in the unique properties of the endothelial cells of the brian capillaries (Figure 1). These cells are joined to one another by rings of tight junctions which restrict solute movement between adjacent cells. The absence of fenestrations in the endothelial cell wall, a relative paucity of pyknotic vesicles and the presence of an astrocytic membrane which surrounds the entire capillary also contribute to the formation of this continuous barrier [5]. The existence of the blood-brain barrier has been confirmed by a number of studies which have demonstrated that intravenously injected aniline dyes such as trypan blue do not penetrate those areas of brain in which capillaries with these morphologic features are found [6]. The principle site of impermeability is the tight junction. In contrast, in certain selected areas of the brain (e.g, choroid plexus, pineal gland) capillaries similar to those found in other tissues of the body, which lack the continuous endothelial barrier, are present. In these areas, a functional barrier to solute movement exists at the level of the tight junctions between parenchymal cells [5]. The blood-brain barrier protects the chemical environment of the brain from indiscriminate penetration by substances within the systemic circulation. Consequently movement from the blood to brain tissue and CSF must occur via the transcellular route, a process regulated by the endothelial cell membrane. This membrane readily permits the entry of small, non-polar, lipid soluble compounds into brain extracellular fluid but restricts transcapillary movement of larger polar, lipid-insoluble and water soluble materials [7]. The permeability of the brain capillaries to a drug may be expressed as a transfer constant, which represents the amount of drug entering the brain during a particular time period [8]. Information regarding such transcapillary movement may be of considerable importance in the selection of a drug for systemic use.

The extent to which the blood-brain barrier is functional within brain tumor tissue and in the area of bran adjacent to tumor is controversial [9]. While some have suggested that the microvasculature in these regions is made up of discontinuous and fenestrated endothelium, others have concluded that the capillary permeability is actually reduced [10, 11]. Although this issue has not been definitively resolved, it is clear that the degree of preservation of blood-brain barrier function has considerable bearing on which systemic agents may be more suitable to treat a particular CNS tumor.

## Anatomic Location of Tumor

The location of a CNS tumor also influences the choice of agents and their route of administration. For example, meningeal spread of CNS malignancy (e.g., meningeal leukemia, carcinomatous meningitis) is treated using the intrathecal approach which bypasses the blood-brain barrier and allows direct instillation of agents such as methotrexate into CSF. In contrast, brain tumors which are present as mass lesions are more optimally approached via the systemic route. This is because systemically administered chemotherapy reaches the tumor by the same vascular channels which supply it. Systemic administration in this situation also is more feasible because lumber punctures are often contraindicated in patients with a CNS mass lesion.

## Physicochemical Characteristics of the Drug

The physicochemical properties of an antineoplastic agent influence its pharmacologic behavior and its antitumor activity. Several characteristics are known to influence the ability of a drug to cross the blood-brain barrier and be delivered to the tumor site. These include lipid solubility, molecular weight, protein binding, and ionization properties.

The influence of lipid solubility in penetration of the CNS was alluded to previously. Log-P values have been used to rank drugs on the basis of their lipid solubility (higher positive Log-P values indicating a higher lipid solubility). For a number of drugs there is considerable correlation between the degree of lipid solubility and CNS penetration (Table 1) [12].

In general drugs which bind less well to protein, have a small molecular weight and exist in an unionized form at physiological pH are likely to exhibit better CNS penetration.

### Drug Distribution

The processes which influence a drug's distribution directly impact on its delivery to its tumor target site. These processes differ depending upon the route of drug administration. CSF bulk flow plays a more significant role in the distribution of intrathecally administered agents; blood flow within the tumor vascular system is more important for systemically administered drugs. However, the ultimate distribution of a drug within the CNS depends not only upon the character of CSF bulk flow (intrathecal administration) or perfusion with blood (systemic administration) but on capillary permeability (see above) as well as on a number of other factors which are listed in Table 2. Distribution of a drug depends upon the presence of a favorable gradient for transport of that drug to the interior of the cell. The rate of diffusion through extracellular fluid, a process largely dependent upon the physical characteristics of the drug and its aqueous diffusion constant is also of crucial import. The concentration of drug achieved in the extracellular fluid of the brain is itself influenced by the degree of drug biotransformation, the amount and rate of cell uptake, diffusion of drug back into capil-

*Table 1.* Relationship of lipid solubility to drug penetration of central nervous system.

| Agent | Dose (mg/kg) and route | Log-P value | Ratio of brain/serum levels |
|-------|------------------------|-------------|-----------------------------|
| DTIC  | 317 i.p.               | −0.24       | 0.10                        |
| 5-FU  | 50 i.v.                | −0.95       | 0.33                        |
| BCNU  | 20 i.p.                | +1.53       | 0.5–1.5                     |
| CCNU  | −                      | +2.83       | 4.0–5.0                     |

Adapted from Mellet [12]. Data presented refer to studies performed in mice with intracutaneously implanted L1210.

(DTIC) Dimethyl triazeno imidozole carboxamide; (5-FU) 5-fluorouracil; (BCNU) 1,3-bis-(2-chloroethyl)-1-nitrosourea; (CCNU) 1-(2-chloroethyl)-3-cyclohexyl-1-nitrosourea; (i.p.) intraperitoneal; (i.v.) intravenous.

Blood-brain barrier – capillary permeability
Activity gradients
Diffusion through extracellular fluid
Diffusion in CSF and other tissue fluids
Cellular uptake

Adapted from Blasberg [8] and Cowles and Fenstermacher [13].

laries, and movement by bulk flow into CSF. The actual movement of drug into tumor cells involves passive diffusion and in some circumstances active transport. A more detailed discussion of those factors which influence drug distribution can be found in recent review articles [8, 13].

## Dose and Schedule of Administration

Dose and schedule considerations play a significant role in the delivery of antineoplastic drugs to the CNS. The dose of drug chosen must be one which achieves therapeutic concentrations at the site of the tumor. Often, because of the inherent difficulties in measuring drug levels at the local tumor site CSF drug concentrations are used to guide therapy. The usefulness of CSF drug levels probably varies depending upon the site of tumor. For example, CSF levels are likely to more accurately reflect the concentrations achieved at the site of a meningeal neoplasm than in an intraparenchymal mass lesion.

Although the drug dose must be high enough to achieve therapeutic concentrations in the CNS, it must also be one which does not produce CNS toxicity. An understanding of the pharmacokinetics of a particular agent within the CNS allows one to optimize drug dose and avoid untoward toxicity.

In addition to identifying a therapeutic, nontoxic dose, the schedule of administration has a significant effect upon the ultimate therapeutic efficacy.

Choice of an appropriate drug schedule requires understanding of tumor cell kinetics as well as knowledge of a drug's metabolism, distribution and pharmacokinetics. For example, there is ample animal and *in vitro* data which suggests that low doses of methotrexate given over a protracted time period are more effective than the administration of a single high dose bolus [14]. This concept has been applied to CNS intrathecal chemotherapy with this agent. Repeated low dose administration of methotrexate via an Ommaya reservoir, a 'concentration × time' approach has been shown to be less neurotoxic and more effective therapy for meningeal leukemia [15, 16].

Studies have also demonstrated the importance of the CSF clearance half-time on drug schedule [8]. Compounds which are rapidly cleared from the CSF (such as the alkylating agent thio-Tepa) are believed best administered by a constant infusion then by a single bolus. In contrast, agents with substantial CSF clearance half-times are more appropriately administered as a single bolus injection. Appropriate scheduling is an important factor in optimizing CNS antineoplastic chemotherapy.

*Route of Administration*

Various routes of administration have been used to deliver antineoplastic chemotherapy to the CNS including the intrathecal, systemic, intra-arterial and intratumor approaches. The two most commonly utilized are the intrathecal and systemic routes. Choice of a particular route varies depending upon the clinical situation in question, the anatomic location of the tumor within the CNS and the physico-chemical properties of the drug being administered.

*Intrathecal chemotherapy*

The intrathecal approach allows direct administration of drug into the CSF, bypassing the blood-brain barrier. The comparatively small initial volume of distribution for an intrathecally administered drug, permits one to achieve significant concentrations of the drug within the CSF, using a relatively small drug dose. This also minimizes the likelihood of significant systemic toxicity. Certain drugs are more appropriate for the intrathecal than for the systemic approach to CNS treatment. For example, cytosine arabinoside is rapidly deaminated in serum when given intravenously and would requires administration in relatively high doses to approach CNS malignancy via the systemic route. In contrast, the disappearance of this drug from the CSF is much slower than from the plasma (because of relatively low levels of cytidine deaminase), making the drug quite suitable for intrathecal use. In addition, the systemic toxicity of certain drugs (e.g., methotrexate) has traditionally precluded their systemic use to treat CNS disease, while they may be administered intrathecally with relative safety.

Although intrathecal administration has a number of advantages there are problems with this approach. Intrathecal administration, in most cases, involves lumber puncture. A drug injected in this region must ascend the spinal subarachnoid space and enter the cerebral ventricles against a unidirectionally oriented CSF flow. This is known to compromise the active drug levels which can be achieved in ventricular CSF. In addition, lumbar punctures frequently are associated with local leakage of CSF at the injection site. Such leakage may alter the pressure, volume and flow of CSF and effect the distribution of the drug within the CSF.

CNS tumors occasionally obstruct CSF flow and interfere with the pharmacokinetics of an intralumbar injected drug. The number and frequency of intralumbar injections are also limited, thus use of a 'concentration × time' administration schedule is not feasible.

Although many of these problems have been circumvented using intraventricular drug administration, via a subcutaneous Ommaya Reservoir (see below), the intrathecal approach still appears more appropriate for meningeal neoplasms than for parenchymal brain tumors. There is considerable evidence which indicates that many intrathecally administered drugs are not capable of penetrating deep enough into brain tissue to reach an intraparenchymal tumor which resides even several millimeters from the CSF-brain interface [17, 18]. Another obvious drawback is that in many situations in which an intraparenchymal mass lesion is present, lumbar puncture is contraindicated because of the possibility of brain herniation. Because of these problems, intrathecal chemotherapy has limited usefulness in the treatment of intraparenchymal CNS tumors.

*Systemic chemotherapy*

The systemic route of administration has been most commonly utilized to deliver antineoplastic chemotherapy to the CNS. Systemic administration has several advantages. First, it is less invasive and more convenient than intrathecal therapy. Second, it is believed to be more physiologic in that drug is carried to the tumor by the same vascular channels which support its growth. Third, systemic administration can be employed even in the presence of large mass lesions which would not permit intralumbar chemotherapy.

However, there are a number of disadvantages to the use of the systemic approach. As mentioned previously a drug given systemically must penetrate the blood-brain barrier. Because the physicochemical characteristics required of a drug for penetration of the blood-brain barrier are stringent, relatively few of the many available systemically administered antineoplastic agents can be used to treat CNS disease. In addition, the systemic route of administration is feasible only in the presence of adequate intratumor blood flow. Because certain areas of many tumors have compromised blood flow, optimal delivery of drugs to the tumor site is frequently not possible [9]. The use of the systemically-administered drug also exposes essentially all systemic tissues to the agent and its attendant toxicity, whereas an intrathecal administration primarily affects the CNS.

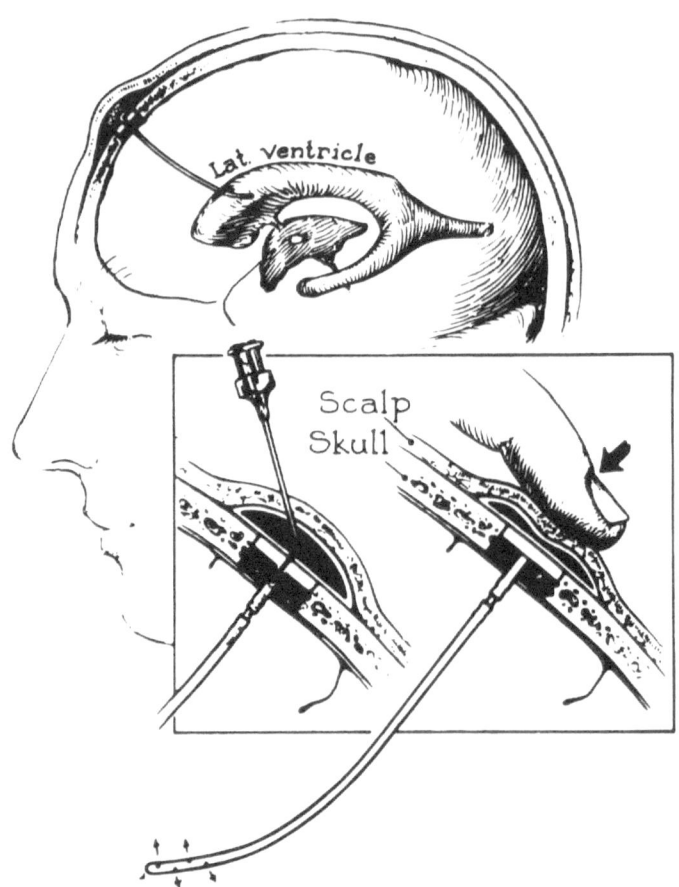

*Figure 2.* Ommaya reservoir. Reservoir is implanted subcutaneously and attached to a catheter, the tip of which sits in the lateral ventricle. This device permits easy, repetitive access to sterile ventricular CSF.

## Methods of Enhancing Drug Delivery to the CNS

As discussed above, both the intrathecal and systemic routes of administration have inherent problems which can hinder optimal drug delivery to the CNS. In addition, the 'blood-brain barrier' represents a formidable obstacle to the chemotherapeutic approach to either intraparenchymal or meningeal malignancy. A number of different techniques potentially able to circumvent many of these problems have been explored. These include use of alternative anatomic approaches, modification of drug structure, reversible perturbation of the blood-brain barrier and high dose systemic chemotherapy. In the following section the advantages and the disadvantages of these relatively new chemotherapeutic approaches will be discussed.

*Alternative Anatomic Approaches*

*Ommaya reservoir*
As mentioned previously, intralumbar injection drugs is associated with a number of technical limitations. One way of improving intrathecal therapy has been to alter the anatomic approach, instilling chemotherapy directly into the ventricular CSF via a subcutaneously implanted Ommaya reservoir. As shown in Figure 2, in this system the reservoir is attached to a catheter, the tip of which lies within the lateral ventricle. Drugs injected via the reservoir are delivered directly into the ventricular CSF insuring a better distribution throughout the ventricular system and normal pathways of CSF flow. In addition to eliminating many of the technical problems associated with lumbar puncture (e.g., CSF leakage into the sub and epidural spaces) intra-reservoir administration is associated with less patient discomfort.

Intraventricular drug administration via the Ommaya reservoir has been primarily used in the treatment of meningeal malignancy. Recent data suggest that this approach may be more effective than intralumbar administration in the treatment of overt meningeal leukemia [16].

An additional advantage of the Ommaya reservoir is that it permits frequent, repetitive administration of chemotherapy to the CNS. As mentioned previously, for many agents, such as methotrexate, the maintenance of a therapeutic drug level for a prolonged period of time provides more optimal tumor cell kill than single bolus administration. This 'concentration × time' approach can be achieved within the CNS via the Ommaya reservoir. For example, the repeated administration of relatively low doses of methotrexate (1 mg at 12-h intervals) provides a cytocidal drug level which can be maintained, without significant toxicity for at least 72 h (total methotrexate dose = 6 mg). This contrasts with the situation following administration of a dose of 12 mg via lumbar puncture which maintains a comparable cytocidal level for less than 32 h. This 'C × T' approach has been shown to be clinically efficacious and devoid of significant neurotoxicity [15].

*Ventriculolumbar CSF perfusion*
Another technique which utilizes an alternative anatomic approach made possible by the availability of the Ommaya reservoir is ventriculolumbar CSF perfusion (Figure 3) [20]. In this system, enhanced perfusion of the CSF is achieved by administering a drug into ventricular CSF via an Ommaya reservoir and removing it via an outflow cannula placed in the lumbar subarachnoid space. During drug infusion CSF pressure is controlled by changing the height of the outflow column at the lumbar end of the infusion system. With this technique the entire volume of CSF is potentially replaced by a simulated CSF fluid containing a desired concentration of drug. The ventriculolumbar perfusion technique enables administration of a

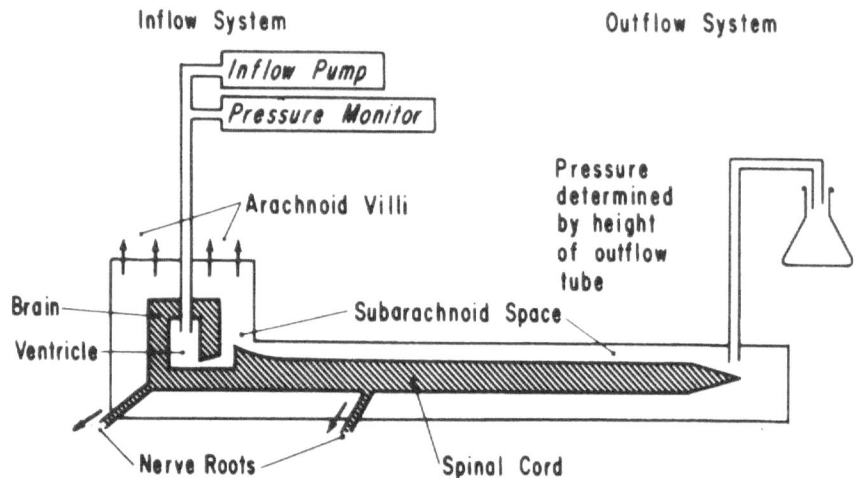

Inflow System                    Outflow System

*Figure 3.* Schematic representation of ventriculolumbar perfusion technique. Perfusate containing drug is administered into ventricular CSF via indwelling subcutaneous Ommaya reservoir and removed via outflow cannula placed in the lumbar subarachnoid space. Reprinted from Poplack et al. [20], with permission.

perfusate which contains higher concentrations of drug than could be administered safely via conventional intralumbar administration. Although results with this technique in refractory meningeal leukemia appear promising, its technical complexity limits its widespread use.

### Intra-tumor injection

Another method for delivering antineoplastic therapy to the CNS which involves an alternative anatomic approach is intra-tumor injection. Intra-tumor injection has been attempted to treat partially resected brain tumors. The original technique utilized a subcutaneous Ommaya reservoir with the tip of the attached catheter inserted directly into the tumor tissue [21]. More recently, drugs have been administered percutaneously through a defect in the bone flap created at the time of tumor resection [22]. Little is known regarding the pharmacology of this approach and clinical experience with this approach has been limited.

### Enhancement of Drug Delivery by Modifying Drug Structure

Few of the available antineoplastic agents possess the physico-chemical properties required for adequate penetration of the blood-brain barrier. A more rational approach than extensive screening for CNS active drugs has been to develop agents with physico-chemical characteristics which facilitate blood-brain barrier penetration. This also has been accomplished by modifying the structure of compounds with known anti-tumor activity in a manner such that they will penetrate the blood-brain barrier.

Perhaps the best example of a family of anti-tumor agents developed as a result of rationale analog research and synthesis are the Nitrosureas. These are among the drugs most commonly utilized to treat brain tumors. Of these agents, BCNI, CCNU and MeCCNU have been extensively evaluated in preclinical and clinical studies [23]. All three compounds share a significant anti-tumor activity and high lipid solubility which facilitates their transport across the blood-brain barrier.

An effort has been made to synthesize drugs with anti-tumor activity which are combined with a carrier compound known to possess those characteristics favorable for penetration of the blood-brain barrier. This approach has been pursued by Peng *et al.* who prepared a series of dilantin-like compounds known to accumulate in human brain tumor [24] and combined them with the alkylating group of nitrogen mustard. The most effective compound identified by these investigators was spirohydantoin mustard. This agent is able to cross into the CSF when administered systemically in dogs [25], and produces cures in at least 50% of mice with intra-cranially implanted ependymoblastoma. It is currently undergoing clinical testing in Phase I trials.

*Reversible Perturbation of the Blood-Brain Barrier using Hyperosmolar Intracarotid Infusions*

A relatively new method of enhancing drug delivery to the CNS involves the use of intracarotid infusion of an hyperosmolar solution which induces reversible osmotic opening of the blood-brain barrier. It is theorized that opening of the blood-brain barrier occurs as a result of an induced shrinkage of the vascular endothelial cells which retract, widening the tight junctions (Figure 4) [26]. This technique has been carefully evaluated in a number of animal models and the conditions for a complete and reversible alteration of the blood-brain barrier have been established [27–29]. The information derived from the animal studies has been utilized to pursue pilot studies on blood-brain barrier disruption in man [11]. In an initial study five patients with primary or metastatic brain tumors underwent intracarotid infusion of a hypertonic mannitol solution (25%), at a rate varying between 4 and 9 ml/second for 25–30 seconds. Blood-brain barrier disruption was monitored by computerized tomography. Under these conditions good to excellent blood-brain barrier disruption was achieved in four out of five patients. In subsequent studies, following initial blood-brain barrier disruption, methotrexate has been infused intra-arterially in an attempt to reach those

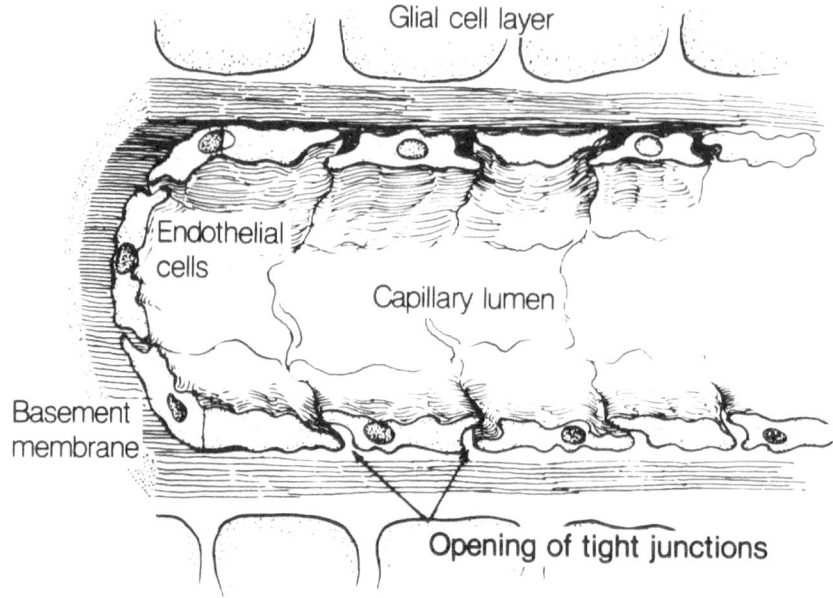

*Figure 4.* Cerebral capillary after hyperosmolar infusion. In a hypertonic environment. endothelial cells shrink and retract, widening the tight junctions. This is the presumed mechanism by which this technique perturbs the blood-brain barrier [28].

tumor cells protected by the previously intact blood-brain barrier. Although it is too early to determine if this approach will be of clinical value, its invasive nature and the short duration of blood-barrier alteration (and drug exposure) achieved will probably limit the applicability of this approach.

*High Dose Systemic Chemotherapy*

Following systemic administration, under steady-state conditions, drugs achieve a specific plasma : CSF ratio. Therefore, it is theoretically possible to increase the delivery of a given drug to the brain and the CSF simply by increasing its systemic dose. However, because most available drugs are used in doses close to those which are maximally toxic, this is not usually feasible. Methotrexate is a unique antineoplastic compound in that its systemic toxicity can be prevented by appropriate use of the 'rescue' agent citrovorum factor. Following I.V. administration of even huge doses of methotrexate, treatment with citrovorum factor within 24–36 h will prevent methotrexate toxicity. High dose methotrexate infusion followed by citrovorum factor rescue was initially utilized to improve the therapeutic index of methotrexate in patients with solid tumors resistant to conventional doses.

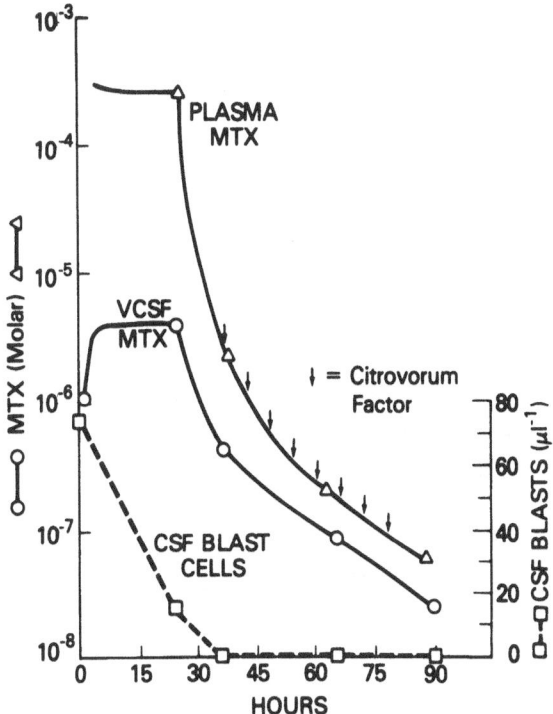

*Figure 5.* Central nervous system (CNS) leukemia responding to a systemic high dose methotrexate infusion. This patient achieved CNS remission with single '3000/600' protracted 24-h
methotrexate infusion. Note that the level of methotrexate achieved in ventricular CSF (VCSF)
is in the therapeutic range.

However, this technique has the potential of increasing the delivery of systemically administered methotrexate to the CNS. In a clinical study we have
explored the utility of treating overt CNS malignancy using high dose, protracted methotrexate infusions. In this approach, methotrexate is given first
in a priming dose as a continuous infusion over the first hour, followed by
1/5th of this initial dose given every hour for the next 23 h. With this regimen, CSF methotrexate levels within the cytocidal range can be achieved
and maintained for an extended period of exposure. Citrovorum factor rescue is utilized to prevent systemic toxicity. This approach has been successfully used to induce remission in patients with overt meningeal leukemia
and as CNS preventive therapy for patients with acute lymphoblastic leukemia (Figure 5) [20, 30, 31].

The high dose, protracted methotrexate infusion has been found to be safe
and has a number of advantages: (1) it provides entrance of the drug at all
levels of the CNS axis and subsequent better distribution throughout the
CSF, (2) it maintains CSF methotrexate levels for a prolonged period of
time so that a large fraction of the leukemic cell population will pass
through the susceptible segment of their cell cycle while methotrexate levels

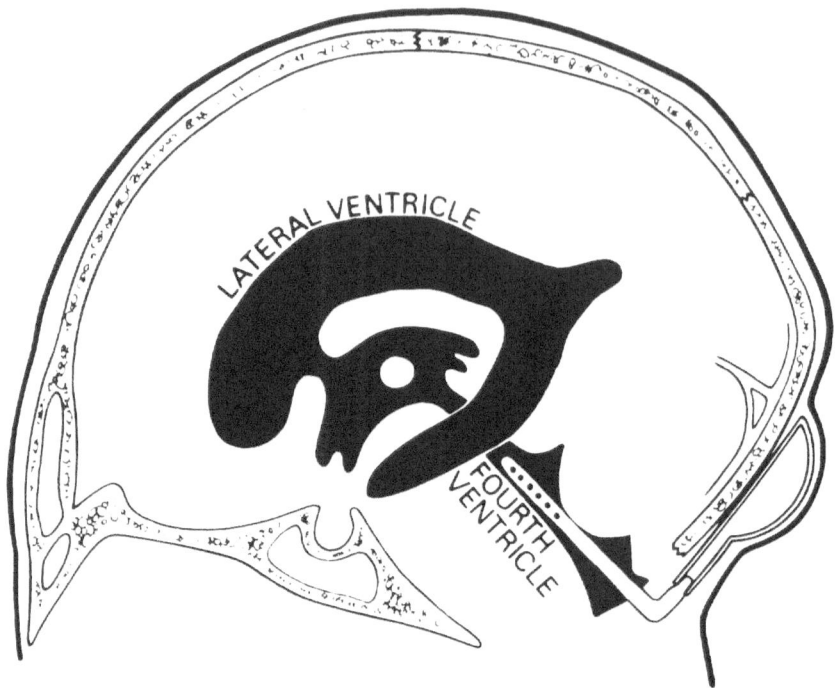

*Figure 6.* Ommayza reservoir implantation in the Rhesus monkey. A Silastic catheter, attached to the subcutaneous CSF reservoir, is passed through the foramen of Magendie and rests in the fourth ventricle [20, 34].

are sufficiently high, and (3) it eliminates the discomfort caused to the patient by frequent lumbar punctures [31].

## Future Directions

The above discussion has detailed some of the problems which prevent optimal delivery of antineoplastic chemotherapy to the CNS. To improve upon these therapeutic approaches current methods of drug delivery must be refined, chemotherapy with existing agents must be optimized and new CNS active drugs must be identified. In an effort to address these issues we have developed an experimental subhuman primate model which provides CNS pharmacokinetic data similar to those obtained in man [33, 34]. In this model, the chamber of an Ommaya reservoir is subcutaneously implanted in the rhesus monkey. The tip of a Pudenz catheter is passed through the foramen of Magendie into the fourth ventricle, and the opposite end attached to the reservoir chamber (Figure 6). This system allows repetitive sterile sampling of CSF over extended periods of time in unanesthe-

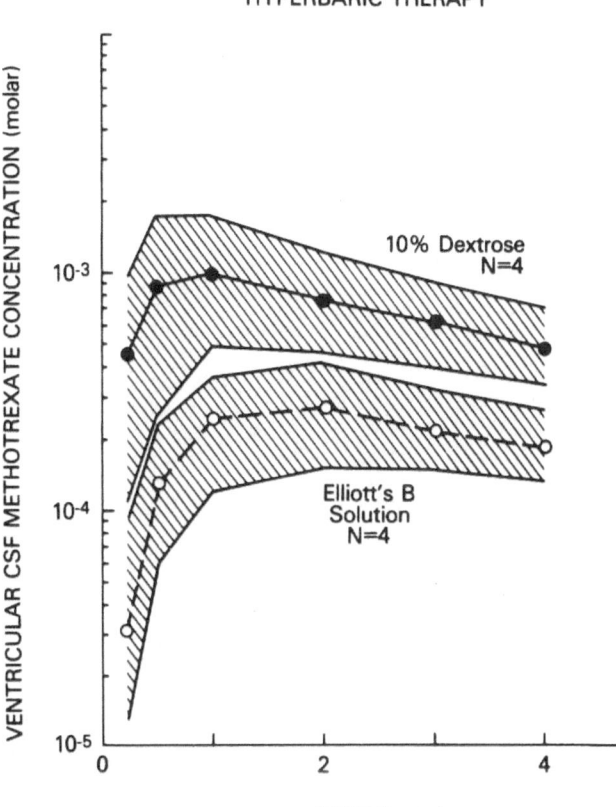

*Figure 7.* Ventricular CSF methotrexate concentrations achieved following intralumbar injection of 13.5 mg/m² of the drug. Higher concentrations were achieved when the methotrexate was administered with 10% dextrose in water (●) than when Elliott's B solution (○) was the diluent [20].

tized animals. The validity of this system as a substitute for human experimentation has been proven [35].

We have used this model to study ways of improving the CSF distribution of intrathecally administered drugs. In one study we examined the effect of hyperbaric intralumbar methotrexate administration on the entry of methotrexate into the cerebral ventricles. Four monkeys were administered methotrexate by lumbar puncture and subsequently placed in the Trendelenburg position at a 45° angle for 4 h. As shown in Figure 7, ventricular CSF methotrexate concentrations were greater when the drug vehicle was a hyperbaric solution (10% dextrose in water) than when a simulated CSF diluent (Elliott's B solution) was used. These results suggest that the hyperbaric technique of intralumbar drug administration has pharmacologic advantages and may be worthy of further clinical study.

152

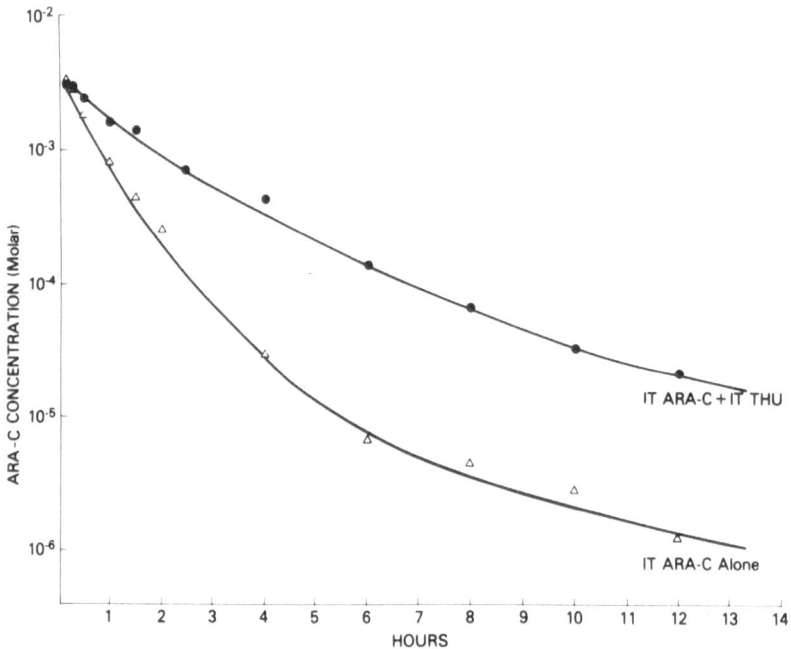

*Figure 8.* Decreased metabolism of cytosine-arabinoside (Ara-C) in CSF induced by tetrahydrouridine (THU). Note that 6 h after combined intrathecal administration of Ara-C (1 mg/kg) and THU (6 mg/kg) (• •) the Ara-C concentration was 20 fold greater than when Ara-C was injected alone (Δ Δ). Experiments were performed in rhesus monkeys (see text for details) [36].

We have also evaluated a number of ways in which chemotherapy with currently available antineoplastic agents can be improved.

In one set of experiments we studied the effect of alteration in drug metabolism upon CSF drug disappearance. There are ample data which indicate that slowing the rate of disappearance of a drug from the CSF can increase its therapeutic effectiveness [8]. One way of affecting a drug's disappearance is by inhibiting its rate of metabolism. We have explored the potential of this relatively new approach by studying the interaction of cytosine arabinoside (Ara-C) and tetrahydrouridine (THU). Under normal conditions, Ara-C is rapidly deaminated by the enzyme cytidine deaminase. Concomitant administration of THU has been shown to competitively inhibit this deamination process. We evaluated the ability of THU to alter the disappearance of intrathecally administered Ara-C in our subhuman primate model. As shown in Figure 8, simultaneous intrathecal administration of THU resulted in higher and more prolonged levels of Ara-C within the CSF [36]. However, it is unclear whether this approach will be of clinical value in man.

The subhuman primate model has also been used to assess the ability of certain potentially active CNS agents to penetrate into the CNS. One group

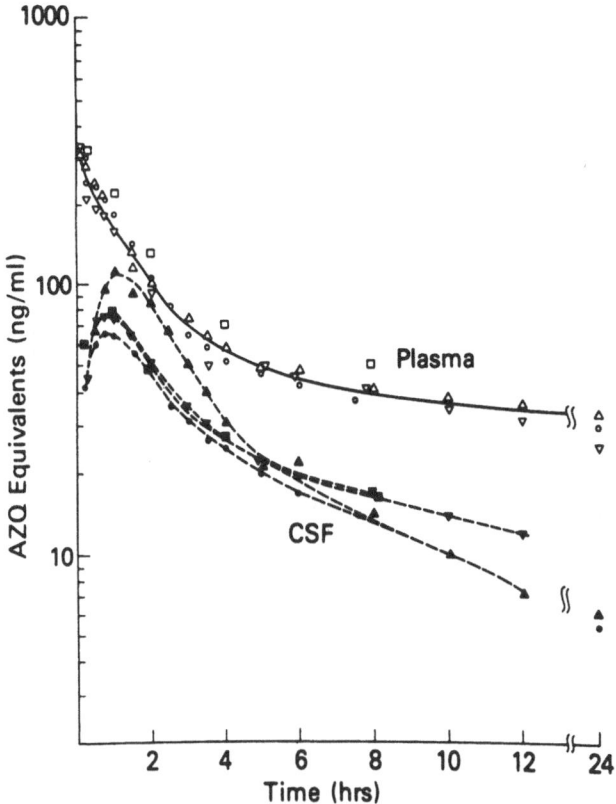

*Figure 9.* Aziridinyl Benzoquinone (AZQ) equivalents as determined by total radioactivity in serum (open symbols) or in CSF (solid symbols). Four monkeys were used. AZQ was given as in intravenous bolus, 0.25 mg/kg. Reprinted from Gormley et al. [38], with permission.

of compounds we have studied is characterized by a unique quinone structure. The quinone structure is believed to be the active site of a number of antineoplastic compounds including adriamycin, daunorubicin and mitomycin C. One of the more lipophilic quinone compounds, aziridinylbenzoquinone (AZQ), has demonstrated significant activity against murine ependymoblastoma [37]. We evaluated this agent in the subhuman primate model (see below) and have confirmed that intravenous administration of AZQ results in significant penetration of this compound into the CSF (Figure 9) [38]. Although some degree of success has been obtained in early clinical studies of systemically administered AZQ the compound may produce significant myelosuppression. One way of circumventing this complication would be to administer AZQ intrathecally, an approach particularly appropriate to treat 'meningeal malignancy'. We have studied intrathecally administered AZQ in the primate model and have demonstrated the feasability of this approach (Figure 10) [39]. A phase I study of intrathecal AZQ (for meningeal malignancies) is currently in progress.

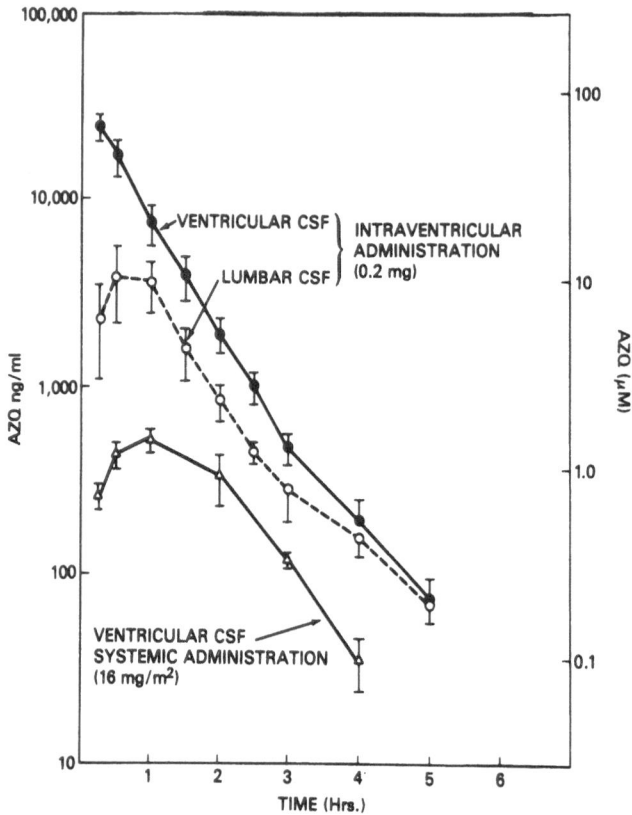

*Figure 10.* Comparison of ventricular CSF levels of AZQ achieved following intraventricular administration of 0.2 mg of AZQ (n = 6) versus I.V. administration of 16 mg/m² (n = 3 in rhesus monkeys (mean ±S.E.) [39].

The above examples illustrate the usefulness of the subhuman primate model in devising new pharmacologic approaches to CNS chemotherapy. It is hoped that future studies in this model will yield information of significant clinical benefit which will improve the outlook for patients with CNS malignancy.

## References

1. Nichol CA: Pharmacokinetics selectivity of action related to physiochemical properties and kinetic patterns of anticancer drugs. Cancer 40:519–528, 1977.
2. Levin VA, Wilson CB: Chemotherapy. The agents in current use. Sem Oncol 2:63–67, 1975.
3. Shapiro WR, Ausman JI, Rall DP: Studies on the chemotherapy of experimental brain tumors. Evaluation of 1,3-bis(2-chloroethyl)1-nitrosourea, cyclophosphamide, mithramycin, and methotrexate. Cancer Res 30:2401–1413, 1970.

4. Poplack DG, Bleyer WA, Horowitz ME: Cerebrospinal fluid pharmacology of antineoplastic agents. Inb: Neurobiology of Cerebrospinal Fluid 1. Wood JH (ed). New York, Plenum Press, 561–578, 1980.

5. Cutler RWP: Neurochemical aspects of blood-brain-cerebrospinal fluid barriers. In: Neurobiology of Cerebrospinal Fluid 1. Wood JH (ed). New York, Plenum Press, 41–51, 1980.

6. Rapoport SI: Blood-Brain Barrier in Physiology and Medicine. New York, Raven Press, 1976.

7. Mayer S, Maickel RP, Brodie BB: Kinetics of Penetration of drugs and other foreign compounds into cerebrospinal fluid and brain. J Pharmacol 127:205–211, 1959.

8. Blasberg RG: Pharmacodynamics and the blood-brain barrier, in modern concepts in brain tumor therapy: Laboratory and clinical investigations. J Natl Cancer Inst 46:19–27, 1977.

9. Vick NA, Bigner DD: Chemotherapy of brain tumors: The blood-brain barrier is not a factor. Arch Neurol 34:523–526, 1977.

10. Levin VA, Clancy TP, Ausman JI, Rall DP: Uptake and distribution of $^3$H-methotrexate by the murine ependymoblastoma. J Natl Cancer Inst 48:875–883, 1972.

11. Neuwelt EA, Frankel EP, Diehl J Vu LH, Rappoport S, Hill S: Reversible osmotic blood-Brain barrier disruption in humans: Implications for the chemotherapy of malignant brain tumors. Neurosurgery 7:44–52, 1980.

12. Mellet IB: Physiochemical considerations and pharmacokinetic behavior in delivery of drugs to the central nervous system. Cancer Treat Rep 61:527–531, 1977.

13. Cowles AL, Fenstermacher JD: Theoretical considerations in the chemotherapy of brain tumors. In: Handbook of Experimental Pharmacology. Sartorelli AC, Johns DG (eds). Springer-Verlag, Berlin and New York, 319–329, 1979.

14. Zaharko DS: Pharmacokinetics and drug effect. Biochem Pharmacol 23:1–8, 1974.

15. Bleyer WA, Poplack DG, Simon RM: 'Concentration × Time' methotrexate via a subcutaneous reservoir: A less toxic regimen for intraventricular chemotherapy of central nervous system neoplasms. Blood 51:835–842, 1978.

16. Bleyer WA, Poplack DG: Intraventricular vs. intralumbar methotrexate for central nervous system leukemia: Prolonged remission with the Ommaya reservoir. Med Pediatr Oncol 6:207–213, 1979.

17. Blasberg RG, Patlak C, Fenstermacher JD: Intrathecal chemotherapy: Brain tissue profiles after ventricular perfusion. J Pharmacol Exp Ther 195:73–83, 1977.

18. Blasberg RG: Methotrexate, cytosine arabinoside and BCNU concentration in brain after ventriculocisternal perfusion. Cancer Treat Rep 61:625–631, 1977.

19. Blasberg RG: Pharmacokinetics and metastatic brain tumor chemotherapy. In: Brain Metastasis. Weiss L, Gilbert HA, Posner JB (eds). G.K. Hall and Co., Medical Publication Division, Boston, 146–164, 1980.

20. Poplack DG, Bleyer WA, Pizzo PA: Experimental approaches to the treatment of CNS leukemia. Amer J Ped Hem Onc 1:141–149, 1979.

21. Ommaya AK: Immunotherapy of gliomas: A review. Adv Neurol 15:337–359, 1976.

22. Neuwelt EA, Diehl JT, Hill SA, Maravilla KR: Use of the metrizamide computerized tomographic cisternography in the evaluation of patients with malignant glioma for immunotherapy. Neurosurgery 5:576–582, 0000.

23. Proceedings of the seventh new drug seminar on the nitrosoureas (Washington, DC, December 15–16, 1975). Cancer Treat Rep 60:645–811, 1976.

24. Peng GW, Marques VE, Driscoll JS: Potential central nervous system antitumor agents. Spirohydantoin mustard. J Med Chem 18:846–849, 1975.

25. Plowman J, Lakings DB, Owens ES, Adamson RH: Initial studies on the penetration of spirohydantoin mustard into the cerebrospinal fluid of dogs. Pharmacology 15:359–366, 1977.

156

26. Riccardi R, Bleyer WA, Poplack DG: Enhancement of delivery of antineoplastic drugs into cerebrospinal fluid. In: Neurobiology of Cerebrospinal Fluid, Vol. II. Wood JH (ed). Plenum Publishing Corporation , New York (in press).

27. Rapoport SI, Hori M, Klatzo I: Testing of a hypothesis for osmotic opening of the blood-brain barrier. Am J Physiol 223:323–331, 1972.

28. Rapoport SI, Thompson HK: Osmotic opening of the blood-brain barrier in the monkey without associated neurological deficits. Science 180:971, 1973.

29. Neuwelt EA, Frenkel E, Rapoport S, Barnett P: The effect of osmotic blood-brain berrier disruption on methotrexate pharmacokinetics in the canine. Neurosurgery, July 1980.

30. Balis FM, Savitch JL, Bleyer WA, Reaman GH, Poplack DP: Remission induction of meningeal leukemia with high-dose intravenous methotrexate. J Clin Oncol 3:485–489, 1985.

31. Poplack DG, Reaman GH, Bleyer WA, Miser J, Feusner J, Wesley R, Hammond D: Central nervous system preventive therapy with high-dose methotrexate in acute lymphoblastic leukemia: A preliminary report. Proceedings Am Soc Clin Oncol 3:204, 1984.

32. Bleyer WA, Poplack DG: Clinical studies on the central nervous system pharmacology of methotrexate. In: Clinical pharmacology of Anti-Neoplastic Drugs. Pinedo HM (ed). Elsevier/North-Holland Biomedical Press, Amsterdam, 115–131, 1978.

33. Poplack DG, Bleyer WA, Wood JH: A primate model for the study of the CNS pharmacokinetics of antineoplastic agents. In: CNS Complications of Malignant Disease. Whitehouse JM, Kay HEM (eds). Macmillan Press Ltd, Hampshire, 397–406, 1979.

34. Wood JH, Poplack DG, Bleyer WA, Ommaya AK: Primate model for long term study of intraventricularly or intrathecally administered drugs and intracranial pressure. Science 195:449–501, 1977.

35. Poplack DG, Bleyer WA, Wood JH, Kostolich M, Savitch JL, Ommaya AK: A primate model for study of methotrexate pharmacokinetics in the central nervous system. Cancer Res 37:1982–1985, 1977.

36. Riccardi R, Chabner BA, Glaubiger DL, Wood JH, Mastrangelo R, Poplack DG: Influence of tetrahydrouridine on cerebrospinal fluid Ara-C levels inthe subhuman primate. Eur J Cancer (in press).

37. Chou F, Khan HA, Driscoll JS: Potential central nervous system antitumor agents. Aziridinylbenzo quinones-2. J Med Chem 19:1302–1308, 1976.

38. Gormley PE, Wood JH, Poplack DG: Ability of a new antitumor agent, AZQ, to penetrate into CSF. Pharmacology 22:196–198, 1981.

39. Zimm S, Collins JM, Curt GA, O'Neill D, Poplack DG: Cerebrospinal fluid pharmacokinetics of intraventricular and intravenous aziridinylbenzoquinone. Cancer Res 44:1698–1701, 1984.

**Use of new agents in children**

# 10. Phase I and II trials in pediatric cancer patients: a rationale

RICHARD S. UNGERLEIDER and SILVIA MARSONI

Childhood malignancies are relatively rare diseases. In the United States, approximately 7,000 new cases of cancer are seen annually in children [1], compared to over 900,000 new cases in adults [2]. Nevertheless, these diseases attract clinical interest far in excess of that predicted by their relative rarity. This is, of course, in large part due to the occurrence of these diseases in the young of our species. Beyond this, however, pediatric oncologists and related scientists are increasingly aware of the unique opportunities to understand the process of malignancy provided by the study of these patients, opportunities afforded by the distinctive characteristics associated with cancer in the young. These characteristics include a generally large kinetic growth fraction and rapid growth [3], origin in mesodermal rather than ectodermal tissue, and occurrence in a growing organism which is continually altering on its way toward biologic maturity, with all the attendant physiologic events associated with development. The increased responsiveness of childhood tumors to current therapeutic strategies is well documented [4], and is one of the major reasons for optimism in the eventual control of malignancy in humans.

Not surprisingly, the relative rarity, the high degree of responsiveness and the differences in the biology of the childhood cancers produce special problems and responsibilities for those oncologists involved in the field of new drug development. These factors affect the design and conduct of both Phase I and Phase II trials, a major area of interest to staff of the Cancer Therapy Evaluation Program (CTEP) of the National Cancer Institute (NCI). As currently defined, Phase I trials determine a safe dose for PHase II trials, describe acute effects on normal tissue, examine the drug's pharmacology, and observe for therapeutic effect. Phase II studies determine whether a drug has antitumor activity and estimate the response rate in a well-defined patient population [5–7].

**Phase I Studies**

The differences in biology between children and adults suggest the desirability of separate Phase I evaluation in children. The relative rarity of childhood malignancies, compounded by their sensitivity to current frontline therapies (thereby further reducing the number of patients available for Phase I trials) makes independent trials highly impractical. Nevertheless, it is CTEP's conclusion that Phase I trials are necessary in children, for reasons which will be explained below.

Since 1948 more than 100 anticancer compounds have been introduced in the United States, and of those, the U.S. Food and Drug Administration has approved 34 for use in adult patients and 18 for use in pediatric patients. Every year the NCI brings to clinical evaluation approximately six new drugs for which a safe and biologically active dose, together with the characterization of the most common associated side effects, must be defined before Phase II evaluation is iniitated. For each drug, several Phase I trials exploring different schedules are conducted in the adult population. The starting dose is calculated on the basis of mouse lethality studies [8]. The modified Fibonacci scale is used for escalating doses [9]. A minimum of three patients who have not previously received the drug are entered at each escalation step.

For the typical drug, a summary of the adult resources involved is as follows: 4 to 6 Phase I trials with different schedules are conducted, each trial evaluating approximately 25 to 30 patients, requiring an average of 6–7 escalations to reach the Maximum Tolerated Dose (MTD), the trial lasting approximately one year. The MTD is the highest dose that can be achieved without producing irreversible toxicity. Because the organs evaluable for toxicity differ (patients with leukemia having abnormal and therefore inevaluable bone marrow function), Phase I trials are conducted separately in leukemia and solid tumor patients. From these figures it is apparent that it would be unrealistic to attempt a parallel effort in the relatively small pediatric population. Furthermore, even a modified effort would be worthwhile only if substantial differences in toxicities and/or MTD's could be found between the adult and pediatric population.

It is reasonable to expect that drug distribution in humans might be affected by age, given the alterations in absorption, metabolism and excretion observed in developing animals. It has been recognized that the disposition of antibiotics and antiepileptics varies considerably between children and adults [10, 12]. Altered distribution might result in different patterns of toxicity, and preliminary data concerning several NCI-sponsored antineoplastic agents suggested age-related differences in relative tolerance to anticancer agents [13]. With the availability of new data on several compounds recently evaluated in Phase I trials, a further analysis of these relationships was undertaken [14].

The anticancer agents for which this analysis was conducted were selected according to the following criteria:

1. independent trials were conducted in children and adults;
2. independent MTD's for solid tumors and leukemia were reached in both children and adults;
3. common schedules and common routes of administration of the drugs were used in both populations.

Seventeen drugs met these criteria, having been evaluated in 14 solid tumor trials and 8 leukemia trials (Table 1). The Dose-Limiting Toxicities (DLT's) were similar in children and adults for 14 of the 17 drugs examined. The major DLT was myelosuppression, or a combination of GI toxicity and myelosuppression. Three drugs induced different patterns of toxicity in children and adults. Cyclocytidine, a slow-release form of cytosine arabinoside resistant to deamination, produced severe postural hypotension in 50% of adult recipients at doses not consistently myelosuppressive [15, 16]. In children, doses up to 60% higher, while inducing prolonged myelosuppression, did not elicit this phenomenon [17]. ICRF-187, a bifunctional alkylating

*Table 1.* Comparison of dose-limiting toxicities of anticancer agents in children and adults.

| Drug | Schedule | Dose-limiting toxicity Children | Adults |
|------|----------|----------|--------|
| AAFC | DX5 | Aplasia[a] | Aplasia[a] |
| Alanosine | DX3 | Mucositis | Mucositis |
| AMSA | | Stomatitis/N & V[a] | Stomatitis/N & V[a] |
| Bisantrene | DX1 | Myelosuppression | Myelosuppression |
| | DX1 | Myelosuppression | Myelosuppression & pheblitis |
| Chlorozorocin | DX1 | Myelosuppression | Myelosuppression |
| | | Myelosuppression | Myelosuppression |
| Diaziquone | DX5 | Hepatotoxicity[a] | Hepatotoxicity[a] |
| DAG | DX5 | Myelosuppression | Myelosuppression |
| | | Renal toxicity[a] | Renal toxicity[a] |
| DGA | DX5 | Myelosuppression | Myelosuppression |
| DON | 2X/W | Myelosuppression N & V | Myelosuppression N & V |
| ICRF-187 | DX5 | Hepatotoxicity | Myelosuppression |
| Indicine | DX5 | Hepatotoxicity | Myelosuppression |
| Mitoxanthrone | DX1 | Myelosuppression | Myelosuppression |
| Rubidazone | DX1 | Myelosuppression | Myelosuppression |
| VM-26 | DX5 | Myelosuppression | Myelosuppression |
| Cyclocytidine | DX10 s.c. | Myelosuppression | Myelosuppression & hypotension |
| 3-Deazauridine | DX5 | Myelosuppression | Myelosuppression |
| 5-Azacytidine | DX5 | Nausea & vomiting | Nausea & vomiting |

[a] DLT in leukemia patients.

agent, produced transient elevation of liver enzymes and prolonged pro-thrombin and partial thromboplastin times in children at non-myelosup-pressive doses which were 2.8 times higher than those which induced severe myelosuppression in adults [18]. Since no adult leukemia patients have been treated with ICRF-187, it is not known whether hepatotoxicity would appear in adult leukemics at higher doses. With indicine N-oxide, severe veno-occlusive disease was observed at non-myelosuppressive doses in chil-dren [19]. Cases of veno-occlusive disease were also observed in adults, but only at higher doses. Although for these three drugs the DLT's differed in adults and children, the mechanism of this phenomenon remains unclear. There is evidence that the volume of distribution for ICRF-187 is much larger in children than adults [18], similar studies have not been performed for indicine N-oxide or cyclocytidine.

In an attempt to quantify the toxicities observed in these trials, ratios of the MTD's reached in adults and children were calculated (Tables 2 and 4).

*Table 2.* Comparison of maximum tolerated dose (MTD) of anticancer agents in children and adults with lymphomas and solid tumors.

| Drug | Schedule | MTD (mg/m$^2$) | | Ratio[a] |
| | | Children | Adults | |
|---|---|---|---|---|
| ICRF-187 | DX3 | 3500 | 1250 | 2.80 |
| Cyclocytidine | DX10 s.c. | 600 | >360 | <1.66 |
| | DX10 i.v. | 600 | 450 | 1.33 |
| 3-Deazauridine | DX5 | 2800 | 1800 | 1.55 |
| VM-26 | DX5 | 45 | 30 | 1.50 |
| Mitoxantrone | DX1 | 18 | 12 | 1.50 |
| Carboplatin | WX4 | >210 | 150 | >1.4 |
| | DX1 | >590 | 440–500 | >1.34–1.18 |
| Bisantrene | DX5 | 120 | 90 | 1.30 |
| | DX1 | 300 | 280 | 1.07 |
| DAG | DX5 | 50 | 40 | 1.20 |
| DON | 2X/W | 520 | 500 | 1.10 |
| Chlorozotocin | DX1 | 150 | 150–200 | 1.00/0.75 |
| Rubidazone | DX1 | 450 | 400 | 1.00 |
| Alanosine | DX3 | 350 | 375 | 0.93 |
| Indicine N-oxide | DX1 | 7500 | 9000 | 0.83 |
| | DX5 | 2000 | 3000[b] | 0.66 |
| Diaziquone | DX5 | 9 | 12 | 0.75 |

[a] Ratio $\dfrac{\text{MTD children}}{\text{MTD adults}}$.

[b] No prior treatment; 2250 if prior Nitrosoureas.

A ratio above 1.0 indicates that children tolerate more drug than do adults, while a ratio below 1.0 indicates that the DLT was observed in children at a dose lower than the adult MTD. For solid tumor patients (Table 2), the MTD ratios varied widely, with a range of 0.66 to 2.80. The median ratio was 1.3, and for five agents it was above 1.5, i.e., the MTD in children was at least 50% higher than in adults. Conversely, for two agents, indicine N-oxide and diazaquone, the ratio was well below 1.0, indicating that children were less tolerant of these agents.

Because of the small number of patients treated in Phase I trials, the MTD is merely an estimation of the dose. Since our primary concern was the comparison of clinically employed doses, we calculated the ratio between Phase II recommended doses for children and adults with solid tumors (Table 3). The distribution had a range identical to that for the MTD (0.66–2.8) with a median of 1.5; the difference between doses in adults and children was statistically significant ($p = 0.002$, Fisher sign test). Only one agent, indicine N-oxide, had a ratio less than 1.0.

*Table 3.* Comparison of recommended Phase II dose of anticancer angents in children and adults with lymphomas and solid tumors.

| Drug | Schedule | Phase II (mg/m$^2$) | | Ratio[a] |
|------|----------|----------|--------|-------|
| | | Children | Adults | |
| ICRF-187 | DX3 | 3500 | 1250 | 2.80 |
| Cyclocytidine | DX10 s.c. | 600 | 360 | 1.67 |
| | DX10 i.v. | Not recommended | | |
| 3-Deazauridine | DX5 | 2000 | 1200 | 1.66 |
| VM-26 | DX5 | 45 | 30 | 1.50 |
| Mitoxantrone | X1 | 18 | 12 | 1.50 |
| Carboplatin | WX4 | Too early | | |
| | DX1 | Too early | | |
| Bisantrene | DX5 | 100 | 80 | 1.25 |
| | DX1 | 280 | 260 | 1.08 |
| DAG | DX5 | 50 | 30 | 1.70 |
| DON | 2X/W | 520 | 300 | 1.73 |
| Chlorozotocin | DX1 | 150 | 120–150 | 1.25/1.00 |
| Rubidazone | DX1 | 300 | 150 | 2.00 |
| Alanosine | Dx3 | 300 | 250 | 1.20 |
| Indicine N-oxide | DX1 | 7500 | 7000 | 1.07 |
| | DX5 | 2000 | 3000 | .66 |
| Diaziquone | DX5 | 9 | 8 | 1.12 |

[a] Ratio $\dfrac{\text{dose children}}{\text{dose adults}}$.

The situation is somewhat different in leukemia, where 50% of the agents had a *lower* MTD in children than in adults (Table 4). This became more striking when the Phase II doses for luekemias were considered, as none of the ratios was significantly greater than 1.0 (Table 5). These data suggested

*Table 4.* Comparison of maximum tolerated dose (MTD) of anticancer agents in children and adults with acute leukemias.

| Drug | Schedule | MTD (mg/m$^2$) | | Ratio[a] |
|------|----------|----------|--------|----------|
| | | Children | Adults | |
| AAFC | Dx5 | 30[c] | 20[c] | 1.33 |
| 3-Deazauridine | Dx5 | 7200 | 6000 | 1.20 |
| Diaziquone | DX5 | 30 | 28 | 1.07 |
| Rubidazone | DX1 | 450 | 450 | 1.00 |
| Indicine | DX5 | 2500 | 3000[b] | 0.83 |
| AMSA | DX5 | 150 | 200 | 0.75 |
| DGA | DX5 | 1500 | 2000 | 0.75 |
| 5-Azacytidine | DX5 | 300 | 400 | 0.75 |

[a] Ratio $\dfrac{\text{MTD children}}{\text{MTD adults}}$ .

[b] Original MTD at 3750, subsequent patient tolerated only 3000.

[c] mg/kg.

*Table 5.* Comparison of recommended Phase II dose in adults and children with acute leukemias.

| Drug | Schedule | Phase II dose (mg/m$^2$) | | Ratio[a] |
|------|----------|----------|--------|----------|
| | | Children | Adults | |
| AMSA | DX5 | 120 | 120 | 1.00 |
| DGA | DX5 | 1500 | 1500 | 1.00 |
| Indicine | DX5 | 2500 | 3000 | 0.83 |
| Rubidazone | DX1 | 300 | 450 | 0.67 |
| 3-Deazauridine[b] | DX5 | 2000 | 3000 | >0.66 |
| 5-Azacytidine | DX5 | 150 | 300 | 0.50 |
| Diaziquone | DX5 | 25 | 24 | 1.04 |

[a] Ratio $\dfrac{\text{dose children}}{\text{dose adult}}$ .

[b] Childhood study: Phase II dose not recommended, severe tox >2000.

that, while children with solid tumors generally appear to tolerate higher doses of anticancer drugs than do adults, this is not true for children with leukemia. The reasons for this difference in tolerance between children with solid tumors and children with leukemia is unclear.

To investigate whether differences in prognostic factors between adult and childhood solid tumor patients were responsible for the increased tolerance to anticancer agents in children with solid tumors, patient characteristics of both cohorts were analyzed in more than 30 Phase I trials in over 2,000 patients treated on NCI-sponsored trials since 1980 (Table 6). Compared with adults, children have similar performance status distribution, with at least 20% being grade 3 or 4; they are more likely to have received prior treatments; and they tend to die on study more frequently than do adults. They are, however, better responders, even at this late stage in the evolution of their disease. If one uses the average pre-treatment renal and hepatic laboratory values as indicators of organ function, no striking differences in

*Table 6.* Characteristics of Phase I patients.

| Characteristics | % Patients | | P value |
|---|---|---|---|
| | Children (n = 267) | Adults (n = 1921) | |
| Performance status | | | |
| 0 | 12 | 8 | |
| 1/2 | 26/33 | 39/31 | N.S. |
| 3/4 | 24/5 | 16/6 | |
| Prior chemotherapy | 100 | 75 | <.005 |
| Died on study | 21 | 15 | <.025 |
| Response (CR+PR) | 7.5 | 1.7 | <.005 |

*Table 7.* Average pre-treatment lab values as indicators of organ functions.

| Age | Renal | | Liver | | |
|---|---|---|---|---|---|
| | Bun | Creat[a] | Bili[b] | SGOT/SGPT | Aph[c] |
| 16 and under (n = 213) | 10 | 0.6 | 0.5 | 47/62 | 191 |
| 17 and over (n = 2389) | 15 | 1.0 | 0.7 | 37/37 | 165 |

[a] creatinine.
[b] bilirubin.
[c] alkaline phosphatase.

these parameters account for the relative intolerance of adults (Table 7). Therefore, patient-selection factors known to affect tolerance to antineoplastic agents, such as prior treatment, performance status or organ dysfunction, seem not to be responsible for the increased tolerance in children, suggesting a biologic basis inherent in youth. It has been demonstrated that the relative volumes of the body water compartment, total body water, and extracellular water decrease progressively from infancy to adulthood [20]. This would lead one to predict a greater tolerance in children; in support of this is the evidence that ICRF-187, the compound with the highest children/adult toxicity ratio, has a larger volume of distribution in children [18]. Greater rates of plasma elimination in children have also been reported for cyclophosphamide [21], methotrexate [22], and VP-16 [23]. It has also been suggested that the increased tolerance of children with solid tumors may simply be a reflection of increased bone marrow reserve associated with youth [13]. Irrespective of the mechanism, the difference in tolerance to anticancer agents between children and adults, coupled with the presumption that the highest tolerable doses are necessary for the adequate assessment of response in Phase II trials, forms the basis of the CTEP recommendation that independent Phase I trials be mounted in children.

The optimum design of Phase I trials in children is still under discussion. Prior to 1980, the starting dose was variously and inconsistently based on animal lethality studies or on some fraction of the adult MTD, varying from 1% to 83%. Escalation was according to the modified Fibonacci scheme, and the number of escalations to reach the MTD likewise varied widely. These practices were subsequently looked upon as wasteful of patient resources, and following an initial review of this experience [13], CTEP recommended that Phase I trials in children commence at 80% of the adult MTD, as the minimum childhood MTD was found to be 83% of its adult counterpart. Escalation procedures were unspecified. Following further review [14], as outlined above, CTEP reconfirmed that Phase I trials in childhood solid tumor and leukemia patients should be based on adult solid tumor trials. The majority of solid tumor trials in children arrived at an MTD above that of adults, providing a margin of safety; this was less often seen in leukemia patients. The data support continuing the entry of both childhood solid tumor and leukemia patients at a dose approximately 80% of the adult solid tumor MTD.

Basing the childhood starting dose on the adult experience should minimize the entry of patients at a biologically inactive dose, thus increasing the probability of response, without placing the patients at undue risk of toxicity. In the absence of non-hematologic toxicity, leukemia patients can then be escalated beyond the childhood solid tumor MTD rather than beginning with some fraction of the adultleukemia MTD which may be intolerable in children. In the event that a particular drug has not been evaluated in children or adults with solid tumors, the starting dose for children with leukemia should be less than 75% of the adult leukemia MTD.

Regarding escalation procedures, those procedures which employ the fewest dose levels between entry and MTD, yet do not escalate into an area of overt toxicity, are obviously preferred. Escalation from the starting dose in children should not follow the conventional Fibonacci schema, with its fixed 33% increment employed in later steps, since the risk of escalation into an area of overt toxicity increases proportionally along the dose-toxicity curve. The efficiency of 33% increments is offset by the increased likelihood of escalating to a dose which produces unacceptable toxicity. It should be remembered that the entry doses for these childhood trials are intended to approximate those which produced overt toxicity in adults, and the margin of safety is accordingly reduced. Escalations at a fixed increment of 20% (starting at 80% the adult MTD and proceeding through 96%, 115%, 138%, 156%, etc.) retains much of the efficiency yet reduces the likelihood of overshoot.

In summary, the NCI is currently recommending that Phase I trials in children:

1. begin in solid tumor and leukemia patients at 80% of the adult *solid tumor* MTD;
2. be escalated at fixed 20% increments, distinguishing between the toxicities observed in leukemia (for whom myelosuppression is a sought-after effect) and solid tumor patients;
3. be designed such that a minimum of three evaluable solid tumor and three evaluable leukemia patients are entered at each level;
4. and in the absence of non-myelosuppressive toxicity, escalating in patients with leukemia beyond the solid tumor MTD.

## Phase II Studies

Phase II studies determine whether a drug has antitumor activity and are employed to estimate the response rate in a well-defined patient population. These trials are disease-oriented. The various tumor types are tested in Phase II as distinct clinical entities, each with differing considerations for patient eligibility and with potentially distinct patterns of responsiveness to any particular drug. These trials serve as a screen for further study, and every effort should be made to optimize the opportunity for obtaining a reliable estimate of the new agent's activity. False negative Phase II trials are particularly wasteful, since the discovery of a useful drug may be significantly delayed or prevented entirely.

For this reason, CTEP has adopted a strict policy concerning the extent of prior treatment with cytotoxic therapy in adult patients entering Phase II studies. CTEP seeks trials which restrict patient eligibility to the minimum extent of prior therapy consistent with ethical medical practice. Specifically, protocols for the initial Phase II trials of a drug in adult patients require the absence of prior cytotoxic chemotherapy except in circumstances where the disease is potentially curable with systemic treatment. Therefore, under current CTEP policy, the following disease categories exclude patients who have had prior chemotherapy: carcinomas of the colon, kidney, liver, pancreas, head and neck, cervix, esophagus, prostate, bladder, stomach, non-small cell lung and malignant melanoma.

Fortunately, there is no comparable list of pediatric malignancies whose outlook is so bleak, as the vast majority of cancers in children are potentially if not actually curable. This creates a problem, however, in defining the appropriate point for introduction of Phase II trials within a given disease category. Foremost, the decision must reflect a balance between that which is ethical or reasonable for the child and that which will afford the best estimate of the activity of the drug in question. It requires an accounting of the nature of the previously administered therapies and the point of relapse during the disease, i.e., during intensive therapy, during maintenance or following completion of treatment.

CTEP currently proposes:

1. no more than two Phase II agents per child;
2. patients who relapse during agressive frontline therapy be eligible for Phase II trials;
3. patients who relapse during maintenance, following completion of therapy, or on frontline therapies which exclude known active agents, may undergo retrieval attempts with known active agents prior to Phase II entry.

Phase II trials in children are otherwise conducted in a manner similar to those in adults. Specifically:

1. patients *must* have measurable disease to allow a quantitation of antitumor activity;
2. patients should be expected to survive a sufficient period of time so that therapeutic observations can be made;
3. activity should be evaluated in discrete diagnostic categories;
4. accrual must be sufficient in *each* diagnostic category such that a reasonably reliable estimate of activity can be arrived at (generally a minimum of 14 patients; no responses among 14 evaluable patients indicates a true response rate of less than 20%).

## Acknowledgement

Our thanks to Jill Johnston for secretarial assistance in preparing this manuscript.

## References

1. Young JL Jr, miller RW: Incidence of malignant tumors in U.S. children. J Pediatric 86:254, 1975.
2. American Cancer Society: Cancer Facts and Figures. New York, 1977.
3. Levine AS: Perspectives on the biology and treatment of cancer in the young: the evolution of our understanding. In: Cancer in the Young. Levine AS (ed). New York, XXV, 1982.
4. Simone J, Cassady JR, Filler RM: Cancers of childhood. In: Cancer: Principles and Practice of Oncology. De Vita VT, Hellman S, Rosenberg S (eds). Lippincott, Philadelphia, 1254–1330, 1982.
5. De Vita VT, Oliverio VT, Muggia FM et al.: The drug development program and clinical trials programs of the Division of Cancer Treatment, National Cancer Institute. Cancer Clin Trials 2:195–216, 1979.
6. Wooley PV, Schein PS: Clinical pharmacology and phase I trial design. In: Methods in Cancer Research. XVII. Cancer Drug Development, Part B. De Vita VT, Busch H (eds). 199–215, 1979.
7. Muggia FM, McGuire WP, Rozencweig M: Rationale, design and methodology of phase II clinical trials. In: Methods in cancer Research. XVII. Cancer Drug Development, Part B. De Vita VT, Busch H (eds). 199–215, 1979.
8. De Vita VT: Principles of chemotherapy. In: Cancer: Principles and Practice of Oncology. De Vita VT, Hellman S, Rosenberg S (eds). Lippincott, 145, 1982.
9. Muggia FM, Rozencweig M, Chiuten DF: Phase II trials: use of a clinical tumor panel and overview of current resources and studies. Cancer Treat Rep 64:1–9, 1980.
10. Morselli Pl (ed): Drug Disposition During Development. Spectrum Publishing, New York, ch 2–6, 1968.
11. Rylance G: Clinical pharmacology. Drugs in children. Br Med J 282:50–51, 1981.
12. Udkow G: Pediatric clinical pharmacology. Am J Dis Child 282:1025–1033, 1978.
13. Glaubiger DL, Von Hoff DD, Holcenberg JS, Kamen B, Pratt C, Ungerleider RS: The relative tolerance of children and adults to anticancer drugs. Front Radiat Ther Onc 16:42–49, 1982.
14. Marsoni S, Ungerleider RS, Hurson SB, Simon RG, Hammershaimb LD: Tolerance to antineoplastic agents in children and adults. Cancer Treat Rep (in press).
15. Lokich JJ, Chawla PL, Jaffe N, Frei E: Phase I evaluation of cyclocytidine (NSC-145668). Cancer Chemother Rep 59:389–393, 1975.
16. Burgess MA, Bodey GP, Minnow RA, Gottlieb J: Phase I-II evaluation of cyclocytidine. Cancer Treat Rep 61:437–443, 1977.
17. Finklestein JZ, Higgins G, Krivit W, Hammond D: Evaluation of Cyclocytidine in children with advanced acute leukemia and solid tumors. Cancer Treat Rep 63:1331–1333, 1979.
18. Holcenberg JS, Tutsch KD, Earhart RH, Ungerleider RS, Kamen BA, Pratt CB, Gribble TJ, Gleubiger DL: Phase I study of ICRF-187 in pediatric cancer patients and comparison of its pharmacokinetics in children and adults. Submitted to Cancer Treat Rep.
19. Miser J, Miser A, Smithson W et al.: A phase I trial of indicine n-oxide in childhood malignancy. Proc ASCO 1:137, 1982.
20. Rare A, Wilson T: Clinical pharmacokinetics in infants and children. Clin Pharmacokinet 1:2–24, 1976.

21. Sladek NE, Priest J, Doeden D et al.: Plasma half-life and urinary excretion of cyclophosphamide in children. Cancer Treat Rep 64:1061, 1980.
22. Wang Y, Sutow WW, Romsdahl MM et al.: Age-related pharmacokinetics in patients with osteosarcoma. Cancer Treat Rep 63:405, 1979.
23. D'Incalci M, Farina PL, Sessa C et al.: Pharmacokinetics of VP-16-213 given by different administration methods. Cancer Chemother Pharmacol 7:141–145, 1982.

# 11. Guidelines for conduct of Phase I studies in children

J. HOLCENBERG

The *primary objectives* of Phase I clinical trials of new anticancer agents are:

1. Determine the MTD which is both predictable and reversible in children on a specific dosage schedule;
2. Determine the qualitative and quantitative toxicity by this schedule in children with drug resistant acute leukemias and malignant solid tumors;
3. Determine the concentration of the new anticancer agents and their metabolites in biologic fluids and tissues and note the influence of inter-patient variability and the influence of other patient characteristics such as age, renal function, hepatic function and disease status on the absorption, drug distribution, metabolism and excretion;
4. Use this information to devise pharmacologically sound Phase II therapeutic trials.

**Eligibility criteria**

1. All patients between two and eighteen years of age with microscopically confirmed diagnosis of malignancy (leukemia or solid tumor) may be eligible for Phase I studies provided they are resistant to all conventional modes of treatment for their malignancies. Generally these patients will have indicators of disease activity evaluated by physical examination, bone marrow aspiration, or radiologic examination;
2. Patients must have a life expectancy of at least eight weeks;
3. Patients or their parents as guardians must sign an informed consent indicating that they are aware of the investigational nature of a particular Phase I study including pharmacokinetic studies;
4. Patients must have recovered from the toxic effects of all prior chemotherapy, immunotherapy, or radiotherapy prior to entering a study;

5. Patients with solid tumors (without bone marrow involvement) must have adequate bone marrow function (defined as a peripheral absolute granulocyte count of equal to or greater than 1500/mm$^3$, and platelet count equal to or greater than 100,000/mm$^3$), adequate liver function (Grade 0 or I toxicity), adequate renal function (creatinine less than 1.2 mg % or BUN less than 20 mg % [Grade 0 toxicity]) and uric acid less than 6 mg %. Patients with leukemia or solid tumors with bone marrow involvement may have granulocytopenia, anemia and thrombocytopenia. The patients must take oral feedings and must not have lost more than 15 % of the optimal weight for age. After the MTD is determined in normal patients, selected patients may be entered with Grade II renal or hepatic toxicity to assess the effect of these abnormalities on the pharmacokinetics and toxicity.

### Rationale for selection of schedule, starting dose and escalation procedure

The schedule of administration are determined according to a number of criteria including the animal and adult pharmacology of the drug, animal data showing whether schedule dependency exists for antitumor effect or toxicity, anticipated clinical uses of the drug and patient convenience. In general, if the adult MTD is not known, the initial dose will be 1/10th of the mouse equivalent 10 % lethal dose (MELD 10) and escalations will be by the standard modification of the Fibonacchi scheme. Usually, an adult MTD will be known. In most cases, the starting dose for a Phase I study will be 75 % of the adult MTD. All subsequent increments usually will be 20 % of the previous dose level. For example, if the adult MTD of a given agent is 400 mg/m$^2$, the dose escalations for a Phase I trial might be

| Level | Dose (mg/m$^2$) |
|-------|-----------------|
| 1 | 300 |
| 2 | 360 |
| 3 | 432 |
| 4 | 518 |
| 5 | 622 |
| 6 | 746 |
| 7 | 896 |

### Definition of MTD

The maximally tolerated dose is the dose that produces predictable and reversible toxicity but is safe for use in Phase II trials.

The evaluation of toxicity in Phase II studies is done using standard toxicity rating scales.

In order to find the MTD, the agent under investigation is administered in a Phase I study with the dose escalation schedule given above. This escalation proceeds independently in groups of patients with and without marrow involvement until a dose is reached at which there is evidence of life threatening toxicity (Grade III or IV) which is attributable to the treatment. This is the minimal toxic dose. Three evaluable patients are then enrolled at the penultimate dose. If there is no evidence of life threatening toxicity among these three patients, the penultimate dose will be considered the maximum tolerated dose. If evidence of life threatening toxicity is noted at this dose, the dose level will be reduced in single steps by its original increments and three evaluable patients enrolled at each dose until no life threatening toxicities are noted. This dose will be considered the MTD.

In solid tumor patients with normal bone marrows the dose limiting toxicity will often be myelosuppression. In leukemic patients with marrow replacement or patients undergoing bone marrow transplantation, myelosuppression cannot be evaluated, so other organ toxicities, such as mucositis, CNS toxicity or hepatic dysfunction often become the dose limiting toxicity. Certain drugs like AZQ, mitoxantrone, and AMSA produce profound, prolonged aplasia of the bone marrow at high doses. With such drugs, a MTD may have to be defined as a dose in leukemic patients that permits marrow recovery in four to six weeks with either normal cells or blasts. This definition is necessary because longer periods of aplasia may be associated with very high mortality rates. This MTD may be lower than the dose that produces other organ toxicity. Certain drugs have primarily non-myelosuppressive toxicity. With these agents, the MTD is the dose that produces the non-marrow toxicity to a reversible and mild enough degree that it is tolerable for Phase II studies.

Thus, the MTD for a drug and dose schedule is determined on an individual basis by careful monitoring of the patients.

**Number of patients per level**

Ordinarily five patients with leukemia or bone marrow compromise and five patients with no bone marrow involvement (and metting other protocol entry requirements) are registered at a specified dose level. Patient accrual is then halted until data from those patients can be evaluated. This number is needed to insure three evaluable patients per dose level. If the MTD has not been reached, patient accrual will resume at the next appropriate dose level. Dose escalations in leukemia or solid tumor groups are usually not carried out until at least three patients (usually 21 days) at the previous dose. If three patients are evaluable prior to five patient entries in each group, escalation can proceed to the next dose.

If consistent grade III or IV myelosuppression is seen at a dose level, three additional patients with normal bone marrows are usually entered at the next lowest dose to insure that this level is safe. If consistent grade III or IV non-marrow toxicity is seen, three additional patients with leukemia or solid tumors are entered at the next lowest dose. The study is terminated as soon as consistent dose limiting toxicity is identified. For practical purposes, this requires consistent, reversible but tolerable toxicity in 4–6 patients with and 4–6 patients without bone marrow compromise. Once the MTD has been determined in both groups, the study is closed.

## Dose escalation in the same patient

Under most circumstances no patient will have dosage escalations from their originally assigned dosage level and no patient, previously admitted to a study will be admitted at a later date for study at a higher dosage level of an investigational new agent.

## Definition of evaluable course for toxicity

An evaluable course is defined as one in which the toxic effects are determined by the assigned treatment schedule. The number of doses and period of observation will depend on the pharmacology of the drug and dosage schedule. In general, drugs administered weekly will be given for four weeks with three weeks of observation. Drugs given daily × 5 or as a single dose are usually followed by 3–4 weeks of observation. Certain drugs with late or prolonged toxicity may require extension of this period to 4–6 weeks. One course of treatment will be sufficient for evaluation of toxicity. Nevertheless patients will generally be given two courses of treatment and continued on therapy as long as no grade III or IV toxicity occurs and the cancer is stable or improving.

Prior to admission to these investigations, patients' histories are reviewed and the patients re-examined. CBC including hemoglobin, WBC, differential counts, reticulocyte and platelet counts are performed. Urinalysis, tests of liver and renal function, uric acid, coagulation factors, chest X-ray and radiographs of other tumor areas along with electro- and echocardiograms are evaluated. Lumbar punctures will be performed for patients with leukemia to determine presence or absence of leukemic infiltration of the leptomeninges. These hemograms and biochemical studies are usually performed at least weekly during the course of administration of the new anticancer agent and appropriate radiographs, cultures, electrocardiograms, and echocardiograms are performed at the time of the end of treatment with new anticancer agents.

All patients are followed for the toxic side effects of the agent including such categories as gastrointestinal toxicity, hematopoietic suppression, abnormalities of hepatic or renal function studies, pulmonary toxicity, cardiotoxicity, neuromuscular complications, skin rashes, allergic manifestations, hypertension or infectious complications. The time of onset of toxicity and the extent of this toxicity are quantitated along with any quantitation of response which might occur. All patients are followed for survival. Autopsy reports obtained at later dates are correlated with the abnormalities of the organ function occurring during life.

*Response criteria*

Although the goal of Phase I studies cannot be evaluation of response, all patients with measurable disease will have serial measurements of such disease. Any responses seen will aid in subsequent Phase II evaluation of the drug. Response criteria are:

1. *Complete response.* The total disappearance of all clinical evidence of disease for at least two measurement periods separated by at least four weeks. Achieveent of M1 marrow in patients with leukemia;
2. *Partial response.* At least a 50% reduction in the size of all measurable tumor areas as measured by the sum of the products of the greatest length and the maximum width. Decrease in the bone marrow involvement by tumor cells by at least 50% on consecutive aspirates. No lesion may progress and no new lesion may appear. Achievement of M2 marrow in leukemia. These parameters must have been present for at least two measurement periods separated by at least three weeks;
3. *No change* (stable disease). Exists when a patient fails to qualify for either a response or progressive disease;
4. *Progressive disease.* An increase of 25% in the size of a measurable tumor as measured by the sum of the products of the greatest length and maximum width or appearance of new lesions.

**Procedures for assuring eligibility**

The best method to assure eligibility in cooperation Phase I trials is insistence on the following commitments by participating institutions:

1. The responsibility for immediate communication in the event of unexpected toxicity;

2. Willingness to enter patients on Phase I trials who have life expectancies sufficient to evaluate the agent under study. The patients must be free of infection and have good nutritional status;
3. An understanding of the necessity of review by the human rights committee at each institution for each drug studied at that institution;
4. A commitment to participate in pharmacokinetic and pharmacodynamics studies.

Participation in Phase I studies involves additional requirements. For any given study, the chairman and an individual at each institution must have experience in the conduct of new agent trials. Prompt submission of data is required of all institutions participating in Phase I trials.

# Pharmacology of antileukemic agents

# 12. Factors affecting the clinical pharmacology of antileukemic drugs

RICCARDO RICCARDI, ANNA LASORELLA and
RENATO MASTRANGELO

## Introduction

In children with newly-diagnosed acute lymphoblastic leukemia (ALL) the current cure rate is approximately 50%. These results are obtained using multiple agent chemotherapy in conjunction with some form of CNS prophylaxis. Induction therapy with prednisone and vincristine results in hematological remission in more than 90% of patients. Maintenance chemotherapy essentially involves administration of daily oral 6-mercaptopurine (6-MP) and weekly or bi-weekly MTX, whereas intensification therapy often includes daunomycin and L-asparaginase [1].

A number of factors have been recognized which influence the clinical pharmacology of antileukemic agents. Drug disposition, metabolism, excretion and interaction at the biochemical level all play a role in the determination of the clinical efficacy of these drugs.

In this chapter we review additional factors that appear to have therapeutic implications, including drug interactions and factors which influence the bioavailability of orally administered drugs.

## Drug interactions

The pharmacokinetics and the biochemical pharmacology of antileukemic agents may be influenced by the concomitant administration of other antineoplastic agents and other drugs. Although a number of studies have reported on drug-drug interactions with antileukemic agents, most of these studies have not been conducted in man and thus their therapeutic implications are not yet known.

We shall limit the present analysis to those interactions which appear to have a clinical relevance.

*Allpurinol*

Allopurinol (AP) is an analogue of hypoxanthine which is frequently used in children with leukemia to prevent hyperuricemia and uric acid nephropathy. In mice, simultaneous administration of 6-mercaptopurine (6-MP) and AP achieved the same antitumor effect as 6-MP but required only 25% of the dose of 6-MP [2].

Because of this a 75% reduction has been recommended when the two drugs are given simultaneously. This phenomenon, however, was not observed in an early study in three patients treated with i.v. 6-MP [3].

A recent study has examined the interaction of AP with both i.v. and oral 6-MP in humans [4]. Although an increase in the AUC and peak plasma levels of 6-MP was observed when AP was simultaneously administered with p.o. 6-MP, an increase was not noted when 6-MP was given intravenously. These data indicate that AP acts via inhibition of the first pass metabolism of 6-MP. The concomitant administration of AP with 6-MP did not prolong the plasma half-life of 6-MP. In accordance with these results, 6-MP dose reduction is recommended when the drug is administered orally with AP, but not when 6-MP is administered intravenously.

*Salicylates*

In humans about 50% of methotrexate (MTX) is usually bound to plasma protein [5]. Therefore a large fraction of the MTX administered is pharmacologically inactive. Salicylates are capable of displacing MTX from plasma proteins increasing the amount of circulating 'free' drug [6]. This may result in increased toxicity in patients in whom MTX and salicylates are administered concomitantly. For example, severe MTX toxicity has been reported in patients with head and neck carcinomas undergoing chemotherapy with intra-arterial MTX who were taking aspirin as pain reliever [7].

Other drugs like sulfonamides, barbiturates and diphenylhydantoin have been shown to displace MTX from plasma proteins; however, the clinical relevance of these interactions has not been determined [8, 9].

Another possible mechanism by which salicylates may increase MTX toxicity is related to the renal excretion of this antileukemic agent. MTX is actively secreted by renal tubules and salycylates compete for the same mechanism of renal excretion. Therefore concomitant administration of salicylates and MTX will also result in a decrease in MTX clearance [10].

*Drug inducers of liver microsomal enzymes*

A large number of drugs including antineoplastic agents are metabolized by liver microsomal enzymes. Any compound able to activate these enzymes may alter the activity of a concomitantly administered antileukemic drug.

Phenobarbital, a widely used anticonvulsant, is a well known inducer of microsomal enzymes. The ability of this drug to increase drug metabolism in the liver may result in a decrease in the pharmacologic activity of antileukemic drugs such as anthracyclines [11] and corticosteroids [12]. In contrast, in the case of cyclophosphamide, only the metabolite posesses antileukemic activity and thus its pharmacologic activity may be increased by concomitant phenobarbital administration [13]. Although, the clinical significance of these interactions are not entirely clear, when possible concomitant administration of phenobarbital and the above mentioned antileukemic drugs should be avoided.

## L-Asparaginase and Methotrexate

L-Asparaginase and MTX have been extensively studied by Capizzi in a murine model both *in vivo* and *in vitro* [14, 15] and in human leukemia cells *in vitro* [16]. It has been shown that these two drugs can be synergistic in terms of antileukemic effect and at the same time L-Asparaginase appears capable of rescuing normal cells from MTX toxicity. The timing of administration of these two drugs appears to be the critical factor.

Data derived from animal studies of the interaction have been utilized to design clinical protocols in the treatment of refractory leukemias [17, 18]. So far the clinical results appear to confirm the results obtained in animal studies.

## 6-Mercaptopurine – Adriamycin

The combination of 6-MP and daunorubicin has been shown to be synergistic against L1210 *in vivo*. Based on these data Rodriguez *et al.* have utilized 6-MP and Adriamycin to treat refractory leukemia in 19 adult patients [19]. Only limited therapeutic efficacy was noted. However, severe toxicity was observed. The most important clinical complication was liver toxicity. Ten patients had cholestasis (mean bilirubin level = 9.1 mg%), two patients had ascending cholangitis and one patient had liver failure with hepatic coma. These observations suggest that the combination of 6-MP and Adriamycin may produce a synergistic effect regarding toxicity.

## Factors affecting drug absorption

Maintenance chemotherapy utilized in the treatment of ALL usually includes orally administered MTX and 6-MP. Both drugs are commonly administered at a starting dose based on body surface area which is subsequently reduced or increased on the basis of ensuing toxicity. However, drug dosing determined clinically by evaluating myelosuppression does not clearly indicate whether MTX or 6-MP have reached adequate plasma levels. Therefore it may well be that leukemic cells may not be exposed to an optimal plasma concentration of either MTX or 6-MP, even in the presence of hematological toxicity. Hence it is important to recognize those factors that may affect the bioavailability of these orally administered drugs by altering their absorption.

### Methotrexate

A study by Pinkerton *et al.* has shown that food intake appears to be an important factor in the absorption of MTX [20]. In that study the influence of food intake was evaluated in ten children with ALL in remission. MTX plasma levels were measured up to 4 h after oral drug administration on three separate occasions when oral MTX was taken (1) in the fasting state, (2) after a milky meal and (3) after a citrus meal. Peak MTX concentrations and the area under the absorption curve were significantly reduced with the milky meal as compared to the fasting state.

### 6-Mercaptopurine

We recently conducted a study to evaluate whether food intake could be one of the factors responsible for 6-MP plasma variability, as has been shown for MTX.

Twelve children, three girls and nine boys, with ALL in complete remission were studied [21]. We administered a single dose of 75 mg/m$^2$ to each patient for two consecutive days, one in the fasting state and the other after a standard breakfast of 250 ml milk and 50 g biscuits, at random. In the non-fasting patients 6-MP was given 15 min after breakfast. Food intake resulted in a longer time to peak in almost all patients. The mean time to peak was 1.2 h (range 0.5–2 h) when the drug was administered in the fasting state and 2.3 h (range 1–4 h) after breakfast. In most of the patients studied a marked decrease in the bioavailability of 6-MP was seen when the drug was given after breakfast. The mean AUC±S.D. of all post fast patients was 407 ng/ml$^{-1}$ h±197, whereas the mean AUC±S.D. of all post breakfast patients was $284 \, ng/ml^{-1} \, h \pm 203$, a difference which is statistically significant ($p < 0.01$).

The exact causes of the reduced bioavailability of 6-MP determined by food intake are not clear and studies are now under way in our institution to gain further insight into these problems.

It is worth noting that only a small amount of food is responsible for the above differences. It is possible that a larger meal could influence the absorption of 6-MP to a greater extent and therefore most patients taking the drug after a meal may not be receiving adequate treatment with this active antileukemic agent. Hence we advise administering oral 6-MP in the fasting state.

# References

1. Poplack DG: Acute lymphoblastic leukemia and less frequently occurring leukemias in the young. In: Cancer in the young. Levine AS (ed). Masson, New York 405–460, 1982.
2. Elion GB, Callahan S, Nathan H et al.: Potentiation by inhibition of drug degradation: 6-substituted purines and xantine oxidanse. Biochem Pharmacol 12:85–93, 1963.
3. Coffey JJ, White CA, Lesk AB et al.: Effect of allopurinol on the pharmacokinetic of 6-mercaptopurine in cancer patients. Cancer Res 32:1283–1289, 1972.
4. Zimm S, Collins JM, O'Neill D, Chabner BA, Poplack DG: Inhibition of first-pass metabolism in cancer chemotherapy: interaction of 6-mercaptopurine and allopurinol. Clin Pharmacol Ther 34:810–817, 1983.
5. Wan SH, Hoffman DH, Azarnoff DL et al.: Effects of route of administration and effusione of methotrexate pharmacokinetics. Cancer Res 34:3487–3491, 1974.
6. Dixon RL, Henderson ES, Rall DP: Plasma protein binding of methotrexate and its displacement by various drugs. Fed Proc 24:454, 1965.
7. Mandel MA: The synergistic effect of salicylates on methotrexate toxicity. Plast Reconstruct Surg 57:733–737, 1976.
8. Reilly MJ: Drug information digest: methotrexate USP (amethopterin) and methotrexate sodium. Am J Hosp Pharm 30:542–548, 1973.
9. Hansten PD: Drug interactions. Lea and Febiger, Philadelphia, 1971.
10. Ziegler DG, Henderson ES, Hahn MA et al.: The effect of organic acids on renal clearance of methotrexate in man. Clin Pharmacol Ther 10:849–857, 1969.
11. Reich SD, Bachur NER: Alterations in adriamycin efficacy of phenobarbital. Cancer Res 36:3803–3806, 1976.
12. Conney AH, Schneidman K, Jacobson M et al.: Drug induced changes in steroid metabolism. Ann NY Acad Sci 123:98–109, 1965.
13. Field RB, Gang M, Kline I et al.: The effect of phenobarbital on 2-diethylaminoethyl-2-2-diphenylvalerate on the activation of cyclophosphamide in vivo. J Pharmacol Exp Ther 180:475–483, 1972.
14. Capizzi RL, Nichols R, Mullins J: Long-term survival of leukemic mice by therapeutic synergism between asparaginase and methotrexate. Fed Proc 31:553, 1972.
15. Capizzi RL: Improvement in the therapeutic index of methotrexate (NSC-740) by L-asparaginase (NSC-109229). Cancer Chemother Rep 6:37–41, 1975.
16. Capizzi RL: Schedule dependent synergism and antagonism between methotrexate and asparaginase. Biochem Pharmacol (Suppl 2) 23:151–161, 1974.

17. Yap BS, McCredie KB, Benjamin RS et al.: Refractory acute leukaemia in adults treated with sequential colaspase and high-dose methotrexate. Br Med J 2:791–793, 1970.
18. Lobel JS, O'Brien RT, McIntosh S et al.: Methotrexate and asparaginase combination chemotherapy in refractory acute lymphoblastic leukemia of childhood. Cancer 43:1089–1094, 1979.
19. Rodriguez V, Bodey GP, McCredie KB et al.: Combination 6-mercaptopurine-adriamycin in refractory adult acute leukemia. Clin Pharmacol Ther 18:462–465, 1975.
20. Pinkerton CR, Welshman SG, Glasgow JFT, Bridges JM: Can food influence the absorption of methotrexate in children with acute lymphoblastic leukemia? Lancet 2:944–946, 1980.
21. Riccardi R, Balis F, Ferrara P et al.: Influence of food intake on the absorption of orally administered 6-mercaptopurine (6-MP). Proc Am Soc Clin Oncol 4:34, 1985.

# 13. Potentiation of 6-mercaptopurine after time and dose-dependent pretreatment with methotrexate in malignant human T- and B-lymphoblasts

JOS P.M. BÖKKERINK, RONNEY A. DE ABREU,
MARINKA A.H. BAKKER and TILLY W. HULSCHER

## Introduction

The combination chemotherapy of methotrexate (MTX) and 6-mercaptopurine (6-MP) has been used for more than 20 years in the maintenance therapy of acute lymphoblastic leukemia (ALL). Although the bioavailability of both drugs after oral administration is very variable [4, 8] and – with respect to 6-MP – very limited [10], empirical studies proved the increased efficacy of the combination chemotherapy in the maintenance therapy of ALL [5].

No mention has been made in the literature with regard to the possible synergistic action of both drugs. Based on the biochemical interactions of both drugs and their effects on purine and pyrimidine metabolism, described below, we will show that this synergism can be anticipated in cells with an active purine de novo synthesis, depending on the sequence and dose of both drugs and on the enzymatic make-up of the cells.

MTX inhibits tetrahydrofolate dependent enzymes, which results in a thymidylate-less state in pyrimidine metabolism. In purine metabolism (see Figure 1) MTX inhibits two formyltransferases: glycinamide ribonucleotide (GAR) formyltransferase and aminoimidazolecarboxamide ribonucleotide (AICAR) formyltransferase. The result will be an inhibition of purine *de novo* synthesis with accumulation of phosphoribosylpyrophosphate (PRPP) [3]. The effect is also a purine-less state, which will be shown in the paper by De Abreu *et al.* (Chapter 14).

6-MP, which is a hypoxanthine analogue, is converted to thio-IMP by hypoxanthine-guanine-phosphoribosyl transferase (HGPRT), using PRPP as a cosubstrate. After further conversion 6-MP is incorporated into RNA and DNA as thioguanine nucleotides.

Preincubation of cells with MTX will result in an increased intracellular availability of PRPP. This can be used for enhanced intracellular uptake and conversion of 6-MP, when 6-MP is added to the cells at that point of time, when PRPP levels are maximal.

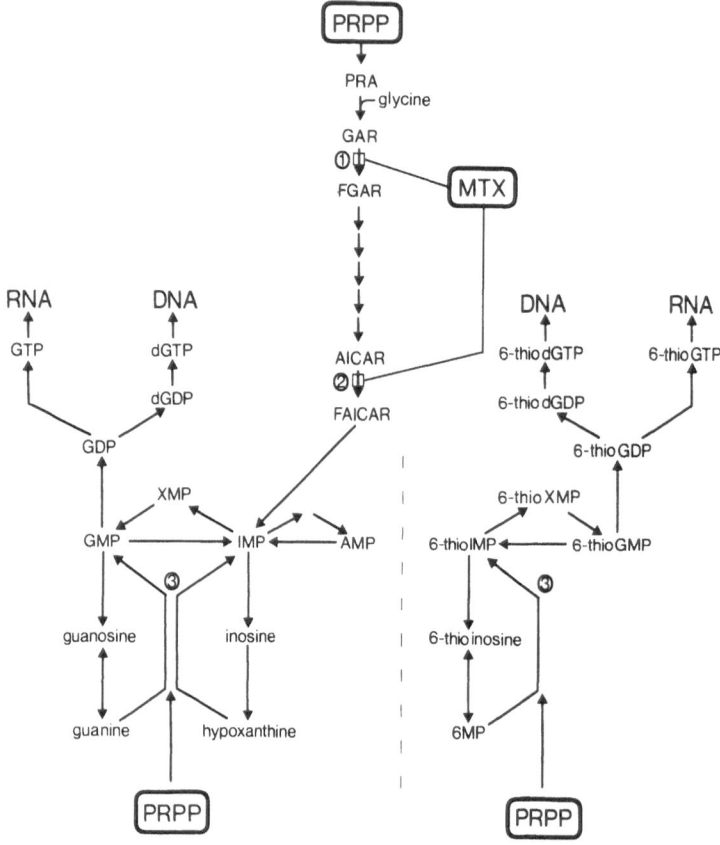

*Figure 1.* Simplified scheme of effects of MTX and 6-MP on purine metabolism. (1) glycinamide ribonucleotide formyltransferase; (2) aminoimidazolecarboxamide ribonucleotide formyltransferase; (3) hypoxanthine-guanine phosphoribosyltransferase.

## Methodology

MOLT-4 cells (T-lymphoblasts) and Raji cells (B-lymphoblasts) were allowed to grow at 37 °C in a water-saturated atmosphere containing 2.5 % $CO_2$ in RPMI Medium 1640 Dutch Modification, supplemented with 10 % fetal calf serum (v/v), sodium pyruvate, penicillin and streptomycin in plastic culture flasks. During the experiments glutamine was added every 24 h to a final concentration of approximately 2 mM. Logarithmically growing cells were suspended in fresh medium in a concentration of $0.3 \times 10^6$ cells/ml 24 h before each experiment. MTX was added to a final concentration of 0.02 μM and 0.2 μM, respectively.

The PRPP assay and incorporation of (8-$^{14}$C) 6-mercaptopurine will be published extensively elsewhere [2]. We modified the PRPP assay described by Peters and Veerkamp [7]. Incubations during 20 min with (8-$^{14}$C) 6-MP

PRPP

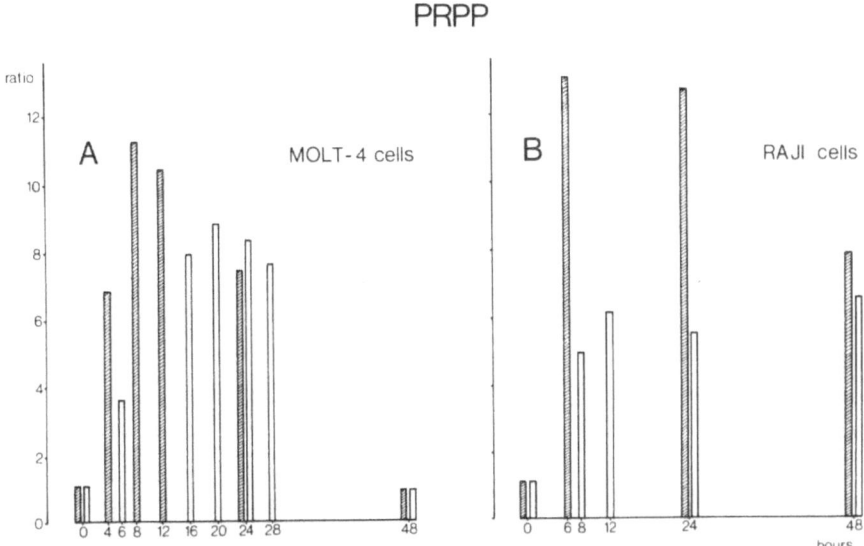

*Figure 2.* Effects of MTX on intracellular PRPP levels in malignant human lymphoblasts in culture. Cells were exposed at t = O to MTX and PRPP levels were determined. The results are expressed as the ratio of the concentration in MTX-treated/untreated cells at each point of time. (A) MOLT-4 cells; (B) Raji cells. Closed bars: 0.2 μM MTX; open bars: 0.02 μM MTX.

in a final concentration of 100 μM and 10 μM, respectively, were performed in aliquots of 0.5 ml of the cell culture at various intervals of time after incubation with MTX. The amounts of incorporated 6-MP in intact cells was determined according to a modified assay described by Müller *et al.* [6].

### Results and discussion

In the experiments, described below, incubations were performed with two concentrations of MTX: 0.02 μM and 0.2 μM. These concentrations were chosen, because they could be reached *in vivo* in patients receiving oral treatment with MTX [4].

The effects of MTX on intracellular PRPP levels in MOLT-4 cells and Raji cells are shown in Figures 2A and 2B, respectively. In MOLT-4 cells 0.2 μM MTX causes a rapid inhibition of purine *de novo* synthesis with accumulation of PRPP with a maximum at 8 h, followed by a decrease of PRPP levels to those of untreated cells at 48 h. In Raji cells this concentration of MTX causes an even more rapid accumulation of PRPP, which continues for a prolonged period of time. The lower concentration of MTX, 0.02 μM, results in a slower increase of PRPP with a maximum between 16

188

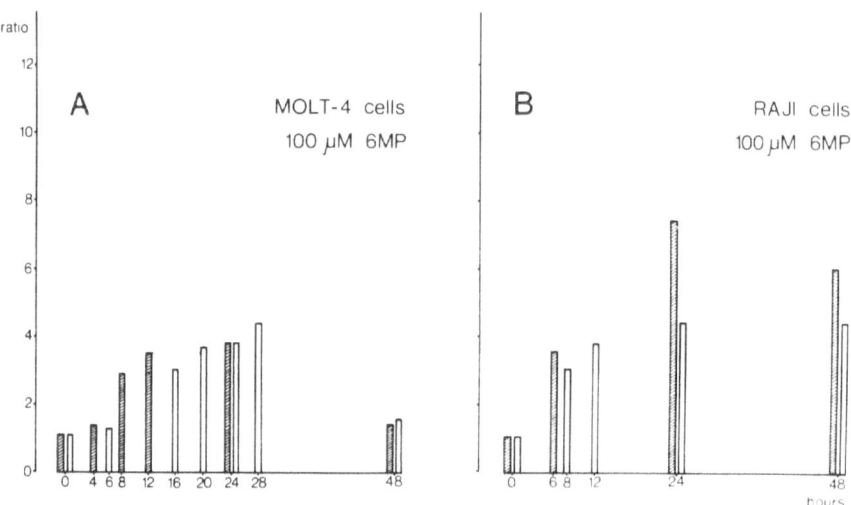

*Figure 3.* Effects of MTX on intracellular incorporation of 100 μM (8-$^{14}$C) 6-mercaptopurine in malignant human lymphoblasts in culture. Cells were exposed at t = O to MTX. at each point of time 0.5 ml of the cell suspension was incubated during 20 min with 100 μM (8-$^{14}$C) 6-mercaptopurine and intracellular incorporation was determined. The results are expressed as the ratio of the concentration in MTX-treated/untreated cells at each point of time. (A) Molt-4 cells; (B) Raji cells. Vlosed bars: 0.2 μM MTX; open bars: 0.02 μM MTX.

and 28 h in MOLT-4 cells, followed by a rapid decrease. Again, in Raji cells the increase of PRPP due to 0.02 μM MTX is more rapid in comparison with MOLT-4 cells and PRPP levels remain elevated.

The inhibition of purine *de novo* synthesis caused by 0.2 μM MTX is almost complete. This could be demonstrated by incorporation of radiolabeled glycine, a cosubstrate in the conversion of PRA into GAR (see Figure 1). In both MOLT-4 and Raji cells the incorporation of glycine at 24 h after incubation with 0.2 μM MTX was almost absent, indicating a complete inhibition of purine *de novo* synthesis, whereas 0.02 μM MTX did show incorporation of radiolabeled glycine, suggesting an incomplete inhibition of purine *de novo* synthesis due to the lower concentration of MTX. This could also be demonstrated by determination of AICAR (see Figure 1). In both cell lines 0.02 μM MTX resulted in elevated AICAR levels (data not shown), suggesting an incomplete inhibition of both formyltransferases. Moreover, there were differences between the two cell lines: AICAR levels in MOLT-4 cells were higher and decreased at 48 h, whereas AICAR levels in Raji cells were lower, but remained elevated in Raji cells. The differences between MOLT-4 and Raji cells with respect to the AICAR levels and to the prolonged accumulation of PRPP, shown in Raji cells in Figure 2B,

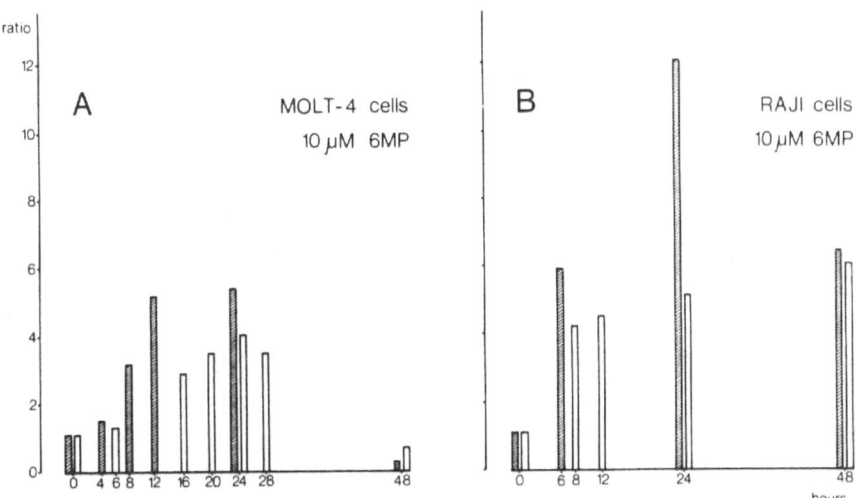

*Figure 4.* Effects of MTX on intracellular incorporation of 10 μM (8-$^{14}$C) 6-mercaptopurine in malignant human lymphoblasts in culture. See legend described in Figure 3. Incubations during 20 min were performed with 10 μM 6MP.

suggest that MTX causes a prolonged and more pronounced disturbance in cell metabolism of B-cells. This could be demonstrated also by a complete absence of dTTP levels in B-lymphoblasts after 24 and 48 h of incubation with both concentrations of MTX (see Chapter 14). These data may be importance in combination chemotherapy of MTX and 6-MP, as will be discussed below.

The increased availability of PRPP due to pretreatment with MTX can be used for enhanced incorporation of 6-MP.

At each point of time after pretreatment with MTX cells were incubated during 20 min with 100 μM 6-MP (Figure 3) and 10 μM 6-MP (Figure 4), respectively. Both figures demonstrate that the incorporation of 6-MP is increased after pretreatment with MTX. The enhanced incorporation of 6-MP follows the increase of PRPP levels, shown in Figure 2. Maximal incorporation of 6-MP is some hours later in comparison with the points of time, where maximal PRPP levels were reached. This could be due to competition of 6-MP with natural purine and pyrimidine bases in the medium.

Again the same differences between MOLT-4 and Raji cells can be demonstrated as were shown in the PRPP levels after incubation with MTX. The increase of 6-MP incorporation in Raji cells is more rapid and the incorporation remains elevated in comparison with MOLT-4 cells. Moreover, these charts demonstrate that 0.2 μM MTX results in earlier peak levels of 6-MP incorporation in comparison with the lower MTX concentration of 0.02 μM.

It should be emphasized that the concentrations of 6-MP used in our experiments, are much higher than those which can be reached in patients after oral administration of 6-MP [9, 10]. On the other hand, the incubations with 6-MP in our experiments lasted only 20 min, whereas the oral administration of the drug in patients causes prolonged exposure. This also resulted in prolonged bioavailability of 6-MP, measured by the presence of 6-MP in plasma during many weeks after cessation of chemotherapy in patients with ALL and suggesting an accumulation of the drug and its metabolites *in vivo* [9].

Our data indicate that a potentiation of 6-MP incorporation and cytotoxicity can be anticipated after pretreatment with MTX. A correlation is demonstrated between the concentration of MTX and the sequence and time dependency of 6-MP incorporation. Moreover, the potentiation is more pronounced in B-lymphoblasts. Our data may lift the veil of the increased efficacy of the combination chemotherapy of MTX and 6-MP in the maintenance therapy of ALL.

It should be stressed that the synergism of MTX and 6-MP will be more effective in malignant lymphoblasts with an active purine *de novo* synthesis. The activity of purine *de novo* synthesis is reflected in the PRPP levels of untreated cells. In normal peripheral blood lymphocytes and normal bone marrow cells the activity of purine *de novo* synthesis is low [1, 7] and we could not demonstrate an elevation of PRPP levels in normal peripheral blood lymphocytes after incubation with MTX. These data indicate that the synergism of 6-MP and MTX will be absent in these cells and that the potentiation of 6-MP by pretreatment with MTX is selective for malignant lymphoblasts with an active purine *de novo* synthesis.

Further studies in patients with ALL are mandatory, using prolonged infusions of MTX followed by prolonged infusions of 6-MP with a sequence of drug administration depending on that point of time where PRPP levels are maximal due to pretreatment with MTX.

## References

1. Becher H, Weber M, Lohr GW: Purine nucleotide synthesis in normal and leukemic blood cells. Klin Wschr 56:275–283, 1978.
2. Bökkerink JPM, bakker MAH, Hulscher MW, De Abreu RA, Laarhoven JPRM van, Schretlen EDAM, De Bruyn CHMM: Sequence, time and dose dependent synergism of methotrexate and 6-mercaptopurine in malignant human T-lymphoblasts. Submitted for publication.
3. Buesa-Perez JM, Leyva A, Pinedo HM: Effect of methotrexate on 5-phosphoribosyl 1-pyrophosphate levels in L1210 leukemia cells in vitro. Cancer Res 40:139–144, 1980.

4. Craft AW, Rankin A, Aherne W: Methotrexate absorption in children with acute lympho-blastic leukemia. Cancer Treat Rep 65(Suppl. 1):77–81, 1981.

5. Frei E III, Freireich EJ, Gehan E, Pinkel D, Holland JF, Selawry O, Haurani F, Spurr CL, Hayes DM, James GW, Rothberg H, Sodee DB, Rundles RW, Schroeder LR, Hoogstraten B, Wolman IJ, Traggis DG, Cooper T, Gendel BR, Ebaugh F, Taylor R: From the acute Leukemia Group B. Studies of sequential and combination antimetabolite therapy in acute leukemia: 6-mercaptopurine and methotrexate. Blood 18:431–454, 1961.

6. Müller MM, Pischek G, Scheiner O, Stemberger H, Wiedermann G: Purine metabolism in human lymphocytes. Blut 38:447–455, 1979.

7. Peters GJ, Veerkamp JH: Concentration, synthesis and utilization of phosphoribosylpyro-phosphate in lymphocytes of five mammalian species. Int J Biochem 10:885–888, 1979.

8. Pinkerton CR, Welshman SG, Glasgow JFT, Bridges JM: Can food influence the absorption of methotrexate in children with acute lymphoblastic leukemia? Lancet ii:944–946, 1980.

9. Schouten TJ, De Abreu RA, De Bruyn CHMM, Van Der Kleijn E, Oosterbaan JM, Schretl-en EDAM, De Vaan GAM: 6-Mercaptopurine: Pharmacokinetics in animals and prelimi-nary results in children. Adv Exp Med Biol 1658:367–370, 1984.

10. Zimm S, Collins JM, Riccardi R, O'Neill D, Narang PK, Chabner B, Poplack DG: Variable bioavailability of oral mercaptopurine. Is maintenance chemotherapy in acute lymphoblas-tic leukemia being optimally delivered? N Engl J Med 308:1005–1009, 1983.

# 14. The effect of methotrexate on purine and pyrimidine deoxyribonucleoside triphosphate pools and on cell viability and cell-phase distribution in malignant human T- and B-lymphoblasts

RONNEY A. DE ABREU, JOS P.M. BÖKKERINK,
MARINKA A.H. BAKKER, TILLY W. HULSCHER and
JOHN M. VAN BAAL

## Introduction

Methotrexate (MTX) and 6-mercaptopurine (6-MP) are widely used in the maintenance treatment of acute lymphoblastic leukemia (ALL) in children. Based on their biochemical interactions there are reasons to support a combination therapy of both drugs. MTX binds tightly to dihydrofolate reductase, the enzyme that catalyses the reduction of dihydrofolate to tetrahydrofolate. Tetrahydrofolate coenzymes are required for one-carbon transfer reactions in purine *de novo* synthesis and thymidylate biosynthesis (Figure 1). As a consequence a purine-less and a thymidylate-less state will occur, ultimately resulting in inhibition of DNA biosynthesis [1–10].

In response to the MTX-inhibition of the purine *de novo* synthetic pathway an increase in the availability of 5-phosphoribosyl-1-pyrophosphate (PRPP) occurs [11]. The subsequent interaction between MTX and 6-MP is dependent on the increased amounts of PRPP due to MTX (Figure 2). The rate limiting step in the intracellular uptake of 6-MP is apparently the formation of thioIMP by the enzyme hypoxanthine-guanine phosphoribosyltransferase in the presence of PRPP. Therefore, the increased intracellular concentration of PRPP, after MTX-treatment, is associated with an increased intracellular accumulation of 6-MP nucleotides (Figure 2).

In the previous paper (Chapter 13), we demonstrated this enhanced intracellular incorporation of 6-MP by pretreatment of malignant human T- and B-lymphoblasts. Therefore, from a clinical point of view there are reasons for investigating possible alterations of intracellular purine and pyrimidine metabolism by MTX under conditions by which potentiation of MTX on 6-MP incorporation occurs and to link the effects on purine and pyrimidine concentrations with effects on cell-phase distribution and cytotoxicity.

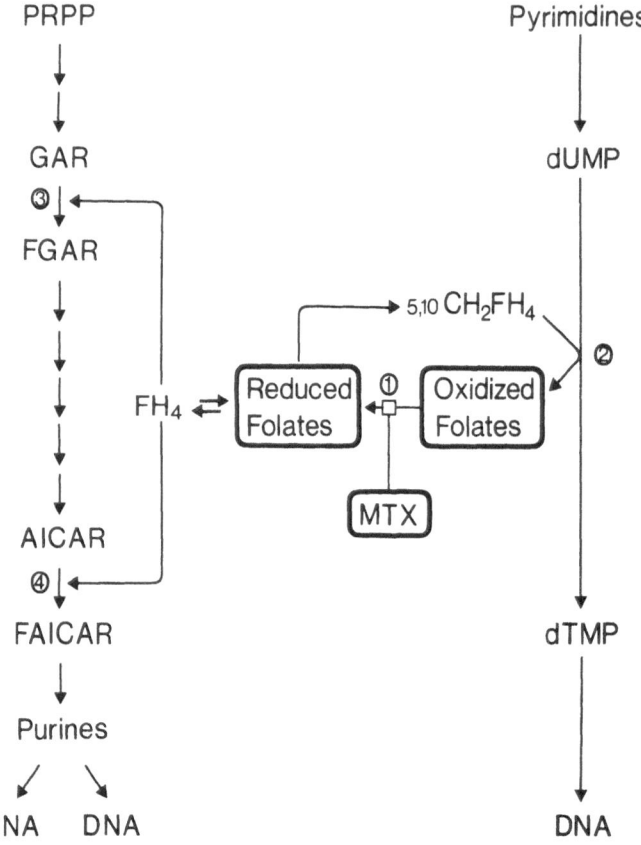

*Figure 1.* Schematic representation of the inhibition of purine *de novo* synthesis and thymidylate biosynthesis by methotrexate (MTX). (1) MTX inhibits dihydrofolate reductase; (2) the result of this inhibition is a depletion of tetrahydrofolates (reduced folates) that are required for the enzymes thymidylate synthetase; (3) GAR formyltransferase; (4) AICAR formyltransferase.

## Methodology

The experiments in MOLT-4 cells and Raji cells were carried out by exposing log phase cells to 0.02 µM and 0.2 µM MTX, respectively. The conditions for cell culture were described in the previous paper.

Experiments were designed to ascertain that the investigations for all data could be performed at the same time and that the results were comparable; e.g., measurements of PRPP, 6-MP incorporation, purine and pyrimidine nucleotide pools, flow cytometry, cell growth and cell viability, achieved from the same cell culture at various time-intervals after incubation with MTX. Purine and pyrimidine nucleotide concentrations were analyzed by high performance liquid chromatography [12]. Deoxyribonucleoside triphosphates were measured after periodate oxidation of ribonucleotides. Cell

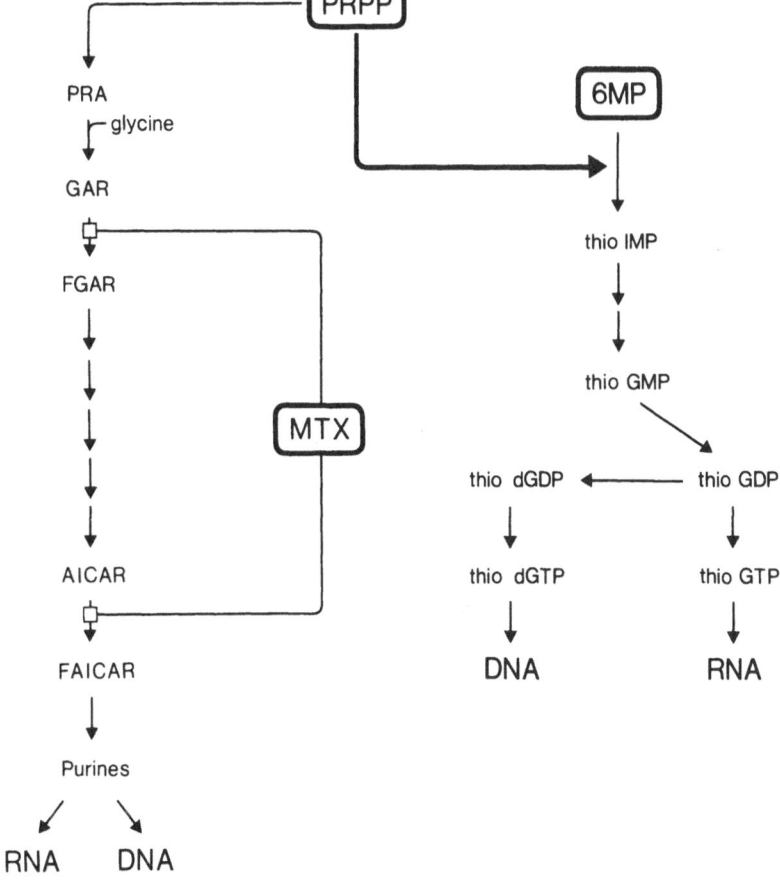

*Figure 2.* The schematic representation of potentiation of 6-mercaptopurine (6-MP) metabolism by methotrexate (MTX). Purine *de novo* synthesis is inhibited by MTX. This leads to increased levels of 5-phosphoribosyl-1-pyrophosphate (PRPP) which results in an enhancement of 6-MP metabolism.

viability was measured by Trypan blue exclusion. Flowcytometry studies were performed according to Hillen *et al.* [13].

## Results and Discussion

The various intracellular deoxyribonucleotides in MOLT-4 cells rapidly decrease when the cells are treated with 0.2 µM MTX (Figure 3). After treatment of MOLT-4 cells with 0.02 µM MTX, no significant decrease of dTTP and dGTP can be demonstrated. A clear decrease of dATP can be observed at 20 and 24 h with 0.02 µM MTX, followed by an increase at 28 h. Even more, treatment of MOLT-4 cells with 0.02 µM MTX results in

196

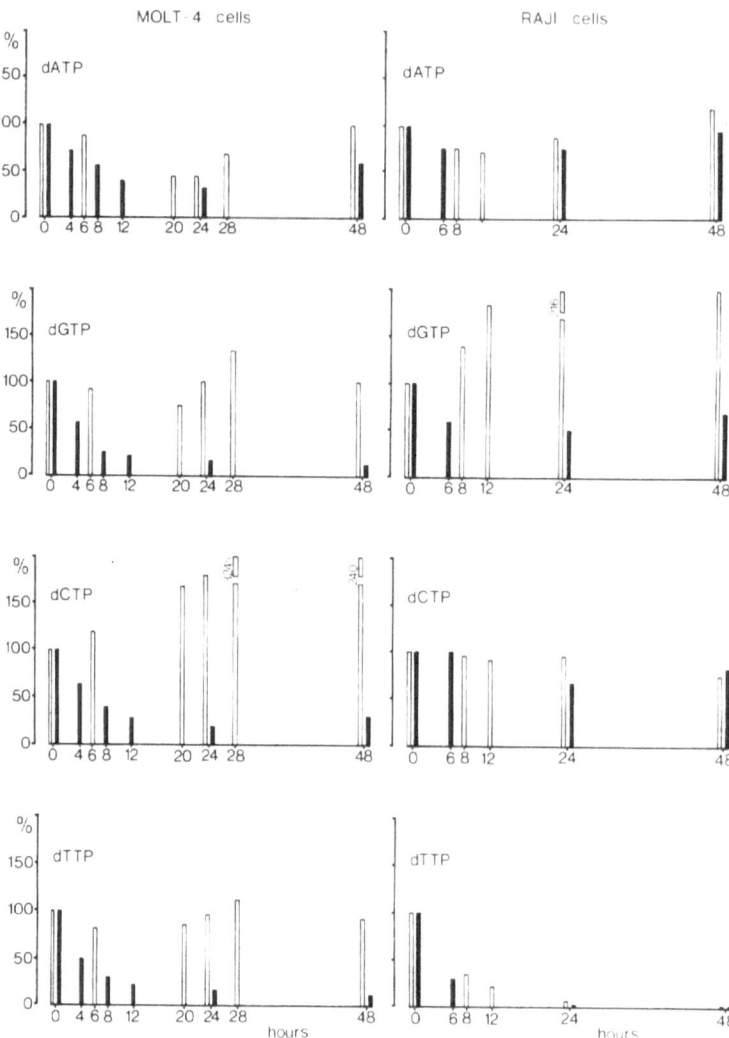

*Figure 3.* Effects of MTX on concentrations of dATP, dGTP, dCTP and dTTP in Molt-4 (left from top to bottom) and raji cells (right from top to bottom). Samples were taken at the indicated times, measured by high performance liquid chromatography and calculated (pmol/$10^6$ viable cells). In this figure the values from MTX-treated cells are expressed in percentage of untreated cells. Closed bars: after treatment with 0.2 µM MTX; open bars: after treatment with 0.02 µM MTX.

an enhancement of intracellular dCTP levels at 28 h to more than three-fold of untreated cells.

The explanation for the rapid decrease of dTTP after treatment of MOLT-4 cells with 0.2 µM MTX must be the maximal inhibitory effect of this MTX concentration on dihydrofolate reductase (Figure 1). Therefore, in response to the MTX-inhibition of this enzyme, the biosynthesis of dTLP and dTTP drops. As a consequence of the lack of replenishment of reduced folates, an inhibition of purine de novo synthesis also can be expected (Figure 1). The decrease of dTTP and purine *de novo* synthesis results ultimately in a decrease of DNA synthesis. Presumably, as a result of the decreased DNA synthesis other deoxyribonucleotide concentrations also are decreasing.

After treatment of MOLT-4 cells with 0.02 μM MTX the inhibition of dihydrofolate reductase is only partial and does not result in a decrease of dTTP levels. This is also reflected in a partial inhibition of purine *de novo* synthesis. Information obtained from data of $^{14}$C-glycine incorporation studies and from PRPP and amidoimidazolecarboxamide ribonucleotide (AICAR) measurements are consistent with these findings. Glycine is incorporated into the purine ring during formation of glycinamide ribonucleotide (GAR) from phosphoribosylamine (PRA) (Figure 2). In both MOLT-4 and Raji cells, with an active purine *de novo* synthesis, radiolabeled glycine can be incorporated by this route into purine nucleotides. After pretreatment for 24 h with 0.2 μM MTX, the $^{14}$C-glycine incorporation is completely inhibited in MOLT-4 cells and almost completely in Raji cells, indicating a complete inhibition of purine *de novo* synthesis. However, after pretreatment for 24 h with 0.02 μM MTX incorporation of radiolabeled glycine is still present suggesting that purine *de novo* synthesis is still active. Similar conclusions can be drawn from the PRPP and AICAR measurements in both cell lines. After preincubation with 0.2 μM MTX, in both cell lines, a rapid accumulation of PRPP can be observed, whereas after preincubation with 0.02 μM MTX a slow accumulation of PRPP and simultaneously of AICAR can be detected. Therefore, with 0.2 μM MTX the first formyltransferase: GAR formyltransferase is completely inhibited in both cell-lines (Figure 1), resulting in elevation of PRPP levels only. With 0.02 μM MTX, however, both formyltransferases, GAR formyltransferase and AICAR formyltransferase are partially inhibited, resulting in enhanced PRPP and AICAR levels.

The opposite effects of the low and the high concentrations of MTX on the dCTP pool in MOLT-4 cells can be explained looking at the effect of MTX on the cell-phase distribution. With 0.2 μM MTX the MOLT-4 cells are arrested in the late G1-phase, followed by a complete prevention of cell progression through the cell cycle, whereas with 0.02 μM MTX the cells are arrested predominently in the early S-phase (Figure 4). Accumulation of dCTP in early S-phase has been described earlier [14, 15] and these considerations seem to be confirmed with our findings that dCTP accumulates after pretreatment of MOLT-4 cells with 0.02 μM MTX and not with 0.2 μM MTX. In Raji cells no accumulation of dCTP is observed after treatment with 0.02 μM MTX, because the distribution of the cells shows an accumulation from late G1- to late S-phase (Figure 4).

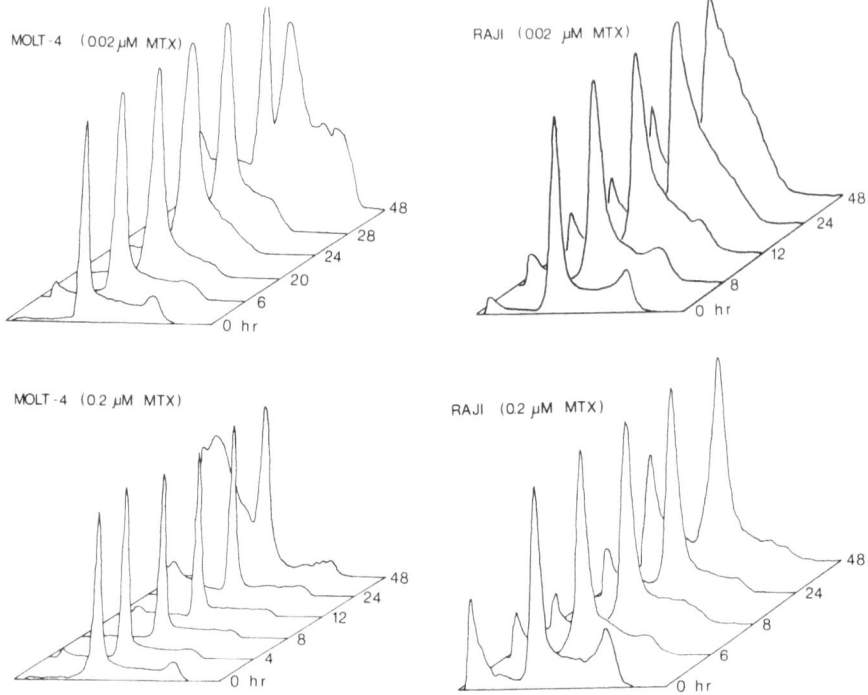

*Figure 4.* DNA histograms of MOLT-4 and Raji calls, before and at indicated times after addition of MTX. Top left: MOLT-4 cells with 0.02 μM MTX; bottom left: MOLT-4 cells with
0.2 μM MTX; top right: Raji cells with 0.02 μM MTX; bottom right: Raji cells with 0.2 μM
MTX.

The dTTP concentrations in Raji cells are more affected by 0.2 μM MTX
than in MOLT-4 cells. A rapid decrease can be observed in both cell-lines
within 6 h which is proceding in Raji cells (Figure 3). Pretreatment with
0.02 μM MTX significantly decreases dTTP synthesis in Raji cells, whereas
dTTP levels in MOLT-4 cells are not affected. These results indicate that
the inhibition of dihydrofolate reductase is more pronounced in Raji
cells.

The results from flowcytometry studies on Raji cells during treatment
with 0.2 μM MTX show a progressive decrease of cells in S-phase and
G2 + M-phase (Figure 4). However, cell proliferation is still present in Raji
cells. This is in contrast with the effects of MTX in MOLT-4 cells. As
mentioned before, treatment with 0.2 μM MTX causes an initial accumulation of MOLT-4 cells in G1, followed by a complete prevention of cell
proliferation. These differences may be explained by the differences in cell
cycle distribution of both cell lines. In untreated MOLT-4 cells the distribution is 60% G1, 32% S and 8% G2 + M, whereas this is in Raji cells:
45% G1, 40% S and 15% G2 + M. Therefore, Raji cells are metabolically

CELL VIABILITY

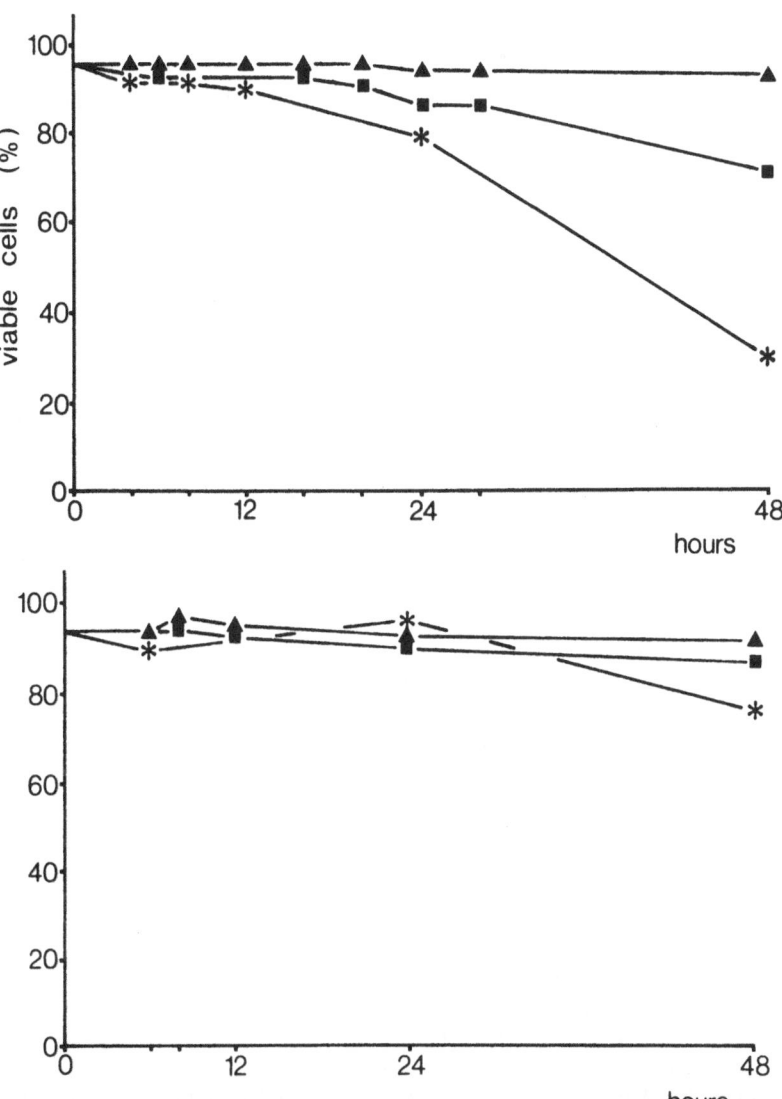

*Figure 5.* The viability of MOLT-4 (left) and Raji (right) Cells following Treatment with MTX. Triangles: untreated cells; squares: cells treated with 0.02 μM MTX; asterisks: cells treated with 0.2 μM MTX.

more active than MOLT-4 cells. This is in concordance with the findings that treatment with MTX causes a prolonged and more pronounced disturbance in cell metabolism in Raji cells, as shown before.

The differences between MOLT-4 and Raji cells are also reflected in the effects of MTX on cell-viability, measured by Trypan blue exclusion. Treatment with 0.2 μM causes a clear cytotoxic effect on MOLT-4 cells: at 48 h only 30% of the cells are viable, whereas in Raji cells 80% of the cells are viable (Figure 5).

In conclusion MTX exhibits a more cytotoxic effect on MOLT-4 cells, whereas Raji cells show a more profound biochemical disturbance. The more profound biochemical effects of MTX on Raji cells suggest that a more enhanced effect can be anticipated in B-cells in comparison to T-cell when 6-MP is administered after pretreatment with MTX. Moreover, the data of our floxcytometry studies indicate that 6-MP preferentially will be incorporated into RNA under these conditions.

## References

1. Sartorelli AC, Le Page GA: Amethopterin on the purine biosynthesis of susceptible and resistant TA3 ascites cells. Cancer Res 18:1336–1339, 1958.
2. Werkheiser WC: The biochemical, cellular and pharmacological action and effects of the folic acid antagonists. Cancer Res 23:1277–1285, 1963.
3. Borsa J, Whitmore GF: Studies relating to the mode of action of methotrexate. II. Studies in sites of action on L-cells in vitro. Mol Pharmacol 5:303–317, 1969.
4. Cohen SS: On the nature of thymidineless death. Ann NY Acad Sci 186:292–301, 1971.
5. Hryniuk WM: The mechanism of action of methotrexate in cultured L5178Y leukemia cells. Cancer Res 35:1085–1092, 1975.
6. Hryniuk WM, Brox LW, Henderson JF, Tamaoki T: Consequences of methotrexate inhibition of purine biosynthesis in L5178Y cells. Cancer TCancer Res 35:1427–1532, 1975.
7. White JC, Loftfield S, Goldman ID: The mechanism of action of methotrexate. III. Requirement of free intra-cellular methotrexate for maximal suppression of $^{14}$C-formate incorporation into nucleic acids and protein. Mol Pharmacol 11:387–297, 1975.
8. Moran RG, Mulkins M, Heidelberger C: Role of thymidylate synthetase activity in development of methotrexate cytotoxicity. Proc Natl Acad Sci USA 76:5924–5928, 1979.
9. Cha S, Kim SY, Kornstein SG, Kantoff PW, Im KH, Nagub FHM: Kinetic parameters of dihydrofolate reductase inhibited by methotrexate, an example of equilibrium study. Biochem Pharmacol 30:1507–1515, 1981.
10. Chabner BA: Methotrexate. In: Pharmacologic principles of cancer treatment. Chabner. Saunders, philadelphia, 229–255, 1982.
11. Buesa-Perez JM, Leyva A, Pinedo HM: Effect of methotrexate on 5-phosphoribosyl-1-pyrophosphate levels in L1210 leukemia cells in vitro. Cancer Res 40:139–144, 1980.
12. De Abreu RA, Van Baal JM, Bakkeren JAJM, De Bruyn CHMM, Schetlen EDAM: High-performance liquid chromatographic assay for identification and quantitation of nucleotides in lymphocytes and malignant lymphoblasts. J Chromatogr 227:45–52, 1982.
13. Hillen HFP, Wessels J, Haanen C: Bone marrow proliferation patterns determined by pulse photocytometry in acute myeloblastic leukemia. Lancet ii:609–611, 1975.
14. Skoog KL, Bjursell G, Nordenskjold BA: Cellular deoxyribonucleotide triphosphate pool levels and DNA synthesis. Adv Enzyme Regul 12:345–354, 1974.
15. Taylor IW, Slowiaczek P, Francis PR, Tattersall MHN: Biochemical and cell cycle pertubations in methotrexate-treated cells. Mol Pharmacol 21:204–210, 1983.

# 15. 7-Hydroxy-methotrexate production after methotrexate therapy

R. ERTTMANN

7-Hydroxy-methotrexate (7-OH-MTX) is the main metabolite following methotrexate (MTX) application in man. It is much less active as a dihydrofolic acid reductase inhibitor compared with the parent compound [1]. A hepatic aldehyde oxidase is assumed to be the converting enzyme.

A few reports focusing on the following questions have been published:

1. What are the characteristics of the serum elimination kinetics of 7-OH-MTX [2–7]?
2. Is there dependence on MTX dose of 7-OH-MTX production [5]?
3. May 7-OH-MTX production be enhanced by enzyme induction following repeated MTX drug cycles [4–6]?

In an effort to examine these questions, we investigated plasma levels of MTX and 7-OH-MTX by a sensitive highly specific reversed phase HPLC method ($C_{18}$-bondapak column $300 \times 4$ mm, $10\,\mu$; bicarbonate buffer ph7/15M/acetonitrile $= 95/5$; UV-detection 313 nm) in children and adolescents with osteosarcoma and leukemia.

## Results

1. 7-OH-MTX plasma elimination from 0 to 44 h after MTX infusion of 93 high dose drug cycles in 19 patients (12 g per $m^2$ MTX as 4 h infusion i.v.; alkaline diuresis, leukovorin rescue) was found to be *monophasic* with a mean $T_{1/2}$ of $5.5$ h (MTX $T_{1/2}$ of the first elimination phase in the same patient group 2.5 h).
2. As shown in Figure 1 peak levels of 7-OH-MTX in plasma are dependent on MTX dose administered. Saturation does not seem to be reached at a dose of 20 g per $m^2$ body surface area.
3. Following repeated high dose cycles we found a decreasing conversion from MTX to 7-OH-MTX. In Figure 2 the 7-OH-MTX/MTX ratio

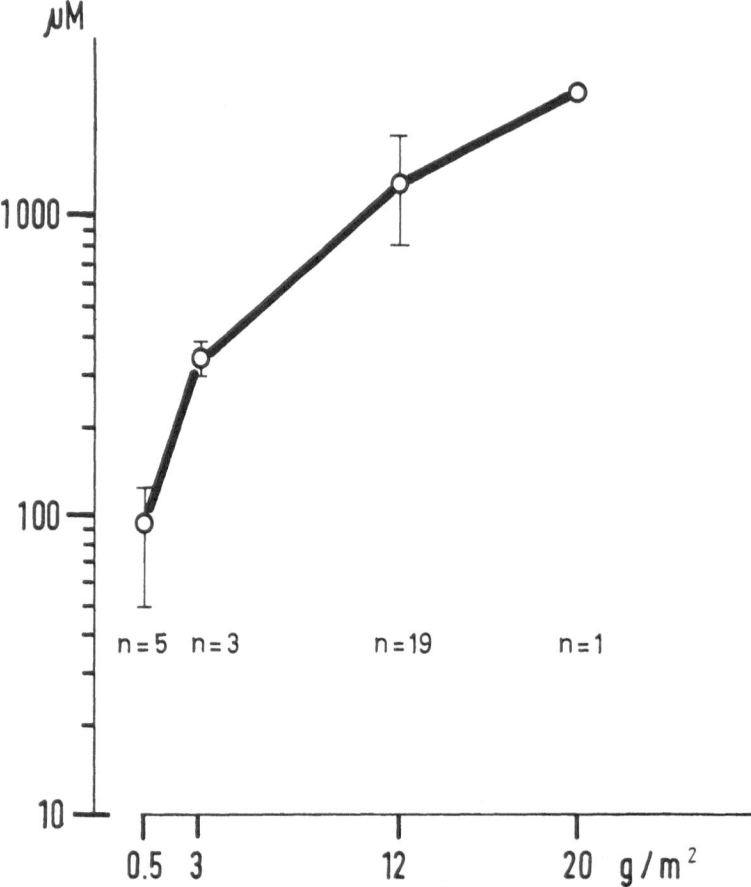

*Figure 1.* Dependence of 7-OH-MTX peak levels on MTX dose administered. The values are given as the mean ±SD of n patients.

obtained from the 12 h post infusion serum levels is shown. There is a significant decrease when the last (14th) value is compared with the first one in each patient undergoing our osteosarcoma protocol (Wilcoxon test, p = 0.01). As the MTX serum values were not different this result reflects decreasing 7-OH-MTX production.

## Conclusions

From our results it may be concluded that 7-OH-MTX is generated in appreciable amounts following MTX therapy. Its serum elimination follows first order kinetics in a monophasic fashion. This finding confirms the observations of Breithaupt *et al.* [2], Chan *et al.* [3], Lankelma *et al.* [4], Milano *et al.* [5], Stewart *et al.* [6] and is in contrast to the results of Wang

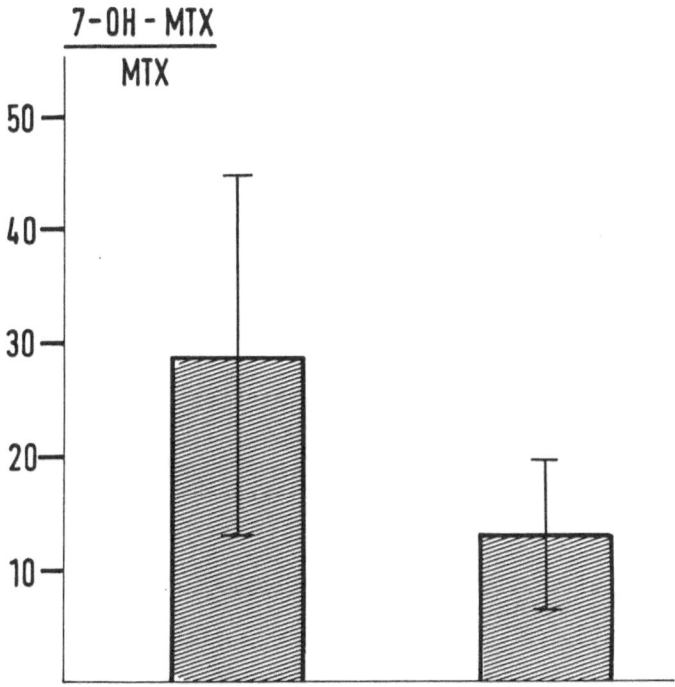

*Figure 2.* The molar quotient 7-OH-MTX/MTX 12 h after MTX infusion (12 g/m² over 4 h i.v.) is compared for the first and last (14th) drug cycle of our protocol. Values are given as the mean ±SD of 19 patients. The difference is significant according to the Wilcoxon test (p = 0.01).

*et al.* [7]. As the $T_{1/2}$ of 7-OH-MTX elimination is longer than that of the parent compound, after 12 h post infusion 7-OH-MTX levels are much higher than those of MTX.

The peak levels of 7-OH-MTX in serum are dependent on MTX dose. This observation confirms the findings of Milano *et al.* [5]. Up to a dose of 20 g/m² the converting enzyme system seems not to be saturated indicating low affinity/high capacity characteristics for the aldehyde oxidase system involved.

As 7-OH-MTX is 200-fold less active as a dihydrofolic acid reductase inhibitor its generation takes part in the detoxification of MTX after administration in man. It acts not only at the target enzyme dihydrofolic acid reductase but also has interacts with the intracellular uptake and polyglutamate formation of MTX [4, 8]. Therefore, our observation of reduced 7-OH-MTX production during consecutive MTX high-dose therapy – which may reflect cumulative hepatic toxicity – may be of clinical importance.

Additional prospective studies are needed to correlate not only MTX levels but also those of its metabolites with observed clinical toxicity as well as with effectiveness of high-dose MTX therapy.

# References

1. Farquhar D, Loo TL, Vadlamudi S: Synthesis and biological evaluation of 7-hydroxymethotrexate, 7-methylaminopterin and 7-methylmethotrexate. J Med Chem 15:567, 1972.
2. Breithaupt H, Kuenzlen E: Pharmacokinetics of methotrexate and 7-hydroxymethotrexate following high-dose methotrexate. Cancer Treat Rep 66:173, 1982.
3. Chan KK, Balachandran N, Cohen JC: Metabolism of methotrexate in man after high and conventional doses. Res Comm Chem Pathol Phamacol 28:551, 1980.
4. Lankelma J, von der Klein E: The role of 7-hydroxymethotrexate during methotrexate anticancer therapy. Cancer Lett 9:133, 1980.
5. Milano G, Thyss A, Renee N, Schneider M, Namer M, Bonseil JL, Lalanne CM: Plasma levels of 7-hydroxymethotrexate after high-dose methotrexate treatment. Cancer Chemother Pharmacol 11:29, 1983.
6. Stewart AL, Margison JM, Wilkinson PM, Lucas SB: The pharmacokinetics of 7-hydroxymethotrexate following medium-dose methotrecate therapy. Cancer Chemother Pharmacol 14:165–167, 1985.
7. Wang YM, Howell SK, Smith RG, Hosoya K, Benvenuto JA: Effect of metabolism on pharmacokinetics and toxicity of high-dose methotrexate therapy in children. Proc Am Soc Clin Oncol 20:334, 1979.
8. Fabre G, Matherly LH, Favre R, Catalin J, Cano JP: In vitro formation of polyglutamyl derivates of methotrexate and 7-hydroxymethotrexate in human lymphoblastic leukemia cells Cancer Res 43:4648, 1983.

# Late effects of chemotherapy

# 16. An overview of adverse late effects of cancer chemotherapy in children

W. ARCHIE BLEYER

## Introduction

It has been estimated that one in every 1000 individuals in the United States reaching their 21st birthday by the year 1990 will be a survivor of childhood cancer and its therapy [1]. As the cure rate increases, and as cancer chemotherapy in children is further intensified in an attempt to augment the cure rate, the potential problem of late adverse effects also increases. Epidemiologically, late effects – both real and potential – will require more and more of our time and attention as more and more children are cured of cancer.

## Adverse late effects of cancer chemotherapy

### Acute versus delayed toxicities

Because most anticancer agents are cycle dependent, their toxicities can be related in general to the proliferation kinetics of individual cell populations. Most susceptible are those tissues or organs with high cell turnover rates: bone marrow, gastrointestinal mucosa, spermatogonia, epidermidis, and liver. Hence it is these tissues that express most, and frequently all, of the *acute* toxicities of chemotherapy.

Least susceptible are those cells that do not replicate or replicate slowly, e.g. neurons, muscle cells, connective tissue and bone. Exceptions to this correlation appear to be the neurotoxicities of the vinca alkaloids, methotrexate and high-dose cytosine arabinoside, the osseous toxicity of methotrexate, and the cardiotoxicity of the anthracyclines. Moreover, injury to tissues with low repair potential often results in a long-lasting or permanent deficit.

*Children versus adults*

Children tolerate the acute toxicities of chemotherapy better than do adults. When expressed on a body weight or surface area basis, the maximally tolerated dose (MTD), is nearly always greater in children. Of 17 anticancer drugs which received phase 1 trials in both children and adults, for example, only three were found to have a higher MTD in adults than in children and the pediatric MTD of all three drugs was 83–90% of the MTD in adults. Thirteen of 14 remaining drugs had higher MTDs in children ranging from 120 to >220% of the MTD in adults [2].

The growing child may be more vulnerable than the adult patient to the *delayed* or *long-term* adverse sequelae of cancer chemotherapy. Just as the embryonic period of fetal development is the most susceptible to deleterious effects of drug exposure, so too the early phase of extra-uterine growth may be the most vulnerable period to the adverse late effects of cancer chemotherapy. Since antineoplastic agents possess the potential for adversely affecting normal tissue and developing organs years later, there is justifiable concern about deleterious effects of such processes on behavioral, psychological, neurologic, and intellectual functions; growth; endocrine status; fertility; teratogenic effects in offspring; second malignancies; etc. In this review I will summarize studies which have addressed this issue, with particular reference to critical target tissues in the growing child.

*Chemotherapy versus radiotherapy and other causes of late effects*

A major problem in evaluating chemotherapy-induced sequelae in children cured of cancer is that the etiology is often confounded by other factors, such as the effects of prior radiation or prior surgery, a genetic predisposition, environmental factors, and residual complications of the cancer itself. In long-term survivors of childhood cancer, the sequelae observed are often due to radiotherapeutic, surgical, genetic or disease-related factors rather than to the chemotherapy *per se*. In general, chemotherapy results in more acute and fewer late adverse effects, whereas with radiotherapy the reverse pattern is true. Hence, the sequelae observed are more often a result of the radiation that was administered rather than of the chemotherapy given [3–5].

Another primary problem is the time interval required for the adverse late sequelae to be expressed. This is particularly true for ionizing irradiation, but it also occurs with chemotherapy – albeit to a much lesser extent. We have yet to learn what today's chemotherapies, which in general utilize more drugs and more aggressive drug combinations than at any time in the past, will produce in the way of adverse late effects in the future.

*Late effects on growth*

Chemotherapy alone may produce an attenuation in linear growth, but the retardation is usually temporary and when the chemotherapy can be discontinued, growth is accelerated and the patient 'catches up' to his or her peers. Prednisone and methotrexate appear to mediate this effect, when given in a high enough dose or for a long enough, time by direct effect on bone growth (cf. section on Bone below). Growth arrest is nearly always symmetrical. Adverse effects of chemotherapy on neurodevelopmental function are outlined in the next section.

*Late effects on neurologic function*

In a cohort of 110 5-year survivors of childhood leukemia, the Late Effects Study Group observed that 21 (19%) had significant sequelae [1]. The most frequently occurring residua were those related to the CNS, with eight patients reported affected. Learning disability was noted in five, encephalopathy in two, and a seizure disorder in one patient. All of these children had received cranial radiation, 2,400 rad, and intrathecal methotexate for prevention of CNS leukemia, and 3 to 5 years of systemic chemotherapy. An example of a severe toxicity is necrotizing leukoencephalopathy. Nearly all of the cases reported have been in children, suggesting that the maturing brain is more susceptible to delayed sequelae [6].

Intelligence quotient (IQ) testing in children regarded cured of acute lymphoblastic leukemia has revealed consistent findings in several studies, whether retrospective [7, 8] or prospective [9], controlled [8, 9] or uncontrolled [7]: long-term survivors of acute lymphoblastic leukemia treated during childhood with cranial irradiation and intrathecal methotrexate have an observed average IQ 13 points lower than expected; and the IQ deficit is greatest in those patients who are the youngest when started on leukemia treatment [7–9].

The primary inciting factor in the pathogenesis of these deficits appears to be an adverse interaction between cranial irradiation and intrathecal methotrexate [6]. Contributing iatrogenic factors may include cerebral thrombosis and hemorrhage from L-asparaginase therapy [10]. In most instances it is impossible to quantitate which factor is the most contributory, although most investigators suspect that radiation is the primary etiology. Recently, a comparison between patients randomized to receive cranial radiation, 1,800 rad, and intrathecal methotrexate during maintenance has suggested that full- and performance-scale IQ and visual-motor integration are lower in the irradiated group (p<.05) and attention, concentration, and short-term memory are lower in the group treated with intrathecal methotrexate during maintenance (p<.10) [11].

In one study of adolescents with cancer histories, 51 % experienced cancer-related problems upon their return to school [12]. Most of the problems resulted from the attitudes and behavior of others, but some were the results of the cancer and its treatment. Nearly half experienced loss of friends, isolation, lack of motor coordination or speech impairment, and 43 % had to eliminate, reduce, or change participation in extra-curricular activities [12].

*Late effects on bone*

Osteopenia, osteoporosis, and temporary cessation of bone growth can be caused by methotrexate or steroids if administered in high doses for a prolonged period. Less commonly, bone pain, aseptic necrosis and pathologic bone fractures may occur with prolonged use of either drug. In 110 children with acute lymphoblastic leukemia who survived more than 5 years and received 3 to 5 years of weekly methotrexate, monthly 5-day pulses of prednisone, daily 6-mercaptopurine, and monthly injections of vincristine, only one had residual osteoporosis [1].

*Late effects on the heart*

Above cumulative doses of 550 mg/m$^2$, both daunomycin and adriamycin are more likely to induce congestive heart failure in children than in adults less than 40 years of age [13, 14]. In a study of 5,613 patients administered daunomycin, the congestive heart failure dose-response curve was steeper in 2,861 children than in 2,752 adults [13]. As with daunomycin, the cumulative threshold dose of adriamycin, below which congestive heart failure rarely occurs, is the same for children and adults. Above the threshold dose, however, patients less than 15 years of age are more likely to develop cardiomyopathy than patients older than 15 years [14].

*Late effects on the liver*

Chronic hepatic disease after cancer chemotherapy during childhood is a rare sequelae [1, 15]. Of 369 5-year survivors of childhood cancer, only two were found by the Late Effects Study Group to have evidence for chronic liver disease [1]. Only one of the 110 5-year survivors of acute lymphoblastic leukemia whose therapy was described above had chronic liver disease [1].

*Late effects on the kidney*

In seven children completing 3 or more years of maintenance therapy for acute lymphoblastic leukemia, renal biopsies revealed only mild toxic effects, which were not associated with elevated blood urea nitrogen or serum creatinine levels [15]. Children are also more likely than adults to recover from the nephrotoxicity of high-dose methotrexate and cisplatin (A. Bleyer, unpublished observations).

*Late effects on gonadal function*

Chemotherapy-induced gonadal dysfunction depends on the age and sex of the patients when the drugs are used, on the dose of the agent, and on the nature of the drug. Alkylating agents such as cyclophosphamide, nitrogen mustard, and busulfan are the drugs most commonly incriminated in gonadal failure. In general, prepubertal boys and girls seem relatively resistant to the effects of chemotherapy, and of combination chemotherapy [16, 17]. The prepubertal girl is clearly less susceptible to these effects than the pubertal or postpubertal woman. The former usually have normal reproductive function after chemotherapy is stopped, whereas the latter may have ovarian failure in as many as 50–60%, when treated with cyclophosphamide, for example [5]. Recovery of ovarian function is not uncommon, but who will and who will not recover is difficult to predict [5].

In a study of 44 boys who were previously treated with combination chemotherapy for acute lymphoblastic leukemia, Shalet and his colleagues observed that with one exception all patients had a normal testosterone response to stimulation with human chorionic gonadotropin, indicating that Leydig-cell function was intact [18]. Subsequent follow-up of these boys has confirmed normal pubertal development in many instances [19]. In a study by Blatt and her coworkers, normal gonadal development was observed in 14 boys with ALL who had been treated for 3 to 11 years with average cumulative doses of vincristine 80 mg/m$^2$, prednisone 40,000 mg/m$^2$, methotrexate 2,000 mg/m$^2$, and 6-mercaptopurine 60,000 mg/m$^2$ [16]. Each demonstrated normal Tanner staging, LH, FSH and testosterone levels throughout the course of follow-up, from 0.2 to 8.5 years and an average of 5 years after discontinuation of chemotherapy [16]. A group in Argentina studied 17 boys after 2 to nearly 6 years of chemotherapy for ALL; in 14 the evaluation included bilateral testicular biopsies [20]. All were prepubertal at the time of diagnosis. Serum testosterone response to human chorionic gonadotropin, intratesticular testosterone concentrations, and the number of germ cells were normal in nearly all patients.

Both germ-cell and Leydig-cell dysfunction can occur, however, in adolescents *during* chemotherapy [17] and improve after chemotherapy is completed [20]. The probability of improvement does not appear to be related to the duration or total dose of therapy [5]. Two of three boys with ALL who had impaired spermatogenesis during chemotherapy subsequently developed normal sperm counts [20]. Gynecomastia as a manifestation of Leydig-cell dysfunction has been associated with alkylating agents, procarbazine, vincristine and nitrosoureas. Procarbazine, mechlorethamine and other alkylating agents are exceptions to the generalization that adverse gonadal effects are reversible. With these agents, gonadal dysfunction may persist [17].

*Teratogenic effects*

To date, the most comprehensive study of fetal effects is the experience reported by Blatt *et al.* on behalf of the United States National Cancer Institute [21]. Twenty-eight children were born to 30 (23 females and 7 males) of 418 patients previously administered intensive chemotherapy at a childbearing age. Prenatal exposures included vincristine in 24, prednisone in 16, methtrexate in 12, cyclophosphamide in 11, 6-mercaptopurine in seven, nitrogen mustard in seven, adriamycin in seven, procarbazine in six, cytosine arabinoside in five, daunomycin in four, a nitrosourea in three and 6-thioguanine in two. Spontaneous abortions were reported in only two pregnancies. Of the 23 females, 19 conceived 1 month to 9 years (median 4 years) after all chemotherapy was stopped, and four became pregnant while on chemotherapy (two during the first 2 months of gestation; one during the second trimester, one during the third trimester). All 28 live births were normal term infants who have had normal growth and development during a median follow-up of 2.5 years. One child has had uncomplicated febrile seizures. No major abnormalities were observed. Minor anomalies were detected in three infants; capillary nevus, pilonidal dimples without spinal bifida, and congenital hip dysplasia [21].

*Oncogenic late effects*

The Late Effects Study Group (LESG) has now registered 292 childhood cancer victims who later developed a second malignant neoplasm [22]. Only 11 (5.5%) had no known genetic predisposition to cancer and had received only chemotherapy such that radiation could not be invoked as an etiologic agent [1]. Only 12 children with acute lymphoblastic leukemia or acute undifferentiated leukemia followed by a second malignant neoplasm have been registered [22]. Two-thirds of the second malignant neoplasms (208/292) developed in a tissue that had been previously irradiated, and one-third (96/292) had certain diseases associated with a predisposition to malignancy (for example, retinoblastoma, neurofibromatosis, xerodermapigmentosa, and nevoid basal cell carcinoma cell syndrome), or had siblings with childhood cancer. In addition, no obvious cause for the development of a second cancer was noted in 5% of the victims (14/292), as they were treated with neither radiotherapy or chemotherapy, and neither their history nor clinical presentation suggested that they might have a predisposition to a malignant disease. Only 49 (17%) had received only chemotherapy for treatment of their primary cancer such that radiation could not be invoked as an etiologic agent. Of these, the majority had a known genetic or familial predisposition to cancer. Hence, only approximately 5% of the 292 children who developed a second cancer were treated with chemotherapy and not radiotherapy, and had no known genetic or familial predisposition.

Moreover, all but two of the 49 patients treated with chemotherapy alone (regardless of other predisposing factors), had been treated with one or more alkylating agents, usually either cyclophosphamide, nitrogen mustard, procarbazine, or a nitrosourea. One patient received vincristine only and another received methotrexate only. The latter patient develop a hepatic tumor in a liver that had undergone chronic pathological changes after 4 years of methotrexate therapy [22]. Because cirrhosis is not an uncommon precursor of hepatocellular carcinoma [23] and methotrexate has been established in clinical studies and laboratory trials not to be a carcinogen, it is probable that the drug was not directly responsible for this patient's cancer. Only 13 children with leukemia followed by a second malignant neoplasm have been reported to the LESG [22]. In the LESG compilation, the most common tumor after acute leukemia was non-Hodgkin's lymphoma or another leukemia [22].

In another report, however, brain tumors were the most common second malignant neoplasm after acute lymphoblastic leukemia. Nine of 11 children with acute lymphoblastic leukemia developed a second neoplasm, and nine of these were brain tumors [24]. All of these children were treated on a single protocol which included cranioradiotherapy, 2,400 rads, in addition to intrathecal methotrexate and three years of systemic chemotherapy. Lifetable analysis of these patients projects a 2–4% incidence of brain tumors within 5 years after completing 3 years of chemotherapy [24]. On balance, however, chemotherapy-induced neoplasms do not appear to be a major late effect of cancer chemotherapy administered during childhood, the vast majority being attributable to radiation, or to familial or genetic factors.

## Conclusion

In conclusion, children generally tolerate both the acute and late effects of cancer chemotherapy better than adults. Exceptions are the neurotoxic sequelae of methotrexate (at least in conjunction with irradiation of the brain) [6], and anthracycline-induced cardiomyopathy [13, 14]. Nonetheless, safer chemotherapeutic regimens are needed, provided that the excellent results currently being achieved with the curative therapies of childhood cancer are maintained. Whether the new drugs, drug combinations and multimodal therapies can be administered without increasing the late effects remains to be ascertained. While continuing surveillance is paramount, delayed tragedies have, on balance, detracted minimally from the current triumphs of cancer therapy in children – at least to date. The potential and real benefits of current chemotherapy are well worth the potential risks, provided that they are applied as skillfully and judiciously as possible.

In order to decrease the potential risk of late effects in as many children as possible, accurate staging systems should be developed in each form of cancer, and each child should be assiduously staged such that therapy can be minimized in those patients with a good prognosis, and the risks of combination therapy be directed to those patients with a poor prognosis. New drugs, more intensive forms of chemotherapy, and chemoradiotherapy combinations should be applied to those subgroups of each malignancy which have the worse prognosis, in whom the risks are more than justified. Accurate staging systems should be developed in each cancer of childhood in order to accomplish this objective and maintain an acceptably low incidence and severity of adverse late effects.

## References

1. Meadows AT, Krejmas NL, Belasco JB: The medical cost of cure. Sequelae in survivors of childhood cancer. In: Status of the curability of childhood cancers. Van Eys, Sullivan M (eds). Raven Press, New York, 263–272, 1980.
2. Glaubiger D, von Hoff DD, Holcenberg JS, Kamen B, Pratt C, Ungerleider RS: The relative tolerance of children and adults to anticancer drugs. Front Radiat Ther Onc 16:42–49, 1982.
3. Byrd RL: Late effects of treatment of cancer in children. Pediatr Ann 12:450–460, 1983.
4. D'Angio GJ: Late sequelae after cure of childhood cancer. Hosp Prac 15:109–121, 1980.
5. Mulne A, Koepke JC: Adverse effects of cancer therapy in children. Pediatrics in Review 6:259–268, 1983.
6. Bleyer WA, Griffin TW: White matter necrosis, mineralizing microangiopathy, and intellectual abilities in survivors of childhood leukemia; associations with central nervous system irradiation and methotrexate therapy. In: Radiation damage to the nervous system. Gilbert, Kagan (eds). Raven Press, New York, 115–174, 1980.
7. Eiser C: Intellectual abilities among survivors of childhood leukaemia as a function of CNS irradiation. Arch Dis Childh 53:391–395, 1970.

8. Moss HA, Nannis ED, Poplack DG: The effects of prophylactic treatment of the central nervous system on the intellectual functioning of children with acute lymphocytic leukemia. Am J Med 71:47–52, 1981.

9. Meadows AT, Massari DJ, Fergusson J, Gordon J, Littman P, Moss K: Declines in IQ scores in children with acute lymphocytic leukaemia treated with cranial irradiation. Lancet 2:1015–1018, 1981.

10. Priest JR, Ramsay NKC, Latchaw RR, Lockman LA, Hasegawa DK, Coates TD, Coccia PF, Edson JR, Nesbit ME, Krivit W: Thrombotic and hemorrhagic strokes complicating early therapy for childhood acute lymphoblastic leukemia. Cancer 46:1548–1554, 1980.

11. Tamaroff M, Salwen R, Miller DR, Murphy ML, Nir Y: Comparison of neuropyschologic performance in children treated for acute lymphoblastic leukemia with 1800 rads cranial radiation plus intrathecal methotrexate or intrathecal methotrexate alone. Proc Am Assoc Clin Oncol 3:198, 1984.

12. Zwartjes WJ: Education of the child with cancer. Proc Natl Conf on the case of the Child with Cancer. Am Cancer Soc, New York, 150–155, 1978.

13. Hoff DD von, Rozencweig M, Layard M, Slavik M, Muggio FM: Daunmomycin induced cardiotoxicity in children and adults. Am J Med 62:200–208, 1977.

14. Hoff DD von, Layard MW, Basa P, Davis HL, Hoff AL von, Rozencweig M, Muggio FM: Risk factors for adriamycin-induced congestive heart failure. Ann Intern Med 91:710–717, 1979.

15. Mahoney DH, Gonzales ET, Ferry GD, Sanjad SA, Noorden GK van, Fernbach DJ: Systemic side effects of chemotherapy in children with acute leukemia in long term remissions. Blood (Suppl 1) 54:196, 1979.

16. Blatt J, Poplack DG, Sherins RJ: Testicular function in boys after chemotherapy for acute lymphoblastic leukemia. New Engl J Med 304:1121–1124, 1981.

17. Sherins RJ, Olweny CLM, Ziegler JL: Gynecomastia and gonadal dysfunction in adolescent boys treated with combination chemotherapy for Hodgkin's disease. New Engl J Med 299:12–16, 1978.

18. Shalet SM, Hann IM, Lendon M, Morris Jones PH, Beardwell CG: Testicular function after combination chemotherapy in childhood for acute lymphoblastic leukaemia. Arch Dis Childh 56:275–278, 1901a.

19. Shalet SM, Lendon M, Morris Jones PH: Testicular function after chemotherapy for acute lymphoblastic leukemia. New Engl J Med 305:518, 1981b.

20. Pasqualini T, Sackmann-Muriel F, Chemes H, Pavlovsky S, Domene H, Rivarola MA: Evaluation of testicular function following longterm treatment for acute lymphoblastic leukemia. Am J Pediat Hemat Oncol 5:11–20, 1983.

21. Blatt J, Mulvihill JJ, Ziegler JL, Young RC, Poplack DG: Teratogenicity of cancer chemotherapy. Am J Med 69:828–832, 1980.

22. Meadows AT, Baum E, Fossati-Bellani F et al.: Second malignant neoplasms in children: An update from the Late Effects Study Group. J Clin Oncol 3:532–538, 1985.

23. Lack EE, Neave C, Vawter GF: Hepatocellular carcinoma: Review of 32 cases in childhood and adolescence. Cancer 52:1510–1515, 1983.

24. Albo V, Miller D, Leiken S, Sather H, Hammond: Nine brain tumors as a late effect in children 'cured' of acute lymphoblastic leukemia from a single protocol study. Proc Am Soc Clin Oncol 4:000, 1985.

25. Mike V, Meadows AT, D'Angio GJ: Incidence of second malignant neoplasms in children: Results of an international study. Lancet 2:1326–1331, 1982.

26. Tucker MA, Meadows AT, Boice JD, Hoover RN, Fraumeni JF (for the Late Effects Study Group): Cancer Risk following treatment of childhood cancer. In: Radiation Carcinogenesis: Epidemiology and biological Significance. JD Boice, JF Fraumeni (eds). Raven Press, New York, 211–224, 1984.

# 17. Focusing on late effects in long-term survivors of childhood leukemia and lymphomas

L. MASSIMO, M.L. GARRE, S. GANDUS, B. CESANA,
R. HAUPT, B. DE BERNARDI, A. COMELLI, E. CASARI,
C. QUERCI, M. COTELLESSA, P. CORNAGLIA,
A. FERRANDO, G.F. GARGANI, G. STELLA, M.L. VITALI
and
A. PELIZZA

## Introduction

Major advances have occurred in the treatment of children with cancer, leading to a high percentage of cure especially in Acute Lymphoblastic Leukemia (ALL), Hodgkin's disease (HD) and non-Hodgkin's Lymphomas (NHL). The remarkable improvement in the prognosis of childhood malignancies has been achieved with the use of combined modalities of treatment [1–4]. Consequently pediatric oncologists are now dealing with an increasing number of long-term survivors of these diseases and with their emerging treatment sequelae [5–9]. Late toxicity attributable to surgery (S) and radiotherapy (RT) is better known than that produced by chemotherpay (CT) or multimodal treatment [10, 11]. The frequency of long-term consequences of antineoplastic drug treatment in the pediatric age group is unknown. In addition there is little information regarding the relationships between their severity and the dose, schedule and duration of therapy [12]. Appropriate investigation of possible late sequelae must include a detailed evaluation of a number of organ systems including the cardiopulmonary, endocrine, hematopoetic, immune, musculoskeletal and central nervous systems [13].

In this study a group of 130 patients who are long-term survivors of childhood leukemias and lymphomas, diagnosed between 1962–1982, were evaluated for late sequelae. The clinical research was performed between February 1983 – September 1984. The main aims of this study were: to obtain detailed information regarding quality of life; to record any relevant medical problems which occurred after the discontinuation of treatment; to evaluate growth and pubertal development; and to assess psychological, immune, cardiopulmonary and musculoskeletal function. We have attempted to correlate our findings with the type of treatment administered. The ultimate goal of this type of study is to provide pediatric oncologists with information which might be of value in selecting less toxic modalities of therapy for children with cancer.

## Materials and methods

This study involved a group of subjects previously affected by Acute Leukemia (AL) and Lymphoma. To be eligibile for evaluation patients must have been in disease-free remission for a minimum of 2½ years from discontinuation of treatment.

One hundred and forty-eight patients were eligible for study; 130 could be properly evaluated (87.8%). The 18 (12.2%) patients who refused to be examined are not included in this study. The status of children with malignancies followed in our Institution from 1962 to 1982 is reported in Table 1.

Table 2 summarizes the diagnoses of the 130 evaluated cases, divided according to sex. The ages at onset and at the time of study are reported in Figure 1; the intervals from discontinuation of treatment ranged between 2½ and 26 years. Table 3 shows the distribution of cases according to the time from cessation of therapy.

The study included:

1. Collection of data regarding desease characteristics (clinical course, acute complications, duration etc.) and treatment (dose, fields, fractionation of radiotherapy; dose and schedule of drugs; type of surgery) by review of the medical records either directly or by correspondence with cooperating hospitals;

*Table 1.* Status of children with malignancies diagnosed at IGG between 1962 and 1982.

|  | No. cases |
|---|---|
| — Total diagnoses | 873 |
| — Long-term survivors | 330 |
| — Deaths occurring in long-term survivors | 5 (1.5%) |
| — Long-term survivors from leukemia and lymphomas | 148 |

*Table 2.* Initial diagnosis by sex in 130 long-term survivors from leukemia and lymphomas.

| Disease | M | F | Total |
|---|---|---|---|
| ALL | 29 | 28 | 57 |
| AnLL | 2 | 4 | 6 |
| NHL | 17 | 8 | 25 |
| HD | 30 | 12 | 42 |
| Total | 78 | 52 | 130 |

*Table 3.* Interval from discontinuation of treatment of 130 long-term survivors of leukemia and lymphoma.

| Years from discontinuing therapy | No. cases |
| --- | --- |
| 2½– 3 | 13 |
| 3– 4 | 41 |
| 4– 5 | 19 |
| 5– 6 | 12 |
| 6– 7 | 17 |
| 7– 8 | 3 |
| 8– 9 | 12 |
| 9–10 | 3 |
| 10–26 | 10 |

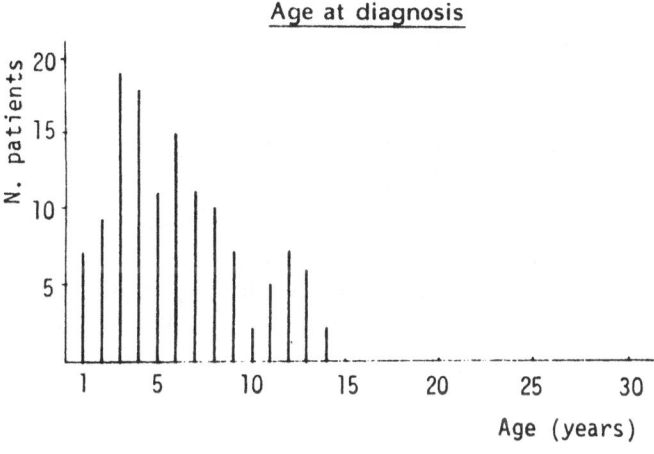

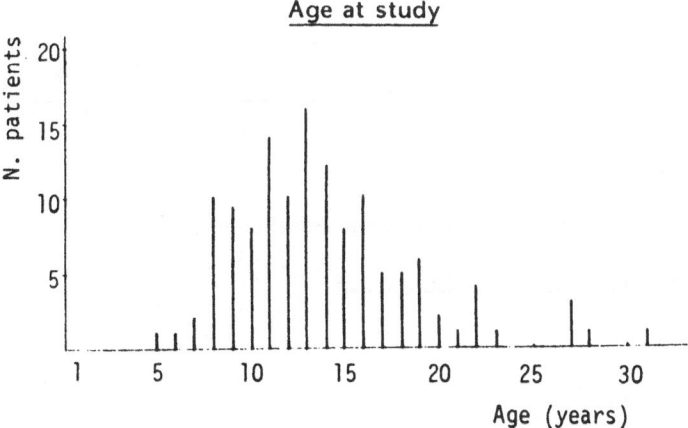

*Figure 1.* Age at diagnosis and age at study of patients evaluated for late effects of treatment.

2. Evaluation of quality of life (education, occupation and marital status) and detailing of any serious diseases, operations, or second tumors which occurred after discontinuation of treatment; all patients had a detailed physical examination;

3. All eligible patients received the following specific studies:
   a. endocrinological evaluation: height evaluation (compared with age standardized growth curves (Tanner's method) [14] and with mid-parental percentile); evaluation of growth velocity and pubertal development (specific hormone levels were tested only if the above evaluation suggested clinical abnormalities);
   b. psychological evaluation: (1) tests for emotional and affective aspects (Harter's Perceived Competence Scale for Children [15], Cattel's 16 Personality Factors and Children's Personality Questionnaire [16, 17], Koch's Baum Test [18], Bellack's Childhood Apperception Test [19]; (2) neuropsychological functions (Raven's Pregressive Matrices [20], Corsi's Block Tapping Memory Test [21], Wechsler's Intelligence Scale for Children, Wechsler's Adult Intelligence Scale [22]; (3) social and family life (Semistructured Interview);

4. Immunological evaluation: (1) clinical evaluation including detailed patient history (regarding frequency and severity of infections, allergy, reumatologic disorders, etc.); (2) laboratory evaluation (including complete blood count, detemrinate lymphocyte subpopulations, serum protein electrophoresis and immunoglobulin levels);

5. Selected groups of patients received the following studies:
   a. evaluation of cardiac function was performed in 122 patients who received anthracyclines and/or cardiac irradiation. They were eva-

Table 4. Severe diseases, operations and second tumors after discontinuation of treatment in 130 study patients.

|  | No. cases |
| --- | --- |
| Transient bone marrow aplasia | 1 |
| Chronic liver disease | 2 |
| Cardiac disease | 3 |
| Major operations (cystectomy, laparotomy for intestinal obstruction, hydrocele) | 5 |
| Skin tumors (basal cell carcinoma, histiocytoma) | 2 |
| Amenorrhea | 2 |
| Acquired cataract | 4 |
| Monolateral blindness | 1 |
| Hearing impairment | 3 |
| Total | 23 |

luated clinically and by noninvasive tests including electrocardiogram (EKG), M-mode echocardiogram (ECHO) and chest X-ray. Cases with abnormal findings were subsequently followed at regular intervals;

b. Evaluation of pulmonary function was performed in 47 patients who received radiotherapy to the lungs (mantle, mediastinal, lung irradiation or total body irradiation (TBI). They were evaluated by chest X-ray and by pulmonary function tests including lung volumes, capacities, forced expiratory volume (spirometry); flow volume loops (Lung Function Analyzer + XY Recorder) and arterial blood gases (oxymeter) [23, 24]. Cases with abnormal findings were subsequently followed at regular intervals;

c. Orthopedic evaluation was performed in 57 cases who received RT to the skeleton; evaluation included physical examination and radiographs if clinical abnormalities were present. The physical examina-

Table 5. Physical examination of 130 long-term survivors from leukemia and lymphomas.

|  | No. cases |
|---|---|
| Skin | |
| Keloid scars | 8 |
| Hyperpigmentation | 3 |
| Alopecia/hair fragility | 3 |
| Skeletal and muscular system | |
| Muscle hypotrophy or atrophy | 28 |
| Structural chest abnormality | 19 |
| Limb length discrepancy | 5 |
| Hip joint motion limitation | 1 |
| Scapular hypoplasia | 1 |
| Head and neck | |
| Microphthalmia and retinal atrophy | 1 |
| Tympanic retraction | 1 |
| Chronic dental and gum disease | 17 |
| Head or face assymmetry | 4 |
| Gonads and endocrine system | |
| Hydrocoele | 1 |
| Gynecomastia | 1 |
| Others | |
| Obesity | 10 |
| Hepatomegaly | 7 |
| Lower limb edema | 2 |
| Splenomegaly | 1 |
| Limping | 1 |

tion included estimating and grading of soft tissue atrophy, scoliosis, kyphosis, limb length discrepancy and epiphyseal changes;
5. Pertinent examinations for patients presenting specific complaints (e.g. cataracts, hearing loss, chronic liver disease, etc.).

All information collected from the analysis of individual cases, were reported in patient record forms, suitable for data managing by computer.

## Results

### General findings

Twenty-four subjects were more than 18 years old: six were married (25%); one had a child. The occupational level of these patients appeared consistent with the status found in a similar age-related group of normals.

Medical problems arising in the groups of long-term survivors are listed in Table 4. Physical examination was normal in 47/130 cases (36%), with minor abnormalities in 32/130 (24%). In 51 subjects (39%) significant residual abnormalities were present (Table 5).

*Table 6.* Growth velocity of prepubertal long-term survivors from leukemia and lymphomas.

| Sex | Normal | Progressive decrease | Total cases |
|---|---|---|---|
| Males | 28 | 3 | 31 |
| Females | 12 | 1 | 13 |
| Total | 40 | 4[a] (9.3%) | 44 |

[a] All cases detected after the beginning of treatment.

*Table 7.* Height evaluation of post-pubertal long-term survivors of leukemia and lymphoma.

| Sex | Normal | Abnormal | Total cases |
|---|---|---|---|
| Males | 20 | 2 | 22 |
| Females | 29 | 1 | 30 |
| Total | 49 | 3[a] (5.6%) | 52 |

[a] Below the 3rd centile and not related to parents' height.

*Disturbances of organ function*

*Growth velocity and height evaluation*
Prepubertal subjects at time of the study were evaluated for growth velocity (Table 6).

Post-pubertal subjects were evaluated for actual height percentile position, considering this as definitive, and compared with both parents and mid-parental percentile position (Table 7).

Subjects in pubertal phase (20 M, 9 F) were excluded, considering the characteristic pubertal growth spurt.

*Pubertal development*
Tables 8 and 9 show pubertal events for evaluable males and females, respectively.

*Central nervous system and behaviour*
Analysis of consciousness showed good psychological adjustment as revealed by the self esteem questionnaires. Projective tests exploring deep uncon-

*Table 8.* Pubertal development of male long-term survivors of leukemia and lymphoma.

|  | No. cases |
| --- | --- |
| Onset |  |
| Evaluable | 47 |
| Normal | 45 |
| Below normal | 2 (4.2%) |
| Completion |  |
| Evaluable | 23 |
| Normal | 21 |
| Below normal | 2 (8.6%) |

*Table 9.* Pubertal development of female long-term survivors of leukemia and lymphoma.

|  | No. cases |
| --- | --- |
| Onset |  |
| Evaluable | 37 |
| Normal | 36 |
| Hormone-therapy induced | 1 (2.7%) |
| Completion |  |
| Evaluable | 30 |
| Normal | 30 |

scious feelings pointed out ego difficulties including, self deficiency aware-ness and the use of ego defense mechanisms such as rigidity and obsessive-ness (Tables 10 and 11).

*Table 10.* Personality assessment of 130 long-term survivors of leukemia and lymphoma.

| | Subjects assessed | | ALL patients vs. control | | |
|---|---|---|---|---|---|
| | No. | Age | | | |
| Projective technique Baum test | 75 | 6–15 | Normal 20% | Slightly pathological 65% | Markedly pathological 15% |
| Self-esteem assessment PCSC | 66 | 8–14 | Overesteem in cognitive competence $X^2 = 7.32$ $p < 0.05$ | Overesteem in physical competence $X^2 = 10.49$ $p < 0.05$ | Overesteem in global competence $X^2 = 7.85$ $p < 0.05$ |
| Anxiety level CPQ 16 PF | 102 | 8–12 >13 | Overanxious in Q3 factor $X^2 = 7.41$ $p < 0.05$ | | Overanxious in Q4 factor $X^2 = 6.66$ $p < 0.05$ |

*Table 11.* Personality assessment of 130 long-term survivors of leukemia and lymphoma.

| | Subjects assessed | | Acute leukemia vs. HD | Age at diagnosis <6 yrs vs. >6 yrs | Duration of treatment <3 yrs vs. >3 yrs |
|---|---|---|---|---|---|
| | No. | Age | | | |
| Projective technique baum test | 75 | 6–15 | No difference | Worse when >6 $X^2 = 7.03$ $p < 0.05$ | Worse when >3 $X^2 = 8.75$ $p < 0.05$ |
| Self-esteem assessment PCSC | 66 | 8–14 | HD overresteem in physical competence $X^2 = 6.81$ $p < 0.05$ | No difference | No difference |
| Anxiety level CPQ 16 PF | 102 | 8–12 >13 | No difference | Subjects >6 yrs old More anxious $X^2 = 7.51$ $p < 0.05$ | No difference |

All subjects showed an abnormal trend in IQ levels. A selective damage in short-term amnestic functions was revealed in the eligible patients assessed, when compared with the control group (Tables 12 and 13).

A more complete analysis was performed on survivors subdivided in subgroups which received a similar treatment. This analysis pointed out that the cluster of children treated with intrathecal chemotherapy and cranial irradiation were responsible for this result. There was generally good acceptance in 75% of long-term survivors among their school peers and in their workplace (Table 14).

*Table 12.* Neuropsychological assessment of 130 long-term survivors of leukemia and lymphoma.

| | Subjects assessed | | ALL patients vs. control |
|---|---|---|---|
| | No. | Age | |
| IQ level<br>  PM  47<br>  PM  38 | 129 | >4 | No difference |
| Verbal fluency<br>  WISC voc.<br>  Wechs voc. | 122 | >4 | Better results than control<br>$X^2 = 10.49 \, p < 0.05$ |
| Memory corsi | 103 | >4 | Worse results than control<br>Subtest fwd $X^2 = 6.45 \, p < 0.05$<br>Subtest bkw $X^2 = 26.46 \, p < 0.01$ |

*Table 13.* Neuropsychological assessment of 130 long-term survivors of leukemia and lymphoma.

| | Subjects assessed | | Acute leukemia vs. HD | Age at diagnosis <6 yrs vs. >6 yrs | Duration of treatment <3 yrs vs. >3 yrs |
|---|---|---|---|---|---|
| | No. | Age | | | |
| IQ level<br>  PM  47<br>  PM  38 | 129 | >4 | No difference | No difference | No difference |
| Verbal fluency<br>  WISC voc.<br>  Wechs voc. | 122 | >4 | Acute leukemia better than HD<br>$X^2 = 6.81 \, p < 0.05$ | No difference | No difference |
| Memory corsi | 103 | >4 | No difference | No difference | No difference |

Evaluation of the family environment revealed that parents were anxious and overprotective of off-therapy subjects and siblings. Sibling rivalry and jealousy appeared to follow prolonged parental detachment. School achievement was declared adequate in 32% and optimal in 54% of subjects. School achievement results probably reflect the overprotective behaviour of both teachers and parents (Table 14).

## Immunological system

The frequency of infections (viral or bacterial) following discontinuation of treatment was higher in long-term survivors from HD. One case (HD)

Table 14. Social behaviour of 130 long-term survivors from leukemia and lymphoma (see text for details).

|  | Inadequate | Adequate, sufficient | Optimal – excellent |
|---|---|---|---|
| Peer's acceptance | 25% | 56% | 19% |
| Parent/child interaction | 44% | 46% | 10% |
| School achievement | 14% | 32% | 54% |

Table 15. Peripheral blood cells and lymphocyte subpopulations in 130 long-term survivors of leukemia and lymphoma.

| Disease | Leuko-penia | Lympho-penia | Granulo-cytopenia | ↓ T lymphocytes | ↓ B lymphocytes |
|---|---|---|---|---|---|
| ALL (56 cases) | 1 | 9 | 8 | 7 | 6 |
| AnLL (6 cases) | – | 1 | 2 | – | – |
| NHL (25 cases) | 6 | 2 | 10 | 5 | 5 |
| HD (42 cases) | 1 | 3 | 9 | 8 | 1 |
| Total (129 cases) | 8 (6.2%) | 15 (11.6%) | 29 (22.4%) | 20 (15.5%) | 12 (8.3%) |

Table 16. Immunoglobulin levels in 130 long-term survivors of leukemia and lymphoma.

| Disease | $\gamma\downarrow$ Glob. | ↓ IgG | ↓ IgA | ↓ IgM |
|---|---|---|---|---|
| ALL (56 cases) | 1 | 5 | 3 | 4 |
| AnLL (6 cases) | – | – | – | – |
| NHL (25 cases) | – | 3 | 3 | 3 |
| HD (42 cases) | 3 | 6 | 2 | 6 |
| Total (129 cases) | 4 (3%) | 14 (10.8%) | 8 (6.2%) | 14 (10.8%) |

experienced severe bone marrow aplasia after a viral infection. Data from laboratory studies are reported in Tables 15 and 16.

*Heart*

The frequency of cardiac impairment according to different diagnostic tests and by diagnosis is reported in Table 17.

The characteristics of the ECHO abnormalities detected and their correlation with therapy are shown in Table 18.

Figure 2 represents the frequency of ECHO abnormalities in three subgroups of patients who received different doses of anthracyclines.

*Table 17.* Cardiac evaluation of 122 study patients who received anthracyclines and/or cardiac irradiation.

| Disease | No. cases | ECG changes | ECHO changes | ECG+ECHO changes + clinical findings |
|---------|-----------|-------------|--------------|--------------------------------------|
| AL | 60 | — | 6 | 2 |
| NHL | 22 | — | 5 | — |
| HD | 40 | — | 6 | 1 |
| Total | 122 | — | 17 (14%) | 3 (2.4%) |

*Table 18.* ECHO changes and correlation with previous therapy in 122 long-term survivors of leukemia and lymphoma.

| ECHO abnormalities | Total anthracyclines (mg/m$^2$) | | | Cardiac Irradiation (32 pts) | Combined therapy (21 pts) | Total |
|---|---|---|---|---|---|---|
| | <250 (18 pts) | 250–400 (28 pts) | >400 (23 pts) | | | |
| LV ↑ | — | 3 | 1 | 2 | — | 6 |
| Hypokinetic IVS | 1 | — | 1 | 1 | — | 3 |
| LPEP/LVET ↑ | — | — | 2 | — | — | 2 |
| RPEP/RVET ↑ | 1 | — | — | 1 | — | 2 |
| PE | — | 1 | — | 1 | — | 2 |
| CMP dil. | — | — | 2 | — | — | 2 |
| Paradoxic IVS | — | — | — | 1 | — | 1 |
| LV ↑, LA ↑ | 1 | — | — | — | — | 1 |
| RV ↑ | — | — | — | 1 | — | 1 |
| Hypokinetic IVS, LV ↑, LA ↑ | — | — | — | — | 1 | 1 |
| Total | 3 | 4 | 6 | 7 | 1 | 21 |

LV = left ventricle; IVS = interventricular septum; LA = left atrium; RV = right ventricle; LPEP = left pre-ejection period; LVET = left ventricular ejection time; RPEP = right pre-ejection period; RVET = right ventricular ejection; PE = pericardial effusion.

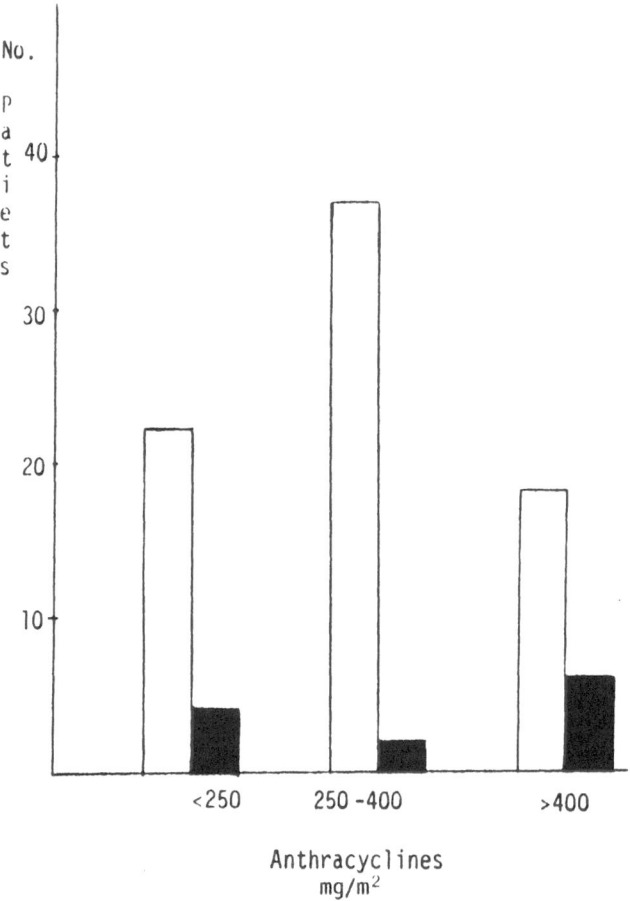

*Figure 2.* ECHO abnormalities correlated with anthracycline doses in 122 long-term survivors of leukemia and lymphoma; □ absent, ■ present.

## Lung

Interstitial lung changes detected by chest X-ray were seen as late sequelae of radiation therapy.

Pulmonary dysfunction of a restrictive type was detected in two subjects. They were not associated with clinical symptoms (Table 19).

## Musculoskeletal system

Orthopedic changes were slight or moderate and rarely required a specific treatment (Table 20). Previous treatment was correlated with these musculoskeletal defects as follows:

Dose:    Consistent bone and/or muscle abnormalities were observed in children who received >3,500 rads of radiation.

*Table 19.* Pneumologic evaluation of 47 study patients who received radiotherapy to the lung(s).

| Disease | No. cases | Restrictive thoracic morphology | x-ray changes | Respiratory function changes |
|---|---|---|---|---|
| ALL | 3 | — | — | — |
| AnLL | 1 | — | 1 | — |
| NHL | 6 | 1 | 5 | 1 |
| HD | 37 | 3 | 26 | 1 |
| Total | 47 | 4 | 32 | 2 |

*Table 20.* Musculoskeletal residual defects in 57 study patients who received RT to the skeleton.

| Disease | No. cases | Soft tissue hypotrophy | Scoliosis Kyfosis Kypho-scoliosis | Limb length discrepancy | Epiphyseal changes |
|---|---|---|---|---|---|
| AL | 5 | — | 1 | 1 | 1 |
| NHL | 13 | 3 | 5 | 3 | — |
| HD | 39 | 12 | 14 | 4 | — |
| Total | 57 | 15 (25.3%) | 20 (35%) | 8 (12.2%) | 1 (1.7%) |

Volume: Hypotrophy of soft tissues, abnormal spinal curvature and limb length discrepancy were correlated with sites of radiotherapy and volume irradiated.

Age: Children under 5 years at diganosis developed significantly more bone and/or muscle abnormalities compared with older children.

## Discussion

The efforts of pediatric oncologists treating children with acute leukemia and lymphoma have led to a dramatic improvement in survival rates. For this reason more attention has recently focused on the consequences of treatment.

This study allowed us to gather the population of our patients who are long-term survivors. Clinical examination was performed in the majority of our patients (87.8%).

The presence of a group of long-term survivors from the early years of pediatric oncology was useful to compare late effects in older versus more recent schedules of therapy.

More severe sequelae were observed in the first group: pericarditis related to high doses of mediastinal irradiation, cystectomy due to hemorrhagic cystitis consequent to prolonged administration of cyclophosphamide, sterility secondary to ovarian irradiation, severe soft tissue atrophy and second tumors.

The analysis of psychological function showed that long-term survivors from cancer could be considered 'out of crisis' subjects [25]. We observed the behaviour of the patient group both in social and family life in order to assess possible adjustment problems. The data showed paradoxically that a prolonged duration of treatment produced a better adjustment than a shorter one.

In spite of selective damage in memory function, general performance was well balanced, as attested by the optimistic evaluation of school achievement (Table 14).

Self-esteem, assessed by direct interview of survivors and questionnaires, appears to be above the normal level [26]. In contrast, a more complete analysis using indirect prospective techniques, revealed unconscious fear, anxiety, negative projections and a low self-esteem in a number of patients. Our data suggest the need for psychological support for the entire population of long-term survivors of malignancies suffered in childhood, particularly in groups treated with short or aggressive schedules [27].

Several factors combined in different modalities (cranial irradiation, intrathecal therapy, prolonged chemotherapy, age at treatment) represent a potential risk to growth and pubertal development of children treated for acute leukemia and lymphomas [28–30]. Endocrinologic investigation in our study, generally showed normal growth and development in most of cases.

Perhaps individual sensitivity to treatment or the disease itself was responsible for those prepubertal and two post-pubertal subjects who underwent a decrease of linear growth rate. The course of puberty was normal in all females, the only exception being one girl who received ovarian irradiation.

Delay in beginning puberty occurred in two males. In one of these cases there was a family history of pubertal delay. Delay in pubertal onset occurred in two males in whom the onset of puberty occured 2 and 5 years respectively from the time of discontinuation of treatment whether the delays were treatment related or not is unclear.

The immunological studies demonstrated dysfunction only in long-term survivors of Hodgkin's disease. These patients had a high frequency of infections. The higher risk of this group appears to be related to splenectomy and to a decreased level of T-lymphocytes, known accompaniments of this disease.

The long-term toxicity of anthracycline drugs and/or cardiac irradiation used in childhood cancer remains undefined [31–33]. In our group of long-term survivors from acute leukemia and lymphomas 84.2% of cases did not present clinical or subclinical cardiac sequelae.

Subclinical ECHO abnormalities were detected in 17 cases (14%) and in three of them they disappeared at follow-up. Three subjects (2.4%) suffered from severe cardiac disease. One boy died 4 years after discontinuation of treatment from cardiac failure.

Cardiotoxicity due to antrhacyclines was related to the cumulative dose of drug. The significant changes observed in patients treated with low doses, suggest an individual sensitivity to anthracyclines [34].

Patients treated with mediational radiotherapy alone showed an increased risk with doses of radiation over 3,000 rads [35, 36]. The future cardiac status of subjects with clinical and subclinical sequelae remains guarded [33, 37].

Pneumological evaluation pointed out a considerable discrepancy between the radiographic evaluation and pulmonary function tests. Interpretation of this data should be cautious considering the fact that the interstitial lung changes on X-ray were minimal in all cases [38].

Residual defects in the musculoskeletal system were found mostly in Hodgkin's disease survivors. Though rarely requiring a specific treatment they significantly affected the image and self-esteem of these subjects.

In conclusion it appears that relatively few of our long-term survivors of acute leukemia and lymphoma demonstrated major abnormalities. The majority of these patients enjoy a good quality of life. However, the finding of several subclinical abnormalities (e.g. cardiac studies) indicate the need for continuing surveillance of this population.

Finally, most of our subjects appear to have generally favorable acceptance among their peers at school and in the workplace and to be coping satisfactorily with their late effects.

### Acknowledgements

This study was supported by the A.I.R.C. (Italian Cancer Research Association). We are grateful to the doctors, nurses and secretaries who helped us to accomplish this research.

# References

1. Van Eys J, Sullivan MP: Status of the curability of childhood cancer. Raven Press. New York, 1980.
2. Kaplan HS: Hodgkin's disease. Harvard University Press, Cambridge, 1980.
3. Wollner N, Burchenal JH, Lieberman PH, Exelby P, D'Angio GJ, Murphy ML: Non Hodgkin's lymphoma in children. Cancer 37:123–134, 1976.
4. Chessells JM: Acute Lymphoblastic Leukemia. Seminars in Hematology 19:155–171, 1982.
5. Meadows AT, D'Angio GJ: Late effects of cancer treatment: methods and techniques for detection. Seminars in Oncology 1:87–89, 1974.
6. D'Angio GJ: Complications of treatment encountered in lymphoma-leukemia long-term survivors. Cancer 42:1015–1025, 1970.
7. Li FP, Myers MH, Heise HW, Jaffe N: J Ped 93:185–187, 1970.
8. Li FP, Stone R: Survivors of cancer in childhood. Ann Int Med 84:551–553, 1976.
9. Pastore G, Antonelli R, Fine W, Li FP, Sallan SE: Late effects of treatment of cancer in infancy. Med Ped Onc 10:369–375, 1982.
10. Trott KR: Chronic damage after radiation therapy: challenge to radiation biology. Int J Rad Onc Biol Phys 10:907–913, 1984.
11. Rubin P: The Franz Buschke lecture: late effects of chemotherapy and radiation therapy: a new hypothesis. Int J Rad Onc Biol Phys 10:5–34, 1983.
12. Schein FS, Winokur S, Macdonald JS, Wooley PV: Long-term survivors complications of cytotoxic and immunosuppressive chemotherapy. In: Cancer Medicine. Holland J, Frei E (eds). Lea & Febiger, Philadelphia, 1982.
13. Philips TL, Fu KK: Acute and late effects of multimodal therapy on normal tissues. Cancer 40:489–494, 1977.
14. Tanner GH: Growth at adolescence. Blackwell Scientific Publications, Oxford, London, Edinburgh, Melbourne, 1973.
15. Harter S: The perceived competence scale for children. Child Development 53:87–97, 1982.
16. Cattel RB: Questionario dei 16 fattori della personalità '16 PF Test', form C. Manuale supplementare. Ed. O.S. Firenze, 1963.
17. Porter RB, Cattel RB: Questionario di personalità per regazzi. Manuale O.S. Firenze, 1981.
18. Koch K: Il reattivo dell'albero. Manuale O.S. Firenze, 1959.
19. Abt C, Bellak L: Projective psychology. Knoff, New York, 1950.
20. Valseschini S, Delton F: Le matrici progressive di Raven. Manuale O.S. Firenze, 1973.
21. Bisiach E, Danes F, Derenzi E, Faglioni P, Gianotti g, Pizzamiglio L, Spinnler HR, Vignolo LA: Neuropsicologia clinica. Franco Angeli Milano, 1977.
22. Blasser AJ, Zimmermann JL: Clinical interpretation of the Wechsler intelligence scale for children. Grune & Stratton, New York and London, 1967.
23. Benoist JR: Esploration functionelle pulmonaire en pediatrie. Flammation, 1979.
24. Evans RF, Sagerman R, Rigrose TL, Auchtincloss JH, Browman J: Pulmonary function following mantlefield irradiation for Hodgkin's disease. Radiology 111:729, 1974.
25. Koocher GP, O'Malley JE: The Damocles syndrome. Mac Graw-Hill, New York, 1982.
26. Holmes H, Holmes AF: After ten years what are the handicaps and life styles of children treated for cancer? Clin Ped 14:819–823, 1975.
27. Jonson WW: Helping the family cope with childhood cancer. Psychosomatic 20:241–251, 1979.
28. Shalet SM, Bearwell CG, Twomay JA, Morris-Jones PA, Pearson D: Endocrine function following the treatment of Acute Leukemia in childhood. J Ped 90:920, 1977.

29. Sklar C, Nesbit M: Summary of workshop on present knowledge of late effects of treatment on endocrine function. Cancer Clin Trials 4(Suppl):21, 1981.
30. Robison LL, Sather ME, Meadows AT, Ortega JA, Hammond GD: Serum gonadotropin levels in long-term survivors of childhood acute lymphoblastic leukemia (ALL). SIOP, XV Annual Conference – York, Sept. 20-24, 1983.
31. Goorin AM, Borow KM, Goldman A, Williams RG, Henderson IC, Sallan SE, Cohen H, Jaffe N: Congestive heart failure due to Adriamycin cardiotoxicity: its natural history in children. Cancer 47:2810-1816, 1981.
32. Kobrinsky NL, Ramsay NKC, Krivit W: Anthracycline cardiomyopathy. Ped Cardiol 3:265-272, 1982.
33. Steinherz L, Murphy ML, Steinherz P, Rosen G, Robins J, Tan C: Cardiac function studies in children 4-11 years follwing cancer chemotherapy (Rx) including anthracyclines (Ant). Proceedings American Society of Clinical Oncology Toronto. May 6-8, 1984.
34. Pratt CB, Ramsom JL, Evans WE: Age related Adriamycin cardiotoxicity in children. Cancer Treat Rep 62:1381-1385, 1970.
35. Gottdiener JS, Katin MJ, Borer JS, Bacharach SL, Green MV: Late cardiac effects of therapeutic mediastinal irradiation. N Engl J Med 308:569-588, 1983.
36. Applefeld MM, Slawson RG, Spicer KM, Singleton RT, Wesley MN, Wiernik PH: Long-term cardiovascular evaluation of patients with Hodgkin's disease treated by thoracic mantle radiation therapy. Cancer Treat Rep 66:1003-1013, 1982.
37. Lewis AB, Crouse VL, Evans W, Takahashi M, Siegel SE: Recovery of left ventricular function following discontinuation of anthracycline chemotherapy in children. Pediatrics 68:67-72, 1981.
38. Paccagnella A, Bevilacqua M, Salvagno L, Venturelli E, Fiorentino M: In: VII corso di aggiornamento in oncologia medica. Deltagraph Editor Padova, 1980.

# High dose chemotherapy

# 18. Purging procedures: a critical step in autologous bone marrow transplantation

THIERRY PHILIP, MARIE FAVROT, IRENE PHILIP,
PIERRE BIRON and ROSS PINKERTON

## Abstract

Autologous bone marrow transplantation (ABMT) provides an effective method of preventing prolonged or permanent aplasia after intensive che-moradiotherapy. Many of the solid tumors in which such 'massive therapy' may be effective, however, metastasize to the marrow and for this reason, although marrow is generally harvested during clinical complete remission (CR), there remains concern about the possibility of reinfusing malignant cells.

For the past 5 years we have been involved in the development of massive therapy strategies for paediatric solid tumors. The problem of marrow contamination has been addressed using Burkitt's lymphoma (BL) and Neuroblastoma as models. The rationale for attempting to purge marrow is based on both laboratory evidence and circumstantial clinical evidence in relation to the pattern of disease relapse post ABMT. Using a liquid culture system we have demonstrated that for BL apparently normal marrow may contain significant numbers of tumor cells.

A variety of purging techniques have been evaluated including ASTA Z, complement lysis and immunomagnetic depletion. At present the most effective method for BL is complement lysis using a cocktail of three monoclonal antibodies. In neuroblastoma, immunomagnetic beads coated with monoclonal antibody are used. In both a reduction of 3–4 logs is achieved estimated by a cell liquid culture assay.

Early clinical results demonstrate clearly the efficacy of massive therapy. It is too early, however, to assess the value of purging clinically, although its lack of toxicity is clear. Further refinements in the laboratory are required, possibly involving a combination of techniques. In addition, the procedure requires further clinical evaluation.

Autologous bone marrow transplantation (ABMT) is not a treatment, but only a rescue from hematopoietic toxicity, a common dose-limiting factor in solid tumor therapy [1]. With ABMT, the graft itself is not a major problem, rather, tumor response, extra medullary toxicity and tumor cell contamination of the bone marrow are the limiting factors [1]. In our group we have performed more than 100 ABMT in a 5-year period mainly in patients with lymphomas [2–4], neuroblastoma [5, 6], Ewing's sarcoma and soft tissue sarcomas [7]. Except for testicular cancer [8] the problem of malignant cells contaminating the bone marrow is always a potential problem. Thus, during these 5 years, the development of effective purging procedures has been a priority.

Burkitt's lymphoma and neuroblastoma have been chosen as models in which to define:

- the role of ABMT in pediatric solid tumors;
- the rationale for purging marrow;
- the different technical approaches for *ex vivo* purging;
- the clinical results of *ex vivo* purging procedures.

*Table 1.* Preparative chemotherapy regimes for autologous bone marrow transplantation.

| | **Bact** | | | | | | |
|---|---|---|---|---|---|---|---|
| Day | 1 | 2 | 3 | 4 | 5 | 6 | 7 |
| BCNU (200 mg/m²) | O | | | | | | |
| ARA-C (200 mg/m²) | | O | O | O | O | | |
| Cytoxan (50 mg/kg) | | O | O | O | O | | |
| 6-Thioguanine (200 mg/m²) | | O | O | O | O | | |
| ABMT | | | | | | | O |

| | **IGR Bact** | | | | | | |
|---|---|---|---|---|---|---|---|
| Day | 1 | 2 | 3 | 4 | 5 | 6 | 7 |
| BCNU (300 mg/m²) | O | O | O | O | O | | |
| ARA-C (200 mg/m²) | | O | O | O | O | | |
| Cytoxan (50 mg/kg) | | O | O | O | O | | |
| 6-Thioguanine (200 mg/m²) | | O | O | O | O | | |
| ABMT | | | | | | | O |

| | **Beam** | | | | | | |
|---|---|---|---|---|---|---|---|
| Day | 1 | 2 | 3 | 4 | 5 | 6 | 7 |
| BCNU (300 mg/m²) | O | | | | | | |
| VP 16 (200 mg/m²) | | O | O | O | O | | |
| ARA-C (200 mg/m²) | | O | O | O | O | | |
| Melphalan (140 mg/m²) | | | | | | O | |
| ABMT | | | | | | | O |

## Role for ABMT in Burkitt's lymphoma and Stage IV neuroblastoma

*Burkitt's lymphoma*

The BACT chemotherapy regimen followed by ABMT was first proposed in 1978 by Appelbaum for relapsed or resistant Burkitt's lymphoma (BL) [9, 10] which at that time had a very bad prognosis (Table 1) [11]. Several teams, including ours, have since confirmed the potential value of this approach [12–14]. Burkitt's lymphoma is, however, now curable by conventional chemotherapy regimens [15, 16] in 75% of cases and despite very good results with ABMT some controversy persists on the precise indication for this procedure. When we initiated our program of ABMT, the overall survival for patients with Burkitt's lymphoma in Lyon by conventional chemotherapy was 42%. CNS relapse was the major problem. In addition, purging procedures prior to ABMT were not ready for clinical use. At the present time, the overall survival in our center by a conventional regimen is 77% [17] and CNS relapse is now a rare event. A purging procedure was developed and was used for 14 of a group of 28 patients. The increasing survival after conventional chemotherapy, however, was observed in parallel with the progress of ablative therapy regimens thus causing a problem in interpreting the value of the latter.

Despite these difficulties in analysis, we think that firm conclusions can be drawn from our initial experience and that massive therapy is indicated in 20% of Burkitt's lymphoma cases. All our patients were children except for three young adults who were included in a pediatric protocol at initial presentation. Thirteen were stage III, ten stage IV (eight $CNS \pm BM$ and two BM alone) and five were stage I or II. They all had received adriamycin-containing regimens prior to ABMT. The median interval between diagnosis and ABMT was 5 months (range 1–26). At the time of ABMT 13 patients (15 courses) were in relapse (all relapses on therapy) but still responding to a rescue protocol (non resistant relapse [2, 3]. Two patients were in resistant relapse and one in progressive disease. Three were in partial remission after first induction therapy and nine in 1st CR (three with a long delay to CR, five with initial CNS disease and one with L3 Burkitt's leukemia).

As shown in Figure 1, patients in resistant relapse and progressive disease are not good candidates for massive therapy. In three cases we observed only 1 PR and all three patients died before day 54 post ABMT. In non-resistant relapses results were good with an overall survival NED of 53.8% despite three therapy-related deaths in CR in this group. Median observation time for the survivors is 295 days post ABMT. All disease related deaths were observed before day 60. Only three patients were submitted to massive therapy when in PR after initial induction therapy and all three are alive NED 1455+, 735+, and 460+ post ABMT. Nine patients were grafted in 1st CR either for long delay to CR or consolidation of those with initial CNS involvement or L3 leukemia. Of those only three are alive NED (33%) including 2/3 with a long delay to CR and only 1/5 with initial CNS disease. The L3 leukemia relapsed day 35 and died day 73 post ABMT.

Seventeen patients were grafted either after isolated CNS relapses (ten cases) or initial CNS involvement (seven cases). No clear difference is observed in the results between CNS relapses (5/10, i.e. 42% survivors NED) and initial CNS involvement (3/7, i.e. 33% of survivors). This group of patients with initial CNS involvement does very badly with conventional therapy [15]. 3/7 are alive NED 277+, 466+ and 735+ post ABMT. All relapses in this group involved the CNS and in 2/3 there was also bone marrow involvement (one died of toxicity in CR). During the 30 courses of massive therapy morbidity was observed in 11 (36%), and mortality in four (14%).

The overall survival NED for the 28 patients is 13/28, i.e. 46%. The median observation time post ABMT for the survivors is 22 months (655 days+). It is well known that in such a group survival is very unlikely with conventional chemotherapy regimens. As previously shown, patients with BL who stay in CR more than 8 months can be considered as cured [11]. Hence it is the case for 80% of our survivors. If we consider the survival for these patients according to the indication for ABMT it appears that the results of ABMT in responding relapse after a CNS or CSF relapse are encouraging with 5/10 long-term survivors. Our very preliminary experience of massive therapy as consolidation for initial CNS involvement in 1st CR is also promising. The observed survival of 3/7 appears better than the 25% survival produced with a conventional regimen [15].

Our conclusion is therefore that the indication of ABMT is restricted to 20% of patients with Burkitt's lymphoma and should be divided in two groups:

- Massive therapy and ABMT are currently the best treatment for BL still in PR after initial induction therapy or in relapse that is responding to rescue protocols. The response rate for this last group in this study was high and 75% of the potential candidates received ABMT. The only question which remains unclear is whether this high rate of efficacy for 'a second line' rescue protocol will continue to be observed for patients who relapse off of more modern protocols. Massive therapy and ABMT must be considered an experimental treatment for BL with initial CNS involvement, a group which is usually not cured with conventional regimens. Results reported here are promising;
- Massive therapy regimens such as BACT or BEAM (Table 1) clearly will not cure patients with progressive disease. For this group of patients new phase II studies are urgently needed and should be set up as multicenter cooperative trials. These studies could be based on conventional chemo-

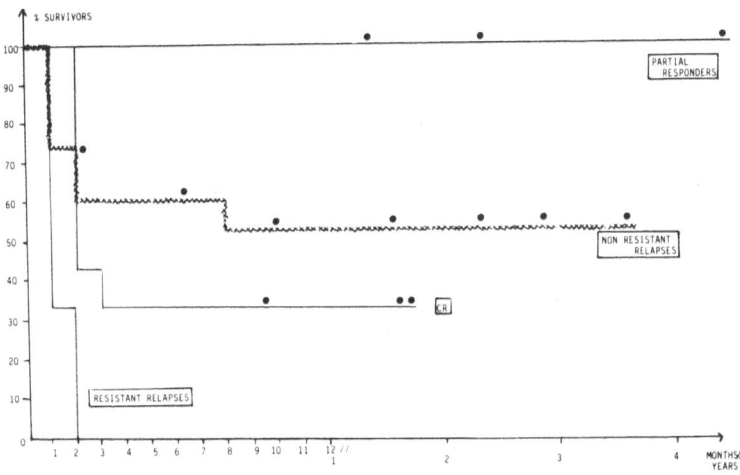

*Figure 1.* Overall disease free survival of the 28 patients according to status at ABMT.

therapy regimens tested with ABMT to define if a dose effect relationship exists which might improve results. New massive therapy combinations including high dose cisplatinum (CCDP), melphalan, isofosfamide, BCNU, cytosine arabinoside and high dose methotrexate should be explored. Combinations of various alkylating agents as proposed by the Baltimore group may be a good avenue to explore [4]. The role of TBI remains unclear in BL despite poor results reported in other lymphomas [4]. However it is clear that such phase II studies will be the basis of any future progress in Burkitt's lymphoma either in conventional or massive therapy regimens.

## Neuroblastoma

Up to March of 1985 our cooperative group has done 30 purged ABMT in very poor prognosis neuroblastoma [6]. Using the very strict criteria used to define CR by O. Hartmann at Villejuif [18] we reviewed all our cases and out of 12 patients previously classified in CR, only four meet these new criteria. Initial chemotherapy consisted of cyclophosphamide, vincristine, doxorubicin, cisplatin, and teniposide (VM-26) [5]. The high dose regimen under study included vincristine 4 mg/m$^2$ as a continuous infusion over 5 days with melphalan 180 mg/m$^2$ on day 6, and total body irradiation with 12 Gy (1,200 rad) (fractionated at 6×2 Gy with lung shielding after 10 Gy).

Disease status varied at the time of high dose therapy so the responses to ablative therapy are described accordingly:

*Progressive disease;* nine patients had progressive disease, five are evaluable. There was a partial response (PR) to massive therapy in two and a complete response (CR) in three. All patients subsequently relapsed (median remission duration 121 days, range 45–192). *Partial remission;* among eight evaluable cases CR was achieved in five, one remained stable and two had progressive disease. Thus out of 13 evaluable cases we observed ten responses, i.e. 76%.

The survival, also according to disease status, was as follows:

*Progressive disease,* one patient is still alive at 352 days with non progressive abdominal disease.

*Non resistant relapses,* two patients are alive NED with a maximum follow up of 2 months post ABMT.

*Partial remission,* 12 were grafted in PR including eight who were evaluable for response and four others. One died of veno-occlusive disease on day 10, one relapsed at 8 months and died in 2nd CR 18 months post ABMT, one relapsed at 7 months in the lung and died, one relapsed at 8 months and died day 358. One progressed under therapy and died day 150 post ABMT, and two not evaluable for response died day 196 and 329 in relapse. Two patients are alive with disease 5 and 13 months post diagnosis and three are alive NED 102 days, 475 days, and 483 days post ABMT. The overall survival post ABMT for this group is 41% but the survival NED is 25% with three survivors (including two more than 1 year post ABMT).

*Very good partial remission (VGPR),* five patients belong to this group. Two died of toxicity day 36 and 60 and three are alive NED 180, 233 and 377 days post ABMT (60%).

*Complete remission,* four patients belong to this group. One died of toxicity day 40 and three are alive NED 178, 205 and 1107 days post ABMT (survival NED 75%).

Thus of 21 patients grafted in PR, VGPR or CR four died of toxicity (19%) and eight relapsed. Nine are alive NED with a median observation time of 10 months post ABMT (3 months to 3 years) i.e. 42.8% of overall survival NED. Our preliminary conclusions are that this massive therapy is effective in very poor prognosis neuroblastoma (76% response rate) and that toxicity is high but often related to the total body irradiation. This unselected group of patients shows a clear improvement compared with the previous series without ABMT [5].

### Rationale for purging procedures in Burkitt's lymphoma and stage IV neuroblastoma

*Burkitt's lymphoma*

We have previously shown *in vitro* that BL cells could grow in a liquid culture system from cytologically and histologically normal marrow [19, 20]. The limit of detection of this test ranged from 1 BL cell in $10^4$ to 1 BL cell in $10^6$ normal ones. The only 'false negatives' in this test are those in which the primitive tumor may not grow in culture.

Two-hundred thirty-four cytologically normal bone marrow samples in 50 patients were studied in the situation of first clinical complete remission and Burkitt cells were found in one, i.e. 2% of the patients [19]. Twenty-one patients were studied prior to ABMT (three 2nd CR, four PR, nine CSF relapses and five other relapses) and of these, eight patients with cytologically normal [7] or suspect [1] marrow were found to have Burkitt cells in culture (0/3 2th CR, 2/4 PR, 5/9 CSF relapses, 1/5 other relapses). Our conclusion is that bone marrow harvested in first CR does not have to be purged. However, the percentage of survivors among CR patients is close to 80% and if all patients were electively harvested at this time 8/10 would be unnecessary. Also such a strategy would be extremely expensive for big centers. We then choose to harvest bone marrow at time of ABMT indication in BL (i.e., PR or relapse) but we then know that we will have to purge it since it is likely to be invaded in at least 40% of cases.

The rationale to purge marrow is then based upon laboratory evidence but in some cases this also correlates with clinical experience, i.e. a 3-year-old boy with stage III BL was grafted in second CR after CSF relapse. At the time of harvesting bone marrow aspiration and biopsy were normal but Burkitt cells grew in culture. The number of Burkitt cells reinjected was of $18 \times 10^6$ maximum (1% of $1.5 \times 10^8$ nucleated cells kg child of 12 kg). The child experienced an explosive relapse day 17 post ABMT (bone marrow, CSF, abdomen, pleural, mediastinal and spinal cord) and died day 25.

## Neuroblastoma

The rationale to purge marrow in stage IV neuroblastoma is less clear because of lack of an *in vitro* clonogenic assay. The only clinical way to define the bone marrow status at harvesting are the classical aspirations and biopsy. We have confirmed Pritchard's data showing that biopsies were more effective than aspirates for tumor detection in 20% of the cases whereas the reverse was the case in 7% [21]. We also confirm the Paris team data showing that extensive straging (seven aspirations and four biopsies) is able to detect at least 30% of patients with minor bone marrow involvement that will not be detected by only one aspiration + one biopsy [18]. As shown in Table 2 a 1% contaminated bone marrow for a 20-kg child will reinfuse 20 million malignant cells. According to Reynolds the proportion of tumor cells that is clonogenic *in vivo* is unknown [22] and may vary for different tumors (as shown *in vitro* with cell lines by Seeger) [23]. Assuming the cloning efficiency ranges [22] from $10^{-1}$ to $10^{-4}$, $2 \times 10^6$ to 2,000 clonogenic

*Table 2.* Potential number of tumor cells infused with autologous bone marrow in Neuroblastoma.

| Total cells | | Tumor cells | = Total reinjected malignant cells |
|---|---|---|---|
| $2 \times 10^9$ | 1/100 | $(10^{-2})$ | $2 \times 10^7$ |
| $2 \times 10^9$ | 1/1000 | $(10^{-3})$ | $2 \times 10^6$ |
| $2 \times 10^9$ | 1/10.000 | $(10^{-4})$ | $2 \times 10^5$ |
| $2 \times 10^9$ | 1/100.000 | $(10^{-5})$ | $2 \times 10^4$ |
| $2 \times 10^9$ | 1/1.000.000 | $(10^{-6})$ | $2 \times 10^3$ |
| $2 \times 10^9$ | 1/10.000.000 | $(10^{-7})$ | $2 \times 10^2$ |

For hematologic and immunologic reconstitution we assume that $10^8$ mononuclear cells/kg will be infused in a 20-kg child (i.e. $2 \times 10^9$).

tumor cells may be infused. This number is probably sufficient to induce neuroblastoma *in vivo* if we compare with the murine lymphoma model in which $10^2$ viable cells kills all recipients [24].

## Techniques for purging Burkitt's lymphoma and neuroblastoma bone marrow prior to ABMT

*Burkitt's lymphoma*

Various techniques are available to purge *in vitro* malignant cells prior to ABMT without harming pluripotential stem cells [5, 24–28]. Considering the published results on the efficiency of an immunodepletion by monoclonal antibodies and complement [29] and our own preliminary results [30, 31], we set up this procedure to clean bone marrow in BL, keeping in mind that we would probably have to combine those techniques [32].

According to our previous analysis of 28 BL cell lines, we selected three monoclonal antibodies, $B_1$, Y29/55 and $AL_2$ (anti-CALLA) to be used with complement to purge bone marrow contaminated by BL cells [30, 31]. We used an artificial model where BL cells from six different cell lines were mixed with excess peripheral blood lymphocytes [29, 33]. We first defined the working conditions, i.e. medium, number of treatments with complement, duration of the treatment, cell concentration, using a quick and reliable method to detect residual malignant cells. The nucleus of BL cells were stained with Hoechst 33258 and the cells then mixed with 10-fold unstained normal cells. This nuclear-staining method allows detection of up to one malignant cell out of 20,000 residual BL cells at the end of the purging procedure [33]. Hence, with optimal defined conditions, we used a cell liquid culture monitoring system to quantify the efficiency of each monoclonal antibody and the 'cocktail' to clean bone marrow contaminated with 1 to 5% BL cells [19]. The following points were clearly shown. First, there was some variability in the efficiency of the whole procedure depending on the cell line used (only five lines out of six were sensitive to the complement lysis). Second, the cocktail of three monoclonal antibodies allowed a constant BL cell cytoreduction of 3 to 4 decimal logs from the five sensitive cell lines, whereas results varied from line to line when only one or two monoclonal antibodies were used. Thirdly, in the sensitive cell lines, the procedure was sufficient to completely inhibit subsequent BL cell growth in liquid culture from BM samples contaminated with 1% BL cells before the purging.

Therefore we conclude that this procedure will be effective in clinical situations to clean cytologically normal or suspect bone marrow. Finally, the procedure produced no major toxicity on normal progenitor cells, as assayed by CFU-GM (colony forming unit-granulocytes monocytes). Tables 3 and 4 summarize the *in vitro* data obtained either with the Hoescht staining or clonogenic assay.

## Neuroblastoma

*In vitro* purging procedures with Asta Z are used by several groups despite questionable evidence of its efficiency *in vitro* [18]. The 6-OH Dopamine purging procedure initiated in 1982 by Reynolds has been shown to be non-toxic even after TBI [5, 34]. *In vitro* data, however, has shown that this

*Table 3.* Efficiency of individual monoclonal antibodies compared to a 'cocktail' of monoclonal antibodies.

| Cell lines (n = number of experiments) | $B_1$ | BL cell elimination (log) | | T Cocktail |
|---|---|---|---|---|
| | | Anti-CALLA | Y29/55 | |
| Raji (n = 5) | 2.66±0.96 | 1.60±0.46 | 1.62±1.05 | 2.46±0.97 |
| $BL_{63}$ (n = 5) | 2.95±0.57 | 1.44±1.20 | 1.34±0.31 | 2.95±0.57 |
| Daudi (n = 6) | 2.71±0.79 | 2.21±0.62 | 2.40±0.59 | 2.87±0.65 |
| $BL_{17}$ (n = 3) | 2 ±0.35 | 1.31±0.63 | 1.23±1.07 | 2.79±0.45 |
| $Ly_{67}$ (n = 3) | 0.76±0.50 | N.D. | 0.56±0.37 | 0.76±0.30 |

$4 \times 10^6$ normal cells were mixed with $4 \times 10^5$ BL cells from each cell line and treated in optimal conditions as previously defined [31, 33] (Hanks medium, two complement treatments at 24°C, with 60' incubation time and 100 µl complement for each treatment, cell concentration: $2 \times 10^7$ cells/ml). Hoechst dye staining enables detection of up to one residual cell per 20,000; results are expressed in logarithms of the initial ratio to the final ratio, malignant cells to normal cells.

*Table 4.* Efficiency of the control procedure determined by the liquid cell culture monitoring system.

| | Treated samples | | | | | | Untreated samples; limits of detection of the test | | | |
|---|---|---|---|---|---|---|---|---|---|---|
| Absolute number of BL cells in the samples (%) | $B_1$ | $Y29/55 + AL_2$ $2 \times 10^5$ (5%) | cocktail | $B_1$ | $Y29/55 + AL_2$ $4 \times 10^4$ (1%) | cocktail | $4 \times 10^3$ (0.1%) | $4 \times 10^2$ (0.01%) | 40 (0.001%) | 4 (0.0001%) |
| **Cell lines** | | | | | | | | | | |
| Raji | 20 | 0 | 50 | 1 | 90 | 0 (4 log) | 61 | | 100 | 90 |
| | | | 65 | | | 0 (4 log) | | | 6 | 0 |
| | | | | | | 0 (4 log) | | | 100 | 60 |
| $BL_{63}$ | 95 | 90 | 0 (3 log) | 0 | 0 | 0 | 100 | 33 | 5 | 0 |
| | | | 0 (3 log) | 0 | 0 | 0 | | 30 | 0 | 0 |
| | | | 0 (3 log) | 5 | 90 | 0 | | 40 | 0 | 0 |
| | | | 0 (3 log) | | | 0 | | 60 | 0 | 0 |
| Daudi | | | 90 | 0 | 50 | 0 (4 log) | | 70 | 20 | 15 |
| | | | 0 (4.5 log) | 6 | 5 | 0 (4 log) | | | 30 | 2 |
| | | | 5 | 1 | 0 | 0 | | | 100 | 90 |
| | | | ND | | | 0 (4 log) | | | 90 | 20 |
| | | | | | | 0 (4 log) | | | 100 | 0 |
| $BL_{17}$ | | | | 0 | 0 | 0 (3 log) | | 60 | 20 | ND |
| | | | | 0 | 0 | 0 (4 log) | | | 80 | 90 |
| $BL_{92}$ | | | 60 | 0 | 95 | 0 (3 log) | 90 | 80 | 50 | ND |

Normal irradiated BM cells were contaminated with 1 % or 5 % malignant cells, treated under optimal conditions and grown 8 days in liquid culture. For each experiment, $4 \times 10^6$ normal irradiated BM cells were contaminated with an increasing number of malignant cells (from 0.0001 % to 0.1 %) and grown in the same conditions without treatment. To avoid errors due to the loss of cells during the purging procedure, $4 \times 10^6$ cells were harvested from untreated and treated samples and poured. Results are expressed in percentages of BL cells at day 10 of the culture, as evaluated by a cytological examination on a smear. Those percentages are correlated with the number of BL cells in the sample. Then, the comparison for each experiment of the percentages of BL cells in treated and untreated samples enables the quantification of residual BL cells after the purging in treated samples. In parentheses, results are expressed in logarithms of the initial ratio (before the purging) to the final ratio (after the purging) of malignant cells to normal cells.

technique alone will not produce more than 1-log reduction of tumor cell load [34]. Complement lysis techniques are unsuitable because of the absence of cytotoxicity with the majority of currently available monoclonal antibodies [27]. In 1982 Kemshead produced an immunomagnetic technique suitable for *ex vivo* treatment [27] and the lack of toxicity of this procedure, even after TBI, is now well established [5, 27]. *In vitro* evaluation, however, has been very preliminary due to the lack of an available technique to detect removal of more than 2 logs of tumor cells [27]. The description in 1984 of the Hoescht dye technique [35] allowed a new definition of the technical parameters [22, 36] and it is now clear that better cell removal can be obtained with several modifications to the initial technique, namely:

- Ficoll is necessary and adds a 1-log depletion to buffy coat marrow [22, 36];
- two successives courses of incubation with the beads and two successive courses in the magnetic system will also add a 1-log of depletion [22, 36];
- the number of beads is dependent not only on the number of malignant cells [27] but also the number of normal cells [36]. A 10-fold increase in the number of beads appears to be necessary over the initial recommended number [27, 36];
- Other technical modifications such as in the medium (PBS instead of albumin), sheep anti-mouse preparation (acidification), dilution of the marrow and the magnet position, may also increase the number of malignant cells removed [36]

With these technical modifications a minimum of 3 logs of depletion can be expected from a 1 % contaminated marrow [22]. At least a 2-logs additional killing is probably necessary and potentially is obtainable by additional techniques such as physical separation, 6-OH Dopamine or chemical purging procedures.

**Clinical results of the marrow purging procedures**

*Burkitt's lymphoma*

In our retrospective data on 30 courses of ABMT in Burkitt's lymphoma the comparison between the marrow purged and unpurged group is difficult because of the predominance of initial CNS disease in the purged group. However, as shown in Figure 2, the overall disease free survival for the two groups is comparable (46 % versus 50 %). A better way to look at this small group is shown in Table 4. If we compare the 5/12 relapses in the unpurged

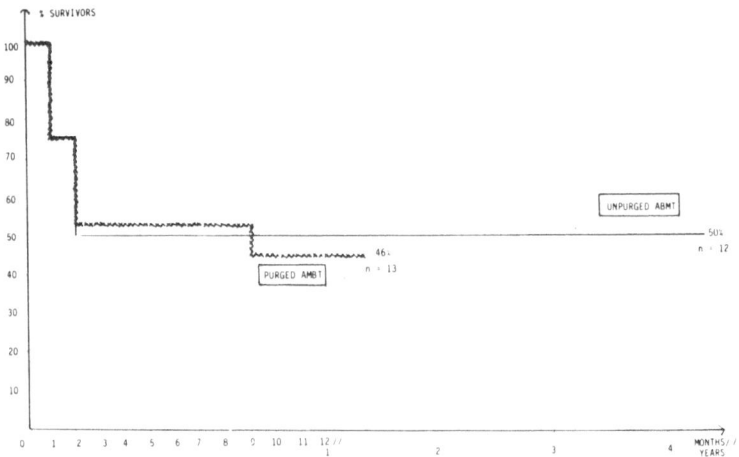

*Figure 2.* Overall disease free survival purged versus unpurged group (See text for details).

group (CR excluded), all relapses were early. Four relapses in group 1 were observed first in the marrow, whereas the two relapses in group 2 are clearly non-marrow relapses. In the group of patients grafted in 1st CR of initial bone marrow involvement, however, 3/4 relapses were bone marrow relapses despite purging of a cytologically normal marrow in all cases.

The continued occurrence of marrow relapse despite purging might lead to the conclusion that such procedures have little to contribute. Evidence of occult infiltration may be revealed using the culture monitoring system. Because each case may manifest different reactivity individual controls are required [20]. We have laboratory evidence that a purging procedure with Y29/55 alone or with $AL_2$ without $B_1$ are incomplete [29, 33]. Only case by case analysis, using a clonogenic assay, can clarify the efficacy of the purging procedure. Our preliminary conclusion is that purging techniques still require perfection at a laboratory level and *the rationale for their use should not be judged on the basis of incomplete procedures* (Table 5).

*Neuroblastoma*

As shown in Figure 3, in our preliminary experience with stage IV neuroblastoma there is a clear difference between patients purged with a cytologically normal or abnormal marrow. When the marrow was cytologically invaded three out of four patients relapsed in the marrow at 2, 4 and 6 months (including malignant interstitial pneumonitis in one patient). In contrast, only 5 out of 13 relapsed in the cytologically normal group (all relapses in marrow). It is possible, however, that such differences in relapse

*Table 5.* Comparison between purged and unpurged marrow prior to ABMT (patients in CR with no initial CNS and the two courses with no ABMT excluded).

| Cases | Unpurged | | | Cases | Purged not in 1st CR | | | Cases | Purged in 1st CR | | |
|---|---|---|---|---|---|---|---|---|---|---|---|
| | Initial BM | BM at harvesting | Site of relapses | | Initial BM | BM at harvesting | Site of relapses | | Initial BM | BM at harvesting | Site of relapses |
| 1 | — | — | Bone marrow CSF abdomen day 17 | 9 | — | — | Died in CR day 223 | 17 | + | — | CSF day 30 |
| 3 | — | — | — | 15 | — | — | CNS day 30 | 18 | + | — | Bone marrow + CSF day 60 |
| 4 | — | — | — | 19 | — | — | Died in CR day 15 | | | | |
| 5 | — | — | Bone marrow day 35 | | | | | | | | |
| 6 | — | — | — | | | | | 23 | + | — | — |
| 7 | — | — | Bone marrow day 60 | 20 | — | — | — | | | | |
| 9 | — | — | CSF day 60 | 25 | — | — | — | 24 | + | — | Died in Cr day 80 |
| 11 | — | — | — | 26 | — | — | — | 28 | + | — | Bone marrow + CSF day 37 |
| 13 | — | — | — | | | | | | | | |
| 14 | — | — | Bone marrow + abdomen day 30 | | | | | | | | |
| 16 | — | — | Died in CR | | | | | 21 | + | — | Head & neck day 30 |
| 22 | — | — | — | 27 | — | — | Bone marrow + CSF day 35 | | | | |

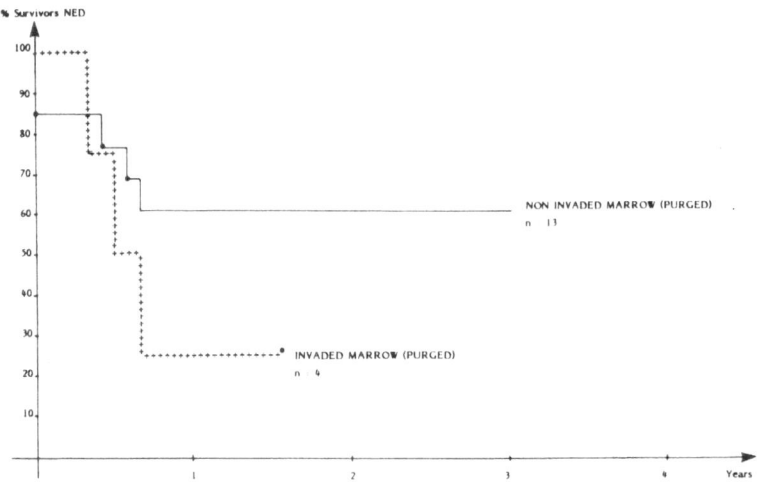

*Figure 3.* Stage IV NEUROBLASTOMA ABMT with purged marrow.

rates simply reflect the extent of disease at time of ABMT rather than a reinfusion of tumour cells.

The major problem with neuroblastoma is the difficulty in accurately assessing purging efficiency *in vitro*. Although the use of monoclonal anti-bodies and more recently the Hoescht dye technique has improved this, it may be necessary to develop highly sensitive culture systems which will detect very low levels of marrow infiltration, as in the case of BL. Only then can methods be refined and assessed in individual patients. It seems prob-able, moreover, that the future lies with a combination of purging tech-niques rather than any single system. For example, new cytolytic monoclon-al antibodies may have a role to play.

Only once the effectiveness of purging systems can be convincingly demonstrated in individual patients, *in vitro*, can a randomized study of purged versus non-purged marrow be of value. It is evident from the fact that patients relapse after allogenic transplantation for neuroblastoma that current massive therapy regimens leave much to be desired, irrespective of the problem of reinfusion of tumour cells. It seems appropriate, therefore, that while purging systems are improved, allogenic grafts should be pursued to search both for improvement in ablative chemotherapy and in the induc-tion regimens which preceed them.

### Acknowledgement

Supported in part by grant from A.D.R.C. and F.N.L.C.C.

# References

1. Philip T, Herve P, Racadot E, Cahn JT, Biron P, Brunat-Mentigny M, Peters A, Mayer M: Intensive cytoreductive regimen and autologous bone marrow transplantation in leukemia and solid tumors. Transpl Clin Immunol 14:86–110, 1982.
2. Philip T, Biron P, Maraninchi D, Gastaut JA, Herve P, Flesh Y, Goldstone ah, Souhami RL: Role of massive chemotherapy and autologous bone marrow transplantation in non Hodgkin's malignant lymphoma. Lancet ii:391, 1984.
3. Philip T, Biron P, Maraninchi D, Goldstone AH, Herve P, Souillet G, Gastaut JL, Plouvier E, Flesh Y, Philip I, Harousseau JL, Le Mevel A, Rebattu P, Linch DC, Freycon F, Milan JJ, Souhami RL: Massive chemotherapy with autologous bone marrow transplantation in 50 cases of bad prognosis non Hodgkin's lymphoma. Brit J Haematol 60, 1985 (in press).
4. Philip T, Biron P, Philip I, Favrot M, Souillet G, Frappaz D, Jaubert J, Bordigoni P, Bernard JL, Laporte JP, LE mevel A, Plouvier E, Marguerite G, Pinkerton R, Brizard LP, Freycon F, Forster k, Brunat-Mentigny M: Massive therapy and autologous bone marrow transplantation in Burkitt's lymphoma (30 courses in 28 patients: a 5 year experience). Blood (submitted).
5. Philip T, Biron P, Philip I, Favrot M, Bernard jl, Zucker JM, Lutz B, Plouvier E, Rebattu P, Carton M, Chauvot p, Dutou L, Souillet G, Philippe N, Bordigoni P, Lacroze M, Clapisson G, Olive D, Trealaven J, Kemshead JT, Brunat-Mentigny M: Autologous bone marrow transplantation for bery bad prognosis Neuroblastoma. In: Advances in Neuroblastoma Research. Evans A (ed). A. Liss Inc., New York, 569–586, 1985.
6. Philip T, Bernard JL, Zucker JM, Souillet G, Favrot M, Philip I, Bordigoni P, Lutz JP, Plouvier E, Carton P, Robert A, Kemshead J: Purged autologous bone marrow transplantation in 25 cases of very poor prognosis neuroblastoma. Lancet ii:576–577, 1985.
7. Philip T, Biron P, Frappaz D, Favrot M, Philip I, Plouvier E, Herve P, Freycon F, Brunat-Mentigny M: Massive therapy and ABMT in children with metastatic or relapsed Ewing's and soft tissue sarcomas. SIOP Meeting, Barcelona 251:252, 1982.
8. Biron P, Philip T, Maraninchi D, Pico JL, Cahn JY, Fumoleau P, Le Mevel A, Gastaut JL, Carcassonne JM, Kamioner D, Herve P, Brunat-Mentigny M, Hayat M: Massive chemotherapy and ABMT in progressive disease of non seminomatous testicular cancer. In: Autologous Bone Marrow Transplantation. Dicke K (ed). Houston, 203–210, 1985.
9. Appelbaum FR, Herzig GP, Ziegler JL, Graw RG, Levine AS, Deisseroth AB: Successful engraftment of cryopreserved autologous bone marrow in patinnts with malignant lymphoma. Blood 52:85–91, 1978.
10. Appelbaum FR, Deisseroth AB, Graw RG, Levine AS, Herzig GP, Ziegler JL: Prolonged complete remission following high dose chemotherapy of Burkitt's lymphoma in relapse. Cancer 41:1063–1068, 1978.
11. Philip T, Lenoir GM, Bryon PA, Souillet G, Freycon F, Gerardmarchand r, Brunat-Mentigny M: Burkitt type malignant lymphoma in France: Individualisation among Caucasian childhood non-Hodgkin's lymphoma. Br J Cancer 45:670–677, 1982.
12. Philip T, Biron P, Herve P, Dutou L, Ehrsam A, Philip I, Souillet G, Plouvier E, Le Mevel A, Philippe N, Vu van O, Bouffet E, Bachmann P, Cordier JF, Freycon F, Brunat-Mentigny M: Massive BACT therapy with autologous bone marrow transplantation in 17 cases of non Hodgkin's malignant lymphoma with a very bad prognosis. Eur J Cancer Clin Oncol 19:1371–1379, 1983.
13. Hartmann O, Pein F, Philip T, Biron P, Lemerle J: The effects of high dose polychemotherapy with autologous bone marrow transplantation in 18 children with relapsed lymphoma. Eur J Cancer Clin Oncol 18:1044–1045, 1982.
14. Baumgartner C, Bleher A, Brun Del Re G, Bucher U, Deubelbeis KA, Greiner R, Hirt A, Imbach P, Luthey A, Odavic R, Wagner HP: Autologous bone marrow transplantation in

the treatment of childhood and adolescents with advanced malignant tumor. Med Ped Oncol 12:104–111, 1984.

15. Patte C, Philip T, Bernard A, Rodary C, Demeocq F, Benz F, LemerleJ: Improvement of survival in advanced stages of B cell non Hodgkin lymphomas of childhood. Proc Am Soc Clin Oncol 937:340, 1984.

16. Philip T: Burkitt's lymphoma in Europe. In: Burkitt's lymphoma: a human cancer model. Lenoir GM, O'Conor G (eds). IARC scientific publications, no. 60, Lyon (in press).

17. Philip T, Lenoir GM, Favrot M, Philip I, Brunat-Mentigny M: Le lymphome de Burkitt en 1985. Pediatrie, Lyon (in press).

18. Hartmann O, Kalifa C, Beaujean F, Bayle C, Benhamou E, Lemerle J: Treatment of advanced neuroblastoma with two consecutive high dose chemotherapy regimens and ABMT. In: Advances in Neuroblastoma Research. Evans A (ed). A. Liss, New York, 565–568, 1985.

19. Philip I, Philip T, Favrot M, Vuillaume M, Fontaniere B, Chamard D, Lenoir GM: Establishment of Lymphomatous cell lines from bone marrow samples from patients with Burkitt's lymphoma. J Nat Cancer Inst 73:835–840, 1984.

20. Philip I, Philip T, Favrot M, Vila G, Frappaz D, Biron P, Lenoir GM: Purging procedures are necessary prior to autologous bone marrow transplantation in Burkitt's lymphoma. In: Autologous Bone marrow Transplantation, Dicke K (ed). Houston, 341–345, 1985.

21. Franklin IM, Pritchard J: Detection of bone marrow invasion by neuroblastoma is improved by sampling at two sites with both aspirates and trephine biopsies. J Clin Pathol 36:1215–1219, 1983.

22. Seeger RC, Reynolds CP, Dai Dany VO, Ugelstad J, Wells J: Depletion of neuroblastoma cells from bone marrow with monoclonal antibodies and magnetic immunobeads. In: Advances in Neuroblastoma Research. Evans A (ed). A. Liss, New York 443–458, 1985.

23. Seeger RC, Ragner SA, Banerjee A, Chung H, Laug WE, Neustein HB, Benedict WF: Morphology, growth, chromosomal pattern and fibrinolytic activity of two new human neuroblastoma cell lines. Cancer Res 37:1364–1368, 1977.

24. Bast RC, Ritz JC: Application of monoclonal antibodies to autologous bone marrow transplantation. In: Biological Responses in Cancer, Vol. 12. Plenum Press, New York, 185–206, 1984.

25. De Fabritiis P, Bregni M, Lipton J, Greenberger J, Nadler L, Rothstein L, Korbling M, Ritz J, Bast RC Jr: Elimination of clonogenic Burkitt's lymphoma cells from human bone marrow using 4 hydroperoxycyclophosphamide in combination with monoclonal antibodies and complement. AACR, C 952, 240, 1984.

26. Dicke KA, Poynton CH, Reading CL: Elimination of leukemic cells from remission marrow suspensions by an immunomagnetic procedure. In: Minimal Residual Disease in Acute Leukemia. Nijfoll M (ed). 209–214, 1984.

27. Treleaven JG, Gibson FM, Ugelstad J, Rembaum A, Philip T, Caine GD, Kemshead JT: Removal of neuroblastoma cells from bone marrow with monoclonal antibodies conjugated to magnetic microspheres. Lancet i:70–76, 1984.

28. Korbling M, Hess AD, Tutschka PJ, Kaiser H, Colvin Mo, Santos GW: 4-hydroperoxycyclophosphamide: a model for eliminating residual human tumor cells and T-lymphocytes from the bone marrow graft. Br J Haem 52:89–93, 1982.

29. Favrot MC, Philip I, Philip T, Lebacq AM, Forster K, Biron P, Dore JF: Set up of bone marrow purging procedure in Burkitt lymphoma with monoclonal antibodies and complement. Quantiticatio by a liquid culture monitoring system. Br J Cancer (in press).

30. Favrot MC, Philip I, Philip T, Portoukalian J, Dore JF: Distinct reactivity of Burkitt cell line with eight monoclonal antibodies correlated with the ethnic origin. J Nat Cancer Inst 73:841–846, 1984.

31. Favrot MC, Philip I, Philip T, Dore JF, Lenoir GM: A possible duality in Burkitt lymphoma origin. Lancet II:745–746, 1984.

32. Vila J, Favrot MC, Philip I, Branger MR, Biron P, Philip T: In vitro cytolytic effects of ASTA-Z 7557 on clonogenic Burkitt cells: potential value for a bone marrow procedure. In: Autologous Bone Marrow Transplantation. Dicke K (ed). Houston, 461–465, 1985.
33. Favrot MC, Philip I, Philip T: Monoclonal antibodies and complement as purging procedure in Burkitt lymphoma. In: Autologous Bone Marrow Transplantation. Dicke K (ed). Houston, 389–401, 1985.
34. Reynolds CP, Reynolds DA, Franhel EP, Smith RG: Selective toxicity of 6 OH Dopamine and ascorbate for human neuroblastoma in vitro: a model for clearing marrow prior to ABMT. Cancer Res 42:1331–1336, 1982.
35. Reynolds CP, Moss TJ, Seeger RC, Black AT, Woody JN: Sensitive detection of neuroblastoma cells in bone marrow for monitoring the efficacy of marrow purging procedures. In: Advances in Nauroblastoma Research. Evans A (ed). A. Liss, New York, 425–441, 1985.
36. Favrot MC, Philip I portukalian J, Philip T: Epuration medullaire immunomagnétique appliquée aux cellules du lymphome de Burkitt. In: Actualités Cancerologiques. Lemerle J (ed). Masson (in press).

# 19. 'High dose' cisplatinum: a phase II study

G. DINI, D. ROGERS, A. GARAVENTA, E. LANINO,
G.P. PERIN, M. STURA, S. DALLORSO, G. SQUAZZINI and
B. DE BERNARDI

Cis-diamino-dichloroplatinum (CDDP) has been shown to be an effective agent in the treatment of pediatric solid tumors. The drug has usually been administered at a maximum dose of 100 mg/sq m either as a single dose or fractionated over 5 days [1–3]. In these schedules the toxicity of CDDP consists of nausea and vomiting, moderate myelosuppression, and cumulative nephrotoxicity and ototoxicity [4, 5]. These toxicities have usually been considered to be dose-limiting. However in a recent report Ozols et al. [6] described good tumor responses to a combination of drugs which included 'high dose CDDP', administered in hypertonic saline to reduce nephrotoxicity [7], in adults with poor prognosis non-seminomatous testicular tumours who had failed to respond to CDDP in conventional doses.

To test the feasibility of this therapeutic approach in children with disseminated neuroblastoma we developed a new combination chemotherapy regimen including 'high dose' CDDP known as OC-HDP.

OC-HDP is a three drug regimen consisting of vincristine (Oncovin, VCR), cyclophosphamide (CPM), and CDDP 200 mg/m$^2$ given as five fractions over 5 days (Figure 1). CDDP is infused in a solution of hypertonic saline over not less than 30 min.

The rationale for the regimen was as follows:

1. The combination of VCR and CPM before CDDP is known to be active in neuroblastoma [2];
2. CDDP has a steep dose-response curve in testicular and ovarian tumors [6];
3. CDDP nephrotoxicity may be reduced if CDDP is administered in hypertonic saline [7].

The aims of this study were to both investigate the toxicity of 'high dose' CDDP in children and to test the efficacy of a drug combination containing 'high dose' CDDP in children with neuroblastoma, most of whom had already been treated with CDDP in conventional dose.

OC-HDP PROTOCOL

VCR
2 mg/m$^2$

CPM
600 mg/m$^2$

CDDP
40 mg/m$^2$
in hypertonic saline

Day

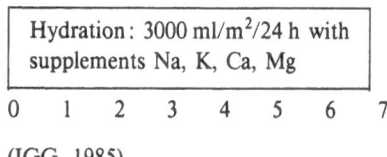

Hydration: 3000 ml/m$^2$/24 h with supplements Na, K, Ca, Mg

| 0 | 1 | 2 | 3 | 4 | 5 | 6 | 7 |

(IGG, 1985)

*Figure* 1.

*Table 1.* OC-HDP: initial therapy and response.

| Child | Initial therapy (cumulative dose mg/m$^2$) | Response | Further therapy (total dose mg/m$^2$) | Response |
|---|---|---|---|---|
| GS | PTC 450, CDDP 180, VM 200 | PD | PTC 450 | PD |
| CK | PTC 450, CDDP 180, VM 200, CPM 200, VCR 0.8, PRED 350 Surgery + 2000 rad | CR 6 mo relapse | PTC 900 | PR |
| DG | PTC 450, 2000 rad | CR 7 mo relapse (local) | Surgery, PTC 45, CDDP 90, VM 100 | CR 4 mo relapse (abdo, marrow) |
| DR | PTC 75, CPM 1800 | PD | — | — |
| CF | PTC 75, CDDP 1800, VM 200 | PR: tumour inoperable | — | — |

PTC: Peptichemio; CDDP: Cis-Platin; VM: VM26; CPM: Cyclophosphamide; VCR: Vincristine; PDN: Prednisone; RT: radiotherapy; ADR: Adriamycin; PD: progressive disease; CR: complete remission; PR: partial remission.

## Patients and methods

Five children aged from 1 year 10 months to 6 years 7 months were treated with OC-HDP. Three had resistant and two had relapsed neuroblastoma (Table 1); all but one had been previously treated with CDDP in conventional doses. Four children received three courses; in one CDDP dose was reduced for the second course because of prolonged myelosuppression after the first course. The remaining child received only two courses because of progressive disease.

Courses of treatment were given every 3 weeks unless delayed by a neutrophil count of less than $1.5 \times 10^9/l$ or a platelet count of less than $100 \times 10^9/l$. Details of fluid and electrolyte therapy are given in Figure 1. Plasma electrolytes including calcium and magnesium and urea and creatinine were measured before, every day during, and after each course.

### Evaluation of toxicity

Vomiting was assessed during each cycle as follows: none, mild (less than 5 episodes), moderate (5 to 10), severe (more than 10). Nephrotoxicity was assessed by means of creatinine clearance corrected for surface area. Ototoxicity was checked by audiometry before every cycle in children aged more than 3 years. Myelotoxicity was assessed by determining the numbers of days after every cycle with polymorphs less than $0,5 \times 10^9/l$ and with platelets less than $50 \times 10^9/l$.

### Evaluation of response

Response to treatment was assessed by change in tumor size using objective measurement by ultrasound and/or computerized tomography or measurement at surgery, by measurement of urinary catecholamine excretion, and by bone marrow aspiration and biopsy at four or more sites.

## Results

### Toxicity

#### Gastrointestinal toxicity
This was acceptable in all children but one, aged 1 year 10 months, who after the third course had persistent vomiting, diarrhea and anorexia of 3 weeks duration.

Vomiting was mild or moderate in the other four children although some vomiting persisted for 2 to 3 days after the cessation of the treatment.

*Nephrotoxicity*
Following treatment the creatinine clearance and glomerular filtration was in the normal range in all patients.

*Ototoxicity*
All the children had high frequency hearing loss (Table 2); some of them also developed it at low frequencies. Otoxicity became progressively more severe after each treatment course.

*Hematologic toxicity*
No child had major problems as a consequence of myelotoxicity (Table 3). Prolonged aplasia was noted in a child with initially heavily infiltrated bone marrow. In three out of four children neutropenia was more severe after the

*Table 2.* High dose cis-platinum: ototoxicity.

| Patient | CDDP dose/m$^2$ (NB-82) | CDDP dose/m$^2$ (high dose) | CDDP dose/m$^2$ (total) | Hearing loss (in db) frequency Hz | | | | |
|---|---|---|---|---|---|---|---|---|
| | | | | 500 | 1000 | 2000 | 4000 | 8000 |
| FA | 600 | 600 | 1200 | 10 | 25 | 40 | 40 | 60 |
| CK | 540 | 400 | 940 | – | 10 | 20 | 40 | 60 |
| CF | 180 | 600 | 780 | – | – | – | 25 | 50 |
| DR | – | 600 | 600 | – | 10 | 30 | 50 | 60 |
| DG | 90 | 500 | 590 | – | – | – | 10 | 60 |

(IGG, 1985)

*Table 3.* OC-HDP: hematological toxicity.

| Child | Cycle | Polymorphs days $< 0.5 \times 10^9/l$ | | | Platelets days $< 50 \times 10^9/l$ | | |
|---|---|---|---|---|---|---|---|
| | | I | II | III | I | II | III |
| GS | | 9 | 5 | 10 | 8 | 4 | 17 |
| CK | | 0 | 0 | – | 3 | 2 | – |
| DG | | 8 | 0 | 18 | 0 | 0 | 0 |
| DR | | 40[a] | 0 | 7 | 17 | 0 | 0 |
| CF | | 4 | 0 | 0 | 0 | 0 | 0 |

[a] Bone marrow initially heavily infiltrated.

(IGG, 1985)

third cycle. Only one episode of candida sepsis was seen in a child whose polymorphs remained less than $0,5 \times 10^9/l$ for 40 days. One child whose platelets were less than $50 \times 10^9/l$ for 17 days had moderate epistaxis requiring platelets support.

## Neurotoxicity
One child developed seizures (after the first cycle) associated with hyponatraemia, as an iatrogenic consequence of diuretic treatment. He received the second course at half dose without any neurological problem and the third course at full dose without additional neurotoxicity.

## Response to treatment

Four out five children showed a good response to OC-HDP treatment; one child after an initial response developed progression of disease after the second cycle. The clinical responses to treatment are shown in Table 4.

## Tumour response
In three children it was possible after OC-HDP to remove completely a previously inoperable abdominal mass. In the fourth child measurable reduction of the mass occurred. All five children had bone marrow disease before OC-HDP. In two the bone marrow was found to be completely clear following OC-HDP. In two only minimal tumour infiltration was present following OC-HDP.

*Table 4.* Tumour, marrow, VMA response.

| | Tumour | Marrow | | VMA | Tumour | Marrow | VMA |
|---|---|---|---|---|---|---|---|
| GS | Inoperable $11 \times 11 \times 10$ cm | + | + | Normal | Complete excision $2.5 \times 3.5 \times 3.5$ | + | Normal |
| CK | Nodes only | + | + | Normal | Progressive disease | +++ | Raised |
| DG | Inoperable $5 \times 4 \times 4$ cm | + | + | Normal | Inoperable $3 \times 2 \times 2$ cm | − | Normal |
| DR | Inoperable $7.5 \times 7.5$ cm | + | + | Raised | Complete excision $4 \times 5 \times 6$ cm | + | Normal |
| CF | Inoperable $7 \times 7 \times 7$ cm | + | + | Raised | Complete excision $7 \times 4 \times 5$ cm | − | Normal |

*VMA response*
Catecholamine excretion was initially raised in two children and fell to normal values after OC-HDP.


## Discussion

The efficacy of CDDP at a maximal conventional dose of $100 \, mg/m^2$ has been established in clinical studies of children with neuroblastoma [1–3]. The importance of the dose-response curve for various alkylating agents has recently been demonstrated in different studies using these agents at higher than conventional doses, some with and some without autologous bone marrow transplantation [8–10]. The experience of Ozols *et al.* [6] who achieved 100% response rate and 80% complete remission rate in a group of adults with poor prognosis testicular disease using CDDP at twice conventional dosage suggested the feasibility of a similar approach in children with poor prognosis neuroblastoma.

The response rate using the protocol described in this report has been encouraging, particularly considering that the majority of the children had previously been treated with CDDP at conventional doses.

From our experience it was not possible to definitively demonstrate a dose-response curve for Cisplatinum, because three out of five patients did not receive VCR and CPM previously. Both these agents were administered with 'high dose' CDDP in our protocol.

Provided that meticulous attention is paid to details of hydration and electrolyte balance, including administration of CDDP in hypertonic saline, avoidance of hyponatraemia, and magnesium supplementation, the protocol was relatively well tolerated without major acute toxicity. The prolonged pancytopenia seen after 'high dose' CDDP administration in a child with heavy tumor infiltration of marrow suggests that protocols of this nature may not be appropriate for treatment of children at initial presentation but should perhaps be reserved for consolidation therapy after an initial response has been obtained with conventional chemotherapy. Nausea and vomiting were moderate, possibly because of fractionation of the dose, although post CDDP hydration frequently was required in some cases.

As with CDDP administration in conventional dosage, chronic toxicity included a significant incidence of ototoxicity and the risk of permanent hearing impairment. However the occurrence of this toxicity has to be set against the poor prognosis seen to date in the majority of children with disseminated neuroblastoma receiving conventional chemotherapy with agents other than CDDP.

Although the number of patients treated in this study is limited, our experience suggests treatment with this regimen may result in measurable and therapeutically useful regression of neuroblastoma even when the disease has previously been resistant to CDDP in conventional doses. CDDP can be given at this dosage without excessive gastrointestinal or haematological toxicity, although as with CDDP administration in conventional dosage, chronic otototoxicity and nephrotoxicity is seen. We suggest that further study of 'high dose' CDDP treatment for disseminated neuroblastoma is warrented.

## References

1. Baum ES, Gaynon P, Greenberg L, Kriwit W, Hammond D: Phase II trial of cisplatin in refractory childhood cancer: Children's Cancer Study Group Report. Cancer Treat Rep 65:815–822, 1981.
2. Shafford EA, Rogers DW, Pritchard J: Advanced neuroblastoma: improved response rate using a multiagent regimen (OPEC) including sequential Cisplatin and VM-26. J Clin Oncol 2:742–747, 1984.
3. Hayes FA, Green AA, Casper J, Cornet J, Evans WE: Clinical evaluation of sequentially scheduled cisplatin and VM26 in neuroblastoma: Response and toxicity. Cancer 48:1715–1718, 1981.
4. Krakoff I: Nephrotoxicity of cis-Dichlorodiamminoplatinum (II). Cancer Treat Rep 63:1523–1525, 1979.
5. Fausti SF, Schechter MA, Rappaport BZ, Frey RH, Mass RE: Early detection of cisplatin ototoxicity. Selected case reports. Cancer 53:224–237, 1984.
6. Ozols RF, Deisseroth AB, Jadvpour N, Ballock A, Messerschmidt GL, Young RC: Treatment of poor prognosis non seminomatous testicular cancer with a 'high-dose' platinum combination chemotherapy regimen. Cancer 51:1803–1807, 1983.
7. Litterst CL: Alteration in the toxicity of cis-dichlorodiamminoplatinum and in tissue localization of platinum as a function of NaCl concentration in the vehicle of administration. Toxicol Appl Pharmacol 61:99–108, 1981.
8. Pritchard J, McElwain TJ, Graham-Pole J: High-dose melphalan with autologous marrow for treatment of advanced neuroblastoma. Br J Cancer 45:86–97, 1982.
9. Sculier JP, Klastersky j: Perspectives for the use of high-dose chemotherapy in the treatment of solid malignant tumors. Eur J Cancer Clin Oncol 20:1335–1337, 1984.
10. Smith IE, Evans BD, Harland SJ, Millar JL: Autologous bone marrow rescue is unnecessary after very high-dose cyclophosphamide. Lancet i:76–77, 1983.

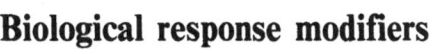

**Biological response modifiers**

# 20. Induction of differentiation: a possible therapeutic approach to the treatment of hematologic malignancy

FELICE GAVOSTO, WANDA PIACIBELLO and
MASSIMO AGLIETTA

## Abstract

The most striking phenotypic abnormality in acute myeloid leukemia is the inability of the cells to differentiate into mature end cells. Because of an apparent uncoupling between proliferation and differentiation the cells remain in the proliferative pool and the neoplastic population greatly expands.

Recently it has been shown that this differentiation block can be overcome using a variety of pharmacological or physiological substances. Leukemic cell lines and fresh leukemic cells have been extensively used as a model to study the biology and effect of these compounds on myeloid differentiation *in vitro*.

This report reviews our study of these agents.

On the basis of the *in vitro* data, some of the inducers of differentiation have been used in the treatment of patients with leukemias or preleukemias. The results, though contrasting, appear somewhat promising.

Hematopoietic development from early pluripotent stem cells to mature end cells involves a progressive loss of self-renewal together with a progression towards terminal differentiation. In this situation the ratio between cell production and cell loss is equal to 1. Because of an uncoupling between proliferation and differentiation, neoplastic cells remain in the proliferative pool and a progressive accumulation of the neoplastic population occurs. In this situation the ratio between cell production and cell loss becomes greater than 1, with a consequent expansion of the tumor mass [1, 2].

In acute leukemia, neoplastic transformation appears to involve an irreversible block in the maturation process and an absolute independence of the cells from normal physiological growth control mechanisms [1]. In contrast, in chronic myeloid leukemia the differentiation potential apparently is maintained and the clonal expansion of the neoplastic transformed multipotent stem cell gives rise to an increased number of apparently normal mature cells. Under this circumstance, the progression of leukemic cell growth derives from an alteration of the regulatory mechanisms which are normally responsible for the increased proliferation of the stem cells. The result is a progressive expansion of both stem cell and mature cell compartments [3, 4].

The proliferative advantage of leukemic cells is two-fold: (1) leukemic cells can specifically inhibit normal stem cell growth by producing leukemic inhibitory activity (LIA), recently identified as AIF (acidic isoferritins) [5]; (2) committed progenitors are not sensitive to growth inhibition by prostaglandin E and acidic isoferritins, which are physiological inhibitors of normal granulopoiesis [6, 7].

A leukemic cell population can therefore be defined by three properties: (1) its retention of a self-renewal potential; (2) its unresponsiveness to normal inhibitory mechanisms; (3) its incapability of normal differentiation and maturation.

Consequently, we can presumably control leukemic expansion by acting on each of the above situations: (1) by inhibiting proliferation (by using chemotherapeutic protocols based or not on cell kinetics); (2) by reinducing responsiveness to normal growth inhibitory factors; (3) by inducing terminal differentiation (i.e., making the cells incapable of further proliferation). From a kinetic point of view the latter means an increased cell loss.

Each of these mechanisms, tends to restore a balance between cell production and cell loss, thus interrupting the expansion of the neoplastic population.

Recently it has been shown that leukemic cells require stimulatory factors for their growth and that the differentiation block, once considered irrever-

*Table 1.* Inducers of leukemic cell differentiation.

| 1. Nonphysiological | |
| --- | --- |
| Phorbol diesters | (TPA and analogues) |
| Indole alkaloids | (Teleocidins) |
| Polar planar drugs | (DMSO, HMBA, Acetamide, Piperidone) |
| Purines, pyrimidines, analogues and chemotherapeutic agents | (Actinomicin D, Methotrexate, Bromo-deoxyuridine, 5-Azacytidine, 6-Thioguanine, Daunomycin, Cytosine Arabinoside, Vincristine) |

2. Physiological

DIF | CSF
Retinoids (Vitamin A and analogues)
Vitamin D metabolites
Interferons

sible, is sometimes reversible. Using certain inducers, both pharmacological or physiological, the block can be overcome and normal differentiated cells produced (Table 1) [8].

Most of the studies on induction of differentiation of myeloid leukemia cells have been conducted with cultured cell lines, both human and murine (Table 2), which, being a homogenous population of neoplastic cells blocked at a certain step of the maturation pathway, greatly simplify the study of cell differentiation [9].

Primary cultures of fresh leukemic cells have been employed only recently, to obtain information on the differentiation of cultured leukemic cells for therapy of human leukemias [8].

Among the nonphysiological compounds, phorbol diesters and indole alkaloids are potent inducers of macrophage-like differentiation of some human myeloid cell lines (HL-60, KG-1, ML-3). Less differentiated cell lines (KG-Ia, K562) are completely resistant to induction of differentiation. These compounds can also induce, *in vitro*, the macrophage-like differentiation of most fresh human leukemia myeloblasts or promyelocytes [9, 10]. However, clinical use of these agents is not feasible for several reasons:

— agents such as TPA can at low concentrations, and in the presence of colony stimulating factor (CSF) stimulate the clonal proliferation *in vitro* of leukemic cells;
— TPA also inhibits human normal CFU-GM growth, while it inhibits leukemic clonal growth *in vitro*, thus indicating little therapeutic advantages;
— both TPA and Teleocidins are very potent tumor promoters;
— phorbol diesters have very strong inflammatory activity;
— they induce differentiation only of the more differentiated myeloid leukemias [11, 12].

Other nonphysiological compounds like DMSO induce differentiation both

*Table 2.* Human and murine myeloid leukemia cell lines

| KG-1 | Myeloblast | Human |
|---|---|---|
| ML-1 | Myelomonoblast | Human |
| ML-3 | | |
| HL-60 | Promyelocyte | Human |
| THP-1 | Monoblast | Human |
| U937 | Monocyte | Human |
| K562 | Early blast, erythroblast | Human |
| WEHI-3B | Myelomonocyte | Mouse |
| M-1 | Myeloblast | Mouse |

of the human leukemic cell line HL-60 and of the murine myeloid leukemia line M-1, thus suggesting that both cell lines have common cellular 'receptors' for these substances. Unfortunately, since they are usually incapable of inducing differentiation of fresh human leukemic cells, no clinical application is indicated [8].

Among purine and pyrimidine analogues, two compounds, already extensively used as chemotherapeutic agents are quite promising: 5-Azacytidine (5-Aza) and Cytosine Arabinoside (ARA-C). At $10^{-5}$–$10^{-6}$ M 5-Aza and its derivative 5-deoxyazacitidine (5-DAza) have been shown to induce the HL-60 cell line to differentiate along the myeloid pathway and the K562 cell line to differentiate terminally into hemoglobin containing erythroblasts.

Recent studies have shown that 5-Aza is capable of triggering globin gene expression when administered *in vivo* to thalassemia and sickle cell anemia patients. These effects could be attributed to the ability of these molecules to cause synthesis of hypomethylated DNA; DNA methylation is believed to control the normal development of the differentiation process. *In vitro,* 5-deoxyazacytidine has been shown to induce terminal differentiation of leukemic blasts from patients with myeloblastic and monoblastic acute leukemias. It is interesting to note that the concentration of 5-deoxyazacytidine used to induce differentiation is significantly lower than that needed to achieve an appreciable clinical cytotoxic effect [13].

Ara-C is a nucleoside analogue that has been used extensively in the treatment of acute myelogenous leukemia. It inhibits DNA synthesis by its incorporation into leukemic cell DNA. Sublethal doses of Ara-C partially slow DNA replication and induce terminal differentiation in human myeloid leukemia cells *in vitro* [14]. Ara-C is only a weak inducer of granulocyte differentiation of the HL-60 cell line. *In vitro* in primary cultures of leukemic cells, Ara-C, at concentrations of $10^{-6}$–$10^{-7}$ M (which are not cytotoxic) induces differentiation and clonal growth inhibition of myeloblastic, myelomonocytic and promyelocytic leukemias [15–17].

In the past few years there have been several reports of the clinical usefulness of low dose Ara-C in the treatment of acute myeloid leukemias, myelodysplastic syndromes and preleukemic states. The results are quite contradictory. Some reports seem to suggest that therapy with continuous infusion of low-dose Ara-C is associated with beneficial responses in from 50 to 75% patients, with very limited toxicity. Other reports state quite the opposite [15, 18, 21]. The mechanisms by which low-dose continuous infusion of Ara-C might induce remission in some of these cases is still unclear. At the present moment, clinical and experimental findings are in keeping with the hypothesis that low-dose Ara-C acts both as a myelosuppressive agent as well as a differentiating agent.

Larger, randomized controlled trials are warranted, however, to definitively determine the clinical utility of low-dose Ara-C.

The group of physiological inducers of differentiation is quite interesting, because it is composed of molecules which are physiological products of normal tissues. Thus, their toxicity should be less than that of nonphysiological compounds.

Vitamin A and its analogues (retinoids) may play an important role in normal and leukemic hematopoiesis. While they appear to enhance normal hematopoietic proliferation, they exert an antiproliferative effect on leukemic cells. The most extensively studied system has been the human promyelocytic leukemic cell line HL-60, which can be induced to differentiate to mature granulocytes following exposure to $10^{-7}$ M retinoic acid. Human U937 and murine WEHI-3B and M1 cell lines can be triggered to maturation, while KG-1, ML-3 and K562 are resistant. Besides their differentiation effect, retinoids exert an antiproliferative effect and have been demonstrated to inhibit the proliferation of HL-60 and KG-1 in vitro [22]. Whereas retinoic acid induces the in vitro differentiation of blast cells from promyelocytic leukemias, it inhibits both the in vitro proliferation of blast cells from patients with AML and the clonal growth and self-renewal potential of granulocyte-monocyte committed precursors from patients with chronic myeloid leukemia [8, 23, 24]. Therefore, it is likely that retinoic acid selectively inhibits leukemic self-renewal independent of activation of the differentiation process in leukemic stem cells. The data from in vitro studies seem to point out that the antiproliferative action of retinoids on leukemic cells is more general than the induction of terminal differentiation.

The potential efficiency of retinoic acid in the treatment of human leukemias is further suggested by the observation that retinoic acid enhances CSF induced clonal growth of normal myeloid stem cells in vitro and that the same dosages which are inhibitory for CML CFU-GM are stimulatory or, at least, not suppressive for normal CFU-GM [23, 24].

Recently, retinoic acid has been administered in vivo. Very few patients have been treated. Therefore, it is not possible, at the moment, to judge its real efficacy. However, it may be of value in treatment of patients with certain myelodysplastic syndromes and perhaps in acute myelofibrosis. Attempts to use retinoic acid in association with chemotherapeutic protocls, as in treatment of CML, in order to prevent the expansion of the $Ph_1$ positive clone are disappointing [25, 26].

The active form of vitamin D and its analogues may also prove of clinical utility in inducing myeloid leukemia cell differentiation. At $10^{-7}$ M Dihydroxyvitamin $D_3$ inhibits the growth of HL-60, KG-1 and ML-3 cell lines. At the same concentration it also induces the maturation to monocyte-macrophages of nearly 85% of HL-60 and ML-3 cells. Recent studies by Moore and his colleagues show that calciferol is capable both of inducing differentiation of WEHI-3B and HL-60 leukemic colonies in an agar system and of mediating a potent and selective inhibition of leukemic clonal proliferation. The selectivity of this action is emphasized by the lack of any inhibition of normal CFU-GM at concentrations of the compound which are strongly inhibitory for leukemic growth [8, 27]. Clinical trials are in progress.

The therapeutic possibility of manipulation of normal regulatory molecules in leukemia has gained interest since the demonstration, *in vitro*, that terminal differentiation and leukemic stem cell suppression can be induced in several mouse and human myeloid leukemic cell lines by normal tissue products.

Increasing attention has been focused on colony stimulating factor (CSF), a known regulator of normal hematopoietic cell growth.

Studies by Moore and Metcalf on murine granulo-monocytic precursors led to recognition of the existence of two distinct molecules which stimulate the proliferation towards macrophage (M-CSF) and granulocyte-monocyte (GM-CSF) pathways. These molecules have been recently purified and characterized in terms of their molecular and functional properties. More recently, an additional type of CSF, antigenically and biochemically different from M-CSF and GM-CSF, was recognized and called G-CSF or GM-DF, because of its ability to stimulate granulocytic colony formation of normal mouse cells and to induce terminal differentiation in mouse leukemia cells [8, 28, 29].

The existence of a similar factor for human leukemias has now been documented; however, the relationship between differentiation-inducing factor (DIF) and CSF is not completely clear. Very recent reports from Moore's laboratories claim that DIF has been purified from the supernatant of a human bladder carcinoma cell line that constitutively produces CSF and BPA. It seem that DIF is present in the same fraction which also possesses GM-CSF, BPA and, probably, multipotent CSF activity [30].

A major source of DIF is post endotoxin sera. Macrophages and lymphocytes are the most likely producers. The ability to induce human GM-DF in patients receiving endotoxin provides the basis for a differential therapy in those leukemias where preliminary *in vitro* studies suggest a sensitivity to GM-DF. Chronic elevated levels of GM-DF could be maintained by administration of an exogenous source of endotoxin or by injecting an inducer of endogenous activity. At the moment, however, no data are available on the effect of GM-DF on fresh human leukemic cells.

The effect of interferons on leukemic and normal myeloid differentiation is not yet clear. Alpha and beta interferons alone do not induce differentiation of HL-60; however, they enhance the induction of differentiation triggered by DIF, TPA and retinoic acid [31]. Human purified gamma interferon induces differentiation of HL-60 and of the human monocytic cell line U937. Recent studies with natural and recombinant gamma interferon show that interferon at low doses acts as a 'biological response modifier' in that it reinduces, in U937 clonogenic cells, responsiveness to several physiological inhibitors of myelopoiesis (i.e. prostaglandin E, AIF, LF) [32].

Induction of remission of acute leukemias by cell differentiation is a new concept and several substances both pharmacological and physiological have been shown to act *in vitro* as differentiating agents.

In comparison to cytotoxic drugs, which inhibit leukemic proliferation, agents which induce terminal differntiation are more selective, but, as yet, less potent. It is unlikely that the administration of a differentiation-inducing factor would be effective *in vivo* as the sole form of therapy, but combinations of biological response modifiers with or without chemotherapy should be considered, mainly to further reduce the leukemic load in the remission phase of acute leukemias and, perhaps, to delay the onset of blastic crisis in CML.

## Acknowledgement

This work has been supported by C.N.R., 'Progetto Finalizzato Oncologia', grant no. 84.00415.44 and by Associazione Italiana Ricerca sul Cancro.

## References

1. Moore MAS, Kurland J, Broxmeyer HE: Regulatory interactions in normal and leukemic myelopoiesis. In: Differentiation of normal and neoplastic hematopoietic cells. Clarkson B, Marks P, Till J (eds). Cold Spring Harbor, New York, 393, 1978.
2. Gavosto F, Pileri A: The cell cycle of cancer cells in man. In: The cell cycle of cancer. Baserga R (ed). Marcel Dekker Inc., New York, 99, 1971.
3. Moore MAS, Spitzer G, Williams N, Metcalf D, Buckley J: Agar culture studies in 127 cases of untreated acute leukemia: The prognostic value of reclassification of leukemia according to in vitro growth characteristics. Blood 44:1, 1974.
4. Moore MAS: Humoral regulation of granulopoiesis. Clin Haematol 8:287, 1979.
5. Broxmeyer HE, Bognacki J, Dörner MH, de Sousa M: The identification of leukemia-associated inhibitory activity (LIA) as acidic isoferritins: A regulatory role for acidic isoferritins in the production of granulocyte and macrophages. J Exp Med 153:1426, 1981.
6. Aglietta M, Piacibello W, Gavosto F: Insensitivity of chronic myeloid leukemia cells to inhibition of growth by prosta-glandin E. Cancer Res 40:2507, 1980.
7. Pelus LM, Broxmeyer HE, Clarkson BD, Moore MAS: Abnormal responsibeness of granulocyte-macrophage committed colony forming cells from patients with chronic myeloid leukemia to inhibition by prostaglandin E. Cancer Res 40:1223, 1980.
8. Koeffler PH: Induction of differentiation of human acute myelogenous leukemia cells: Therepeutic implications. Blood 62:709, 1983.
9. Lotem H, Sachs L: Regulation of normal differentiation in mouse and human myeloid leukemic cells by phorbol esters and mechanisms of tumor promotion. Proc Natl Acad Sci USA 76:5158, 1979.
10. Koeffler PH, Bar Eli M, Territo M: Phorbol ester effect on differentiation of human myeloid leukemia cell lines blocked at different stages of maturation. Cancer Res 41:919, 1981.

11. Koeffler HP: Human myelogenous leukemia: enhanced clonal proliferation in the presence of phorbol diesters. Blood 57:256, 1981.

12. Pegoraro L, Bagnara G, Bonsi L, Biagini G, Garbarino G, Pagliardi G: Different responsiveness of colony-forming cells from normal subjects and chronic leukemia patients to 12-O-tetradecanoylphorbol 13-1cetate (TPA). Cancer Res 41:5049, 1981.

13. Pinto A, Attadia V, Fusco A, Ferrara F, Spada OA, Di Fiore PP: 5-Aza-2'-Deoxycytidine induces terminal differentiation of leukemic blasts from patients with acute myeloid leukemias. Blood 64:922, 1984.

14. Major PP, Egan EM, Herrick DJ, Kufe DW: The effect of Ara-C incorporation on deoxyribonucleic acid synthesis in cells. Biochem Pharmacol 31:2937, 1982.

15. Wisch JS, Griffin MD, Kufe DW: Response of preleukemic syndromes to continuous infusion of low-dose cytarabine. N Engl J Med 309:1599, 1983.

16. Kufe DW, Major PP, Egan EM, Beardsley GP: Correlation of cytotoxicity with incorporation of Ara-C into DNA. J Biol Chem 255:8997, 1980.

17. Griffin J, Munroe D, major P, Kufe D: Induction of differentiation of human myeloid leukaemia cells by inhibitors of DNA synthesis. Exp Hematol 10:774, 1982.

18. Housset M, Daniel M, Degos L: Small doses of Ara-C in the treatment of acute myeloid leukemia: differentiation of myeloid leukemia cells? Br J Haematol 51:125, 1982.

19. Castaigne S, Daniel MT, Tilly H, Herait P, Degos L: Does treatment with Ara-C in low dosage cause differentiation of leukemic cells? Blood 82:85, 1983.

20. Michalewicz R, Lotem J, Sachs L: Cell differentiation and therapeutic effect of low doses of cytosine arabinoside in human myeloid leukemia. Leukemia Res 8:783, 1984.

21. Hagenbeek A, Sizoo W, Löwenberg B: Treatment of acute myelocytic leukemia with low dose cytosine arabinoside: results of a pilot study in four patients. Leukemia Res 7:443, 1983.

22. Breitman TR, Selonie SE, Collins SJ: Induction of differentiation of the human promyelocytic leukemia cell line (HL-60) by retinoic acid. Proc Natl Acad Sci USA 77:2936, 1980.

23. Douer D, Koeffler HP: Retinoic Acid enhances colony-stimulating factor induced clonal growth of normal human myeloid progenitor cells in vitro. Exp Cell Res 138:193, 1982.

24. Aglietta M, Piacibello W, Stacchini A, Sanavio F, Gavosto F: Invitro effect of retinoic acid on normal and chronic myeloid leukemia granulopoiesis. Leukemia Res (in press).

25. Flynn PJ, Miller WJ, Weisdorf DJ, Arthur DC, Branda RF: Retinoic acid treatment of acute promyelocytic leukemia: in vivo and in vitro observations. Blood 62:1211, 1983.

26. Arlin Z, Berman E, Gee T, Mertelsman R, Kempin S, Moore M, Itri L, Kurland E, Clarkson B: 13 cis-retinoic acid (RA) does not improve the true remission rate or the duration of the true remission (induced with cytostatic chemotherapy) in chronic myeloid leukemia. Blood 62(Suppl 1, abstr):700, 1983.

27. Miyaura C, Abe E, Kuribayashi T, Tanaka H, Konno K, Nishii Y, Suda T: 1,25-dihydroxyvitamin $D_3$ induces differentiation of human myeloid leukemia cells. Biochem Biophys Res Commun 102:937, 1981.

28. Moore MAS, Sheridan APC: The role of proliferation and maturation factors in myeloid leukemia. In: Maturation factors and cancer. Moore MAS (ed). Raven Press, NY, 361, 1982.

29. Metcalf D: Clonal analysis of the response of HL60 human myeloid leukemia cells to biological regulators. Leukemia Res 7:117, 1983.

30. Gabrilove J, Platzer E, Welte K, LuL, Levi E, Moore MAS: Constitutive production and biochemical purification of leukemia differentiation factors, by a human epithelial bladder carcinoma cell line. Exp Hematol 12(6) (Abstr):47, 1984.

31. Tomida M, Jamamoto Y, Hozumi M: Stimulation by interferon of induction of differentiation of human promyelocytic leukemia cells. Biochem Biophys Res Commun 104:30, 1982.

32. Piacibello W, Broxmeyer HE: Modulation of expression of Ia(HLA-DR)-antigens on human monocyte cell line U937 by gamma interferon and prostaglandin E and responsiveness of U937 colony forming cells to inhibition by lactoferrin, transferrin, acidic isoferritins and prostaglandin E. Blood 62(Suppl 1, abstr):246, 1984.

# 21. The development of 9-substituted purines as immunomodulators

A. GINER-SOROLLA and J.W. HADDEN

Antineoplasic and antiviral therapy has been centered in recent decades on the study and application of cytostatic agents of synthetic origin such as alkylating agents, steroids and antimetabolites or natural occurring substances such as alkaloids and antibiotics. With these drugs, a certain percentage of malignant tumors have responded with more or less prolonged remissions. Unfortunately, many human neoplasias do not respond to this kind of therapy. In addition, the use of these agents is accompanied by toxic effects and by the appearance of the phenomenon of drug resistance. Also paradoxically, a high proportion of these agents are carcinogenic in animals. In man this fact is reflected in an incidence of secondary cancers in those patients who survive chemotherapeutic treatment and may be attributed to the intrinsic immunosuppressive nature of these chemotherapeutic agents. Alkylating agents, for example, act by inhibiting protein synthesis, including that of antibody formation which results in a profound humoral immunosuppression. As had been observed with the use of most chemotherapeutic agents, suppression of the cellular immune response is also very evident. To circumvent these obstacles, immunotherapy aims at augmenting natural body responses against the attack of cancer cells by the use of non-toxic and non-carcinogenic substances. This 'pro-host' approach, led to the development of two series of 9-substituted purines: one consisting of 9-alkyl-hypoxanthines and the other of 7,8-dihydrothiazolo-hypoxanthines. Their development and action on the immune system will be discussed.

The study of the immune system has experienced an extraordinary growth in recent years; one of the discoveries responsible for the progress attained was the association of cases of congenital immunodeficiency with defects in enzymes which are involved in the metabolism of components of nucleic acids such as purine nucleosides. The first finding of a relationship between congenital immunodeficiency and altered functions of an enzyme intimately related to the metabolism of components of nucleic acids, was made by Giblett and coworkers [1]. These authors noticed that one case of congenital deficiency of adenosine deaminase (ADA) was accompanied with a severe dual system immunodeficiency. This defect involves an absence of ADA in children who showed a marked susceptibility to infections and was related to a dysfunction in T and B cells. It is well known that T cells are not active by themselves, acting upon factors, e.g., interleukins, lymphokines, etc. which in a non-specific form augment their proliferative and cytotoxic activity. Also macrophages possess the capacity of recognizing and destroying neoplastic cells *in vivo* and can be activated by a variety of immunostimulants *(Corynebacterium parvum,* BCG [2–4], among those of biological origin; polynucleotides, nucleosides and purines, among the chemically defined agents, see [5] for review). These findings helped focus attention on the study of components of nucleic acids as factors related with immunological processes.

## 9-Substituted purines as immunomodulators

### 9-Alkylpurine derivatives

The enzyme ADA is widely distributed in the mammalian organism and functions to convert upon deamination, adenosine (or adenylic acid) into inosine (or inosinic acid). The finding that a polymer of ionisic-cytidylic acids (poly-I:C) has an immunopotentiating effect, as well as the presence of inosinic acid in transfer factor stimulated our interest towards the development of derivatives containing the hypoxanthine moiety. The chemical structure of transfer factor has been recently partially unraveled; in addition to inosinic acid it contains an oligopeptide which may be responsible for informational function [6]. To these facts, we have to add the extensive work carried out with a complex containing inosine, inosiplex or methisoprinol (the salt of p-acetaminobenzoic acid, N,N-dimethylamino-2-propanol and inosine in a 3:1 molar ratio) (Figure 1). By a diversity of physicochemical data it has been shown that the three components of Inosiplex form a complex which exerts biological effects either not manifest or weakly so when the components are used separately. Inosiplex is endowed with a mild to modest antiviral activity *in vivo* and has been used throughout more than 70 countries for the treatment of a variety of viral or viral-related disorders [7]. Inosiplex does not exhibit a detectable mitogenic activity for lymphocytes at pharmacological concentrations; it does enhance their proliferative responses to a variety of stimuli. The mechanisms of these actions are not clear. Inosiplex also induces T-cell differentiation [8]. This effect is only weakly mimicked by inosine alone. Inosiplex partially [9] restores the inhibited proliferation of lymphocytes cultured in the presence of 2'-deoxycoformycin, an irreversible ADA inhibitor [10]. Hadden [11] has shown

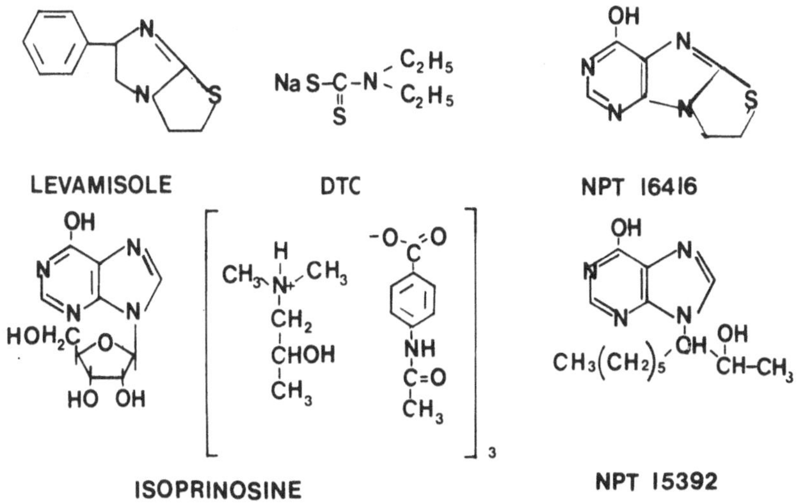

*Figure 1.* Synthetic Immunomodulators.

that the *in vitro* profile of action of isoprinosine on lymphocyte proliferation is mimicked by inosine and concluded that complex formation potentiates inosine effects. An action of Inosiplex to stimulate RNA synthesis has been described [12], perhaps mediated by the effects of inosine on orotic acid incorporation into RNA.

Inosiplex (50–600 mg/kg) has been shown to be active in murine tumor systems, to increase vaccine protection in L1210 leukemia, to potentiate interferon therapy in sarcoma 180, and to reduce tumor development in rabbits infected with Shope virus and NZB mice with autoimmune disease. Inosiplex therapy has promoted restoration of depressed immunological responses in humans with gynecological cancer treated with radiation and decreased infections in chemotherapy-treated patients.

The effect of Inosiplex can be best explained by its action on the immune system; it induces lymphocyte differentiation comparable to thymic hormones and augments lymphocyte, macrophage and natural killer cell activities in an immunopotentiator mode of action. In addition, inosiplex among other effects has shown a promotion of restoration of depressed immune responses in humans with cancer and in the early phases of acquired immunodificiency syndrome (AIDS).

Results described above prompted the investigation of molecules related to inosine and among the several derivatives obtained in a first series of 9-alkylpurines. We found that a compound related to the ADA inhibitor *erythro*-9 (2-hydroxy-3-nonyl) adenine, (EHNA) developed by Schaeffer, namely, *erytrho*-9 (2-hydroxy-3-nonyl) hypoxanthine (NPT 15392) (Figure 1) having less ADA inhibitory activity *in vitro*, shared each of the immunopharmacological properties of inosiplex [7]. However, NPT 15392 is effective at 1/10th to 1/1000th of the concentration of inosiplex. A number of differences in the degree of activity suggests that NPT 15392 may have clinical activities that will be complementary to those of inosiplex. Specifically, NPT 15392 at 0.01 1 μg/ml induces prothymocyte differentiation [14] and augments rosettes of T cells and modulates their proliferative, helper, and suppressor functions [15–18]. It also potentiates lymphokine effects on macrophages [15, 16]. At therapeutic doses of 0.1–1 mg/kg, side effects in animals and man have been neglible and animal toxicity studies indicate oral $LD_{50}$ of more than 500 mg/kg. *In vivo* immunopharmacological effects have included significant augmentation of antibody and cellular immune responses in mice. NPT 15392 augments natural killer-cell activity in mice *in vivo* but not *in vitro*. This effect is apparently not mediated by interferon and the effect of the combination of interferon and NPT 15392 is additive.

In murine models, NPT 15392 (0.1 mg/kg) has shown effects that partially reversed tumor-, virus- and chemotherapy-induced immunosuppression in eight of nine studies. Correlation of immunorestoration with increased survival or decreased metastasis formation has been observed in T241 fibrosarcoma, sarcoma 180, Lewis lung carcinoma, AH41c, 44, 66, and 130 tumors, and P388 leukemia. No effect alone was observed in L1210 leukemia or NF sarcoma. In immunopharmacological trials in humans with cancer under the aegis of the EORTC, NPT 15392 showed effect to augment lymphocyte counts, active rosettes, and natural killer cells in some but not all patients.

At concentrations above 1 μg/ml NPT 15392 is a relatively selective cGMP phosphodiesterase inhibitor, and while it is 100 times more active than inosiplex or inosine in this regard, this effect probably does not account for its immunopharmacological effects, observed at 0.01–0.1 μg/ml. It does not influence adenosine effects on cAMP levels [19]. Low concentrations (0.1 μg) partially inhibit PNP (<20%) [20] and this observation, of the several mentioned, is the only which correlates on a dose-response basis with biological activity. Touraine [21] has shown that NPT 15392 can potentiate inosiplex indicating that NPT 15392 action may involve an inosine sparing effect, perhaps through the action of NPT 15392 to partially inhibit nucleoside phophorylase. Thus, an inosine-sparing activity, if documented, could be an explanation for the action of this drug.

### 9-Thiazolylpurine compounds

A second series of immunomodulators developed in our laboratory consist of thiazolyl compounds of hypoxanthine. Initially we synthesized a variety of 8-(4′-thiazolyl)purines [22] as the analogs of thiabendazole, a potent antihelmintric drug, ((4′-thiazolyl)benzimidazole), which was independently found by Renoux and Lundy to act as an immunopotentiator by increasing the cellular and humoral immune responses in animals. The potential immunostimulant activity of the thiazolyl derivatives as analogs of thiabendazole was determined in our laboratory; and the hypoxanthine, adenine, 6-chloro and 6-mercaptopurine derivatives with the thiazolyl ring covalently bond to the c-8 were found to have no significant immunostimulating effect. We turned our attention then to levamisole, a tetrahydro-6-phenylimidazothiazole derivative [23] which was originally used as an antihelmintic and, like thiabendazole, was found to augment cellular immune response in animals and also clinically in cancer patients [24, 25]. In parallel to the analogy used in the synthesis of 8-(4′-thiazolyl)purines, we explored the possibility of synthesizing purine analogs of levamisole. Thiazole fused to purines such as several thiazole derivatives of xanthine and theophylline were synthesized by Todd and Ochiai, respectively [26, 27], as potential purine antagonists. Other similar compounds were described by Gordon [28] and Montgomery [29] and coworkers.

We have synthesized the prototype/purine analog of levamisole, namely 7,8-dihydrothiazolo [3,2-e] hypoxanthine, (NPT 16416) (Figure 1) by interaction of 8-mercaptohypoxanthine with 1,2-dibromoethane, which gives two isomers (N-9 and N-7 substituted) or by other novel methods which lead to the N-9 compound exclusively. Unlike levamisole, NPT 16416 is relatively nontoxic ($LD_{50}$ in mice in excess of 500 mg/kg per os). This compound at submicrogram per milliliter doses increases 'active' rosettes of human T cells. At these concentrations it has an intermediate effect to induce T-cell differentiation in the Komuro and Boyse assay. This effect is approximately one-half that of isoprinosine and NPT 15392 and compares directly to effects of similar concentrations of adenosine and inosine. These findings indicate further that the purine configuration independent of the 9-substitution is responsible for this activity. NPT 16416, like levamisole and NPT 15392, shows little or no effect on mitogen responses of human lymphocytes in the concentration range 0.001–1 µg/ml. Above 5 µg/ml it stimulates pokeweed and LPS responses but not PHA or Con A responses, indicating a possible selective effect on B cells in this concentration range unlike any of the other substituted purines. *In vivo,* like all the 9-substituted purines, it augments sheep erythrocyte plaqueforming cell responses. While much is needed to be learned about this agent, it appears to share some properties with the purines and some with levamisole, in addition to the unique effect on B-cell mitogen responses [30].

NPT 16416 acts to increase cGMP in lymphocytes in a parallel way to imidazole and levamisole [31]. While imidazole-like effects to increase cGMP phosphodiesterase and to inhibit cGMP phosphodiesterase, as described in the brain, might be involved, rapid reversible increases of cGMP observed with NPT 16416 are more reminiscent of agonists of the guanylate cyclase system. Other actions of this compound remain to be explored.

## Discussion

We discussed at the Advanced Course in Immunopharmacology and Immunotherapy held in Erice in 1983 [32] the polyvalent and often paradoxical properties of several purines and nucleosides which we developed in the past as potential antitumor and antiviral agents. It was a common feature of the C-6 and C-2,6 substituted purines to exert, along with their inhibitory activity on tumor growth in experimental animals, a potent carcinogenic effect, which is also found with the majority of clinically used antitumor agents. In contrast, the corresponding N-9 ribosyl or arabinosyl purine derivatives which had antitumor or antiviral activity, did not show any carcinogenic effect, but they were toxic in clinical trials. This toxicity and carcinogenicity can be attributed to the enzymatic activity of ADA and also to the immunosuppressing effect inherent to the antimetabolite mode of action of these compounds.

It is impossible at this time to offer a unified hypothesis to explain the action of these 9-substituted hypoxanthines, and obvious differences in the actions and mechanisms might mitigate against this. Certain similarities, however, make it enticing to speculate. All of the compounds share a hypoxanthine structure and since hypoxanthine is inactive in the assays of lymphocyte differentiation and proliferation and inosine is active, it seems likely that inosine forms the basis for the active site. Because the biological actions differ from those of adenosine actions via cAMP and because inosine is inactive on the adenylate cyclase system, they do not appear to act on a purine receptor for adenosine. Their actions probably do not involve modification of function through a direct contribution to substrate levels since; except for isoprinosine the compounds are active only at low concentration (0.01–10 µg/ml).

The evidence points to an inosine receptor linked to allosteric modification of an unknown enzymatic pathway. All the compounds have activity to induce T-cell differentiation and while the mechanism by which thymic hormones induce the differentiation is not known, it seems logical to suggest the mechanism for these compounds will be the same as that of the thymic hormones.

We have tested more than 80 9-substituted hypoxanthines and it is clear they offer a spectrum of action. It might be suggested that, in parallel argument to the adenosine analogs, the ribose-like substitutions modify the affinity of the hypoxanthine moiety for an inosine P-type receptor, so it might be that these compounds will bind and be agonists for an inosine P receptor; alternatively, like the methylxanthines, these compounds may turn out to be antagonists for R-type receptors.

It is possible that 9-substituted components of the purine ring have individual activities under certain circumstances. For example, NPT 16416 has an imidazole-like activity in that it induces, like levamisole and imidazole [11], early increases in cGMP. It is not clear how an exposed imidazole may occur. If the action is, indeed, mediated by imidazole, the cyclic nucleotide-related effects may be explained directly or indirectly either by action on phosphodiesterases or other enzymes related to cyclic nucleotide formation (e.g., cyclo- and lipooxygenases or cyclic nucleotide cyclases, etc.). This imidazole-like activity is not shared by the other compounds, as far as we know.

The 9-substitutions may offer activities on different enzymes in lymphocytes or even on different cells. It is clear that the action of NPT 15392 compares favorably to the methylxanthines for inhibition of cyclic nucleotide phosphodiesterase; this action is imposed with the 9-*erythro* moiety. We do not know yet if EHNA, NPT 16416, are active in this regard. We do know that the potency of NPT 15392 for this effect is 100 times greater than inosine itself.

The sulfur-containing ring apparent in the structure of NPT 16416 is envisioned to confer levamisole-like activities to inhibit suppressor cell function and induce *in vivo* a thymic hormones-like substance as described by Renoux for levamisole and other sulfur-containing compounds.

The alkyl chain of NPT 15392 may confer properties that simulate the ribose moiety of inosine and favor a mimicry of inosine. Alternatively, the chain may confer yet-to-be-defined properties of its own. With the addition of a terminal arginine on an alkyl chain, as in the PCF compounds [33], a new characteristic is apparently acquired. A direct activation of guanylate cyclase is suggested, based on indirect evidence [34]. Notably, the target cells involved may change and tuftsin-like actions on phagocytes [35] become included in the repertoire of immunopharmacological effects.

The actions of NPT 15392 on NP and ADA are provocative in suggesting that these enzymes might be regulatory in lymphocyte function. While it is clear that marked inhibition (or absence) is destructive for lymphocytes, mild or transient inhibition may be stimulatory. The notion that these compounds are allosteric modifiers of inosine- or hypoxanthine-utilizing enzymes is thought-provoking. Through metabolic conversion, hypoxanthine-containing compounds may give rise to active analogs of xanthine and uric acid. Uric acid is an antioxidant which has been hypothesized to be a pro-host, anticancer, antiaging agent [8, 36], and it could conceivably be that these compounds, as has been shown for isoprinosine, increase urate levels. Finally, allosteric modification either with induction of increased or decreased activity of ADA, PNP, 5'-nucleotidase inosine dehydrogenase and HGPRT must be considered as possible enzymatic targets of action [37].

## Conclusions

The foregoing indicates that purines, particularly inosine-containing or inosine-like compounds, offer a variety of structures having diverse immuno-pharmacological properties. Insofar as tested, the compounds are remarkably nontoxic, potentially immunosuppressive only at very high concentrations, and if antiviral, not potently so and not carcinogenic. They generally share, where examined, the capacity to mimic thymic hormones action, to induce precursor T-cell differentiation and to potentiate functional responses of mature T cells. They also act to augment macrophage functions. The biochemical information on their mechanisms of action would indicate some are linked to cyclic nucleotides in their actions but others are not: one common mechanism of action may be through a proposed inosine receptor. The different structures here described as well as other new derivative currently under development show promise to attain a goal of obtaining compounds with clinically useful applications.

*Table 1.*

| Class 1: Thymmommetic drugs | Indirect T-cell induction[a] | Active rosettes | CMI | T-dependent B-cell response |
|---|---|---|---|---|
| Sulphur-containing compounds | | | | |
| Levamisole | + | + | + | + |
| Diethyl dithocarbamate | + | NT | + | + |
| NPT 16416 | NT | + | NT | + |
| Thiabendazole | + (+Ag) | NT | + | NT |
| Thiazolobenzimidole | NT | + | + | + |
| Cimetidine | NT | + | + | + |

| Class 2: Thymommetic drugs | T-cell induction | Active rosettes | CMI | T-dependent B-cell response |
|---|---|---|---|---|
| Purine containing compounds | | | | |
| Isoprinosine | + | + | + | + |
| NPT 15392 | + | + | + | + |
| NPT 16416 | + | + | NT | + |
| PCF compound | + | NT | NT | NT |
| Transfer factor | + | + | + | NT |

[a] Via a serum factor induced *in vitro*.

# References

1. Giblett E, Anderson J, Cohen F et al.: Lancet II:1067, 1972.
2. Scott MT: J Natl Cancer Inst 55:65, 1975.
3. Old LJ, Clarke DA, Benacerraf B: Nature 184:291, 1959.
4. Mathé G: Br Med J iv:7, 1969.
5. Hadden JW, Delmonte L, Oettgen HF: In: Comprehensive Immunology and Immunopharmacology. Hadden JW, Coffey RG, Spreafico F (eds). Plenum Publishing, New York, 279, 1977.
6. Kirkpatrick CH, Burger DR: In: The lymphokines: Biochemistry and Biological Activities. Hadden JW, Stewart II WE (eds). Humana Press Clifton NJ, 261, 1982.
7. Hadden JW, Giner-Sorolla A: In: Augmenting agents in Cancer Therapy. Current Status and Future Prospects. Chirigos M, Hersh E (eds). Raven Press, New York, 497, 1981.
8. Ames BN, Cathcart R, Schwiers E, Hochstein P: Proc Natl Acad Sci USA 78:5858, 1981.
9. Hadden JW, Pahwa R, Unpublished data.
10. Ballet JJ, Morin A, Schmitt C, Agrapart M: Int J Immunopharma 4:151, 1982.
11. Hadden JW, Chedid L, Mullen P, Spreafico F: In: Advances Immunopharmacology. Pergamon, Oxford, 1981.
12. Gordon P, Brown ER: Can J Microbio 18:1463, 1972.
13. Schaeffer HJ, Schwender CF: J Med Chem 17:1, 1974.
14. Ikehara S, Hadden JW, Good RA, Pahawa R: Thymus 3:90, 1981.
15. Hadden JW, Hadden EM, Spira T, Settineri R, Simon L, Giner-Sorolla A: Int J Immunopharmacol 4:235, 1982a.
16. Hadden JW, Giner-Sorolla A, Hadden EM, Ikehara S, Pahwa R, Coffey R, Castellazi AM, Jones C, Maxwell K, Simon L: Int J Immunopharmacol 4:287, 1982b.
17. Merluzzi VJ, Walker MM, Williams N, Susskind B, Hadden JW, Faanes RB: Int J Immunopharmacol 4:219, 1982.
18. Florentin I, Taylor E, Davigny M, Mathé G, Hadden JW: Int J Immunopharmacol 4:225, 1982.
19. Coffey RG, Hadden JW, in preparation.
20. Sordillo M, Trotta P, Hadden JW, unpublished data.
21. Touraine JL, Ferret GG, Sandji L, Othmane O, Fournie GJ, Touraine R: In: Current Concepts in Human Immunology and Cancer Immunomodulation. Serrou B (ed). Elsevier, Amsterdam, 491, 1982.
22. Giner-Sorolla A, Segarra JT, Brooks MH: J Med Chem 21:344, 1978.
23. Verhaegen H, DeCree J, DeCock W, Verbruggen F: N Engl J Med 289:1148, 1973.
24. Renoux G, Renoux M: CR acad Sci 278:1139, 1974.
25. Hadden JW, Coffey RG, Hadden EM, Lopez-Corrales E, Sunshine GH: Cell Immunol 20:98, 1975.
26. ToddAR, Bergel F: J Chem Soc 1559, 1936.
27. Ochiai E: Ber 69B:1650, 1936.
28. Gordon M: J Am Chem Soc 73:984, 1951.
29. Montgomery JA, Holum LB: J Am Chem Soc 79:2184, 1957.
30. Hadden JW, Cornaglia-Ferraris P, Coffey RG: In: Progress In Immunology, Fifth International Congress of Immunology. Yamamura Y, Tada T (eds). Academic Press, New York, 1393, 1984.
31. Hadden JW, Doffey RG: unpublished experiments.
32. Giner-Sorolla A: Proc. of Advanced Course of Immunopharmacology, Erice, Italy. In: EOS, Rivista di Immunologia ed Immunofarmacologia 4:129, 1983.
33. Cornaglia-Ferraris P, Coffey RG, Hadden JW: Proc of Advanced Course of Immunophar-

macology, Erice, Italy. In: EOS, Rivista di Immunologia ed Immunofarmacologia 4:134, 1983.

34. Deguchi T, Yoshika M: J Biol Chem 257:10147, 1982.
35. Phillips JH, Babcock GF, Nishioka K: J Immunol 126:915, 1981.
36. Hovi T, Allison AC, Raivio KO, Vaheri A: Ciba Found Symp 48:225, 1973.
37. Brosh S, Boer P, Kupfer B, DeVries A, Sperling o: J Clin Invest 58:289, 1976.

# 22. Immunopharmacologic profile of an L-Arginine hypoxanthine derivative: PCF/01

P. CORNAGLIA-FERRARIS

## Summary

The pharmacologic activity of a new hypoxanthine derivative, PCF/01, is described. This compound induces differentiation of θ-negative lymphocytes from nu/nu mice, modulates lymphocytes mitogen or antigen responsiveness and activates phagocytosis *in vitro*. Balb/c mice challenged with Pseudomonas Aeruginosa or with a transplantable methylcholanthrene-induced sarcoma (CE-2), survived when treated with this drug.

PCF/01 belongs to a new series of compounds which have been synthesized to expand the repertoire of N-9 substitutions of hypoxanthine. Evidence indicates that these compounds represent a new series of synthetic immunomodulators retaining some properties of inosine and hypoxanthine derivatives as Isoprinosine, also mimicing the action of immunoactive peptides, as Tuftsin.

## Introduction

Minute alterations of the purine structure yields compounds with different pharmacologic effects: anti-viral, anti-tumoral, carcinogenic, mutagenic, immunosuppressive, immunostimulant, etc.

The presentation of Giner-Sorolla in this section makes it clear that derivatives retaining an intact hypoxanthine moiety usually lack cytotoxicity and antitumor activity often showing immunomodulatory properties. Interest in some of these compounds such as isoprinosine [1], poly-I, poly-C [2] and erythro-9 (2-hydroxy-3-nonyl)hypoxanthine (NPT 15392) [3] is largely centered around their ability to modulate T-cell function resulting in various pharmacologic effects [4]. Isoprinosine (also known as methisoprinol) is actually under clinical investigation in acquired immune deficiency syndrome (AIDS) due to its capability to increase both IL-2 synthesis and TAC positive T-cells in such patients [5].

The mechanism of action of these synthetic immunomodifiers is still not completely understood (see Table 1 for summary). However it seems to be clear that the different functions induced by the various compounds of this family imply highly specific regulatory responses of immunocompetent cells in terms of both proliferation and differentiation. Variation at the N-9 site chain modifies the immunomodulatory properties while retaining some purine related activities [4].

In order to expand on the repertoire of the hypoxanthine derivatives we developed an original series of compounds characterized by a terminal amino acid substitution at the N-9 side chain [6]. Experimental evidence conducted both *in vitro* and *in vivo* indicates that these substances represent a unique series of drugs which, while retaining immunomodulatory properties of some of the inosine derivatives, such as isoprinosine, differ in action and mechanism (Table 1). A prototypic structure of this series is a N-9-alkyl-arginine derivative (PCF/01, Figure 1). In this paper we describe its pharmacologic properties emphasizing its potential application in clinical oncology.

*Table 1.* Mechanism of action of purines having immunomodulatory properties.

| Lym-phocyte diff. | Lym-phocyte prolif. | Immunomodulator | Cyclic AMP | Cyclic GMP | Other | Comments |
|---|---|---|---|---|---|---|
| + | − | Thymic humoral factor | ↑ | − | Adenosine or Adenosine-like | |
| + | − | Poly I: Poly C | ↑ (?) | − | | Poly I more active than Poly C |
| ? | + | Transfer factor | − | ↑ | | Cyclic GMP effect, result of contaminant? |
| + | + | Methisoprinol | − | − | ↑ RNA synthesis | |
| + | + | NPT 15392[a] | − | ↑ | | Inhibits cGMP >cAMP phosphodiesterase |
| + | + | NPT 16416[b] | − | ↑ | | Compares to imidazole, levamisole |
| + 0 | + | PCF compounds[c] | − | ↑ | | ? Arginine effect |

[a] 9-erythro 2 nonyl 3 hypoxanthine.

[b] 7,8-dihydrothiazole (3,2e) hypoxanthine.

[c] See Figure 1.

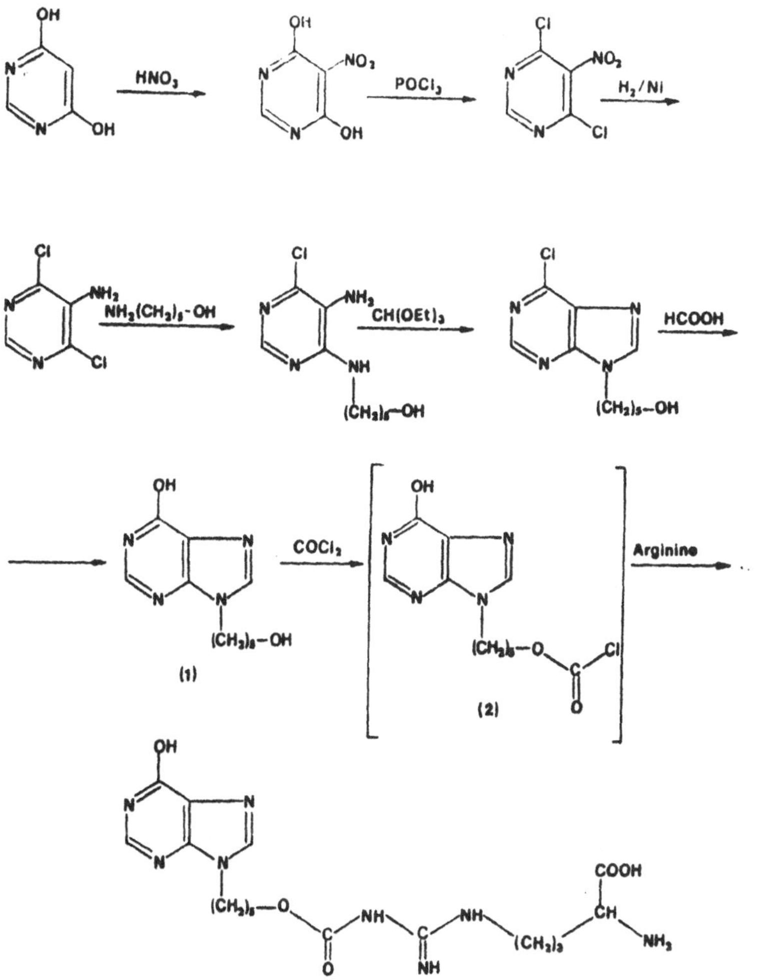

PCF/01

Synthesis of PCF/01: N⁷-/:/:b-(1,6-dihydro-6-oxo-9-purinyl)
pentyloxy:/carbonyl:/L-Arginine

*Figure 1.*

## Materials and methods

### PCF/01: Synthesis, chemical and physical properties

The synthetic pathway of PCF/01 is summarized in Figure 1; Figure 3 also reports the chemical and physical properties of this substance. Briefly the N-9 position of hypoxanthine has been conjugated (by a uretanic bond) with an L-Arginine which is the terminal amino acid of several peptides having pro-phagocyte activity, such as Tuftsin and Substance P [7–9].

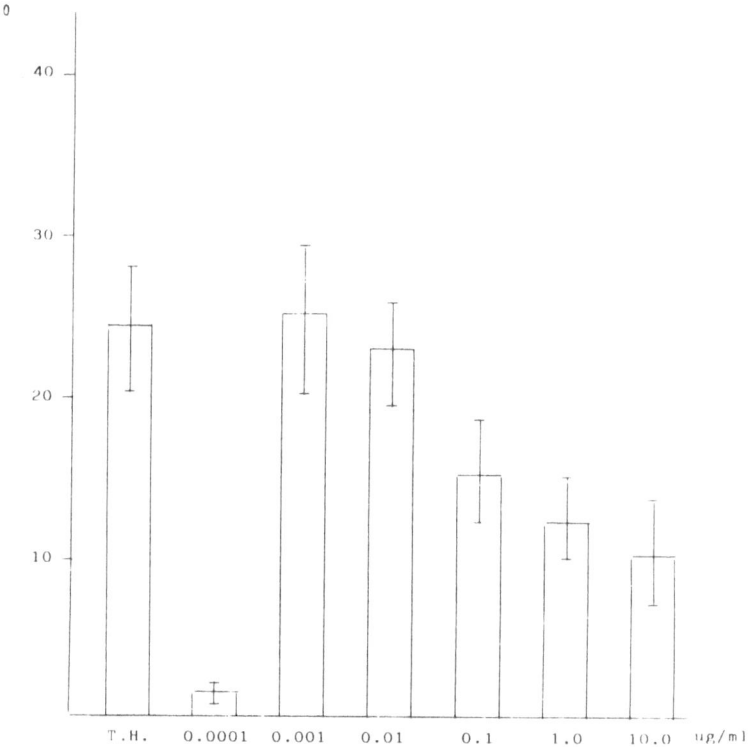

*Figure 2.* Fragmentation pattern from electron impact spectrum of PCF/01.

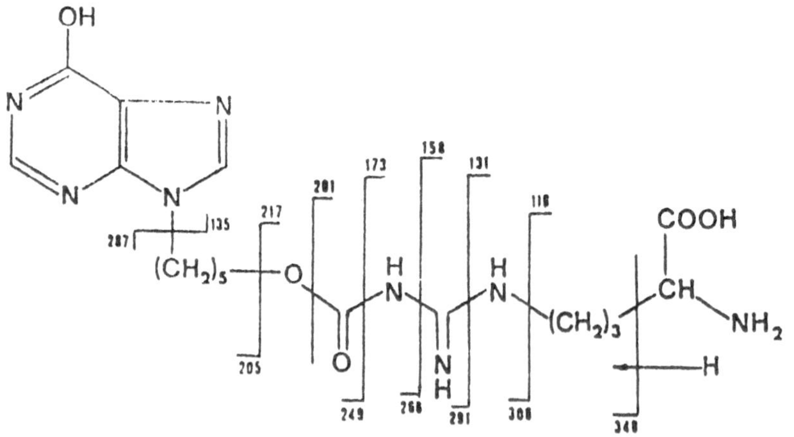

*Figure 3.* Fragmentation pattern from electron impact spectrum of PCF/01. Elemental analysis, infrared, proton magnetic resonance, 13 C nuclear magnetic resonance and mass spectra are in agreement with the proposed structure. Empirical formula: $C_{17}H_{26}N_8O_5$; Molecular weight: 422,442; melting point: 167°C; UV: 228.

*Pharmacologic activity* in vitro

The pharmacologic profile of PCF/01 will only be summarized in this section. PCF/01 has been tested at various concentrations *in vitro* for cytotoxicity (Table 2) and anti-viral activity (Table 3) with negative results.

The immunomodulatory properties have been tested *in vitro* with two cell targets: lymphocytes (both murine and human) and human polymorphonuclear leukocytes (PMN-L).

*Table 2.* PCF/01 toxicity on different cellular lines.

| PCF/01 (µM) | No. of viable cells after 72 h[a] | | | |
|---|---|---|---|---|
| | VERO | HEp-2 | W138 | MDCK |
| 0 | $1.5 \times 10^6$ | $2.4 \times 10^6$ | $2.1 \times 10^6$ | $2.8 \times 10^6$ |
| 500 | $1.0 \times 10^6$ | $2.0 \times 10^6$ | $2.0 \times 10^6$ | $2.6 \times 10^6$ |
| 250 | $1.3 \times 10^6$ | $2.2 \times 10^6$ | $2.1 \times 10^6$ | $2.7 \times 10^6$ |
| 125 | $1.4 \times 10^6$ | $2.6 \times 10^6$ | $2.0 \times 10^6$ | $2.8 \times 10^6$ |
| 62.5 | $1.4 \times 10^6$ | $2.3 \times 10^6$ | $2.2 \times 10^6$ | $2.7 \times 10^6$ |
| 31.2 | $1.3 \times 10^6$ | $2.4 \times 10^6$ | $2.1 \times 10^6$ | $2.5 \times 10^6$ |
| 15.6 | $1.5 \times 10^6$ | $2.5 \times 10^6$ | $2.3 \times 10^6$ | $2.6 \times 10^6$ |

[a] The different types of cells have been plated at the concentration of $3 \times 10^5$ cells/plate. After 24 h PCF/01 was added to the cultures at the concentrations indicated. After 3 days the number of viable cells were counted by Trypan blue esclusion test.

*Table 3.* Lack of antiviral activity of PCF/01[a].

| PCF/01 (µM) | HEV-1[b] | HSV-2[b] | Vaccinia[c] | Poliovirus[d] | A/PR/8/34[e] |
|---|---|---|---|---|---|
| — | $5.2 \times 10^7$ | $9.3 \times 10^6$ | $1.8 \times 10^8$ | $2.4 \times 10^8$ | $2.3 \times 10^5$ |
| 500 | $4.6 \times 10^7$ | $8.2 \times 10^6$ | $1.8 \times 10^8$ | $2.2 \times 10^8$ | $2.0 \times 10^5$ |
| 250 | $4.9 \times 10^7$ | $8.6 \times 10^6$ | $2.0 \times 10^8$ | $2.5 \times 10^8$ | $2.2 \times 10^5$ |
| 125 | $5.3 \times 10^7$ | $8.6 \times 10^6$ | $2.3 \times 10^8$ | $2.3 \times 10^8$ | $2.4 \times 10^5$ |
| 62.5 | $5.3 \times 10^7$ | $9.4 \times 10^6$ | $1.9 \times 10^8$ | $2.1 \times 10^8$ | $2.5 \times 10^5$ |

[a] Antiviral activity has been evaluated by Viral reduction test.
[b] Number of plaque forming units (PFU) of HSV-2 developed in VERO after 24 h of infection. Multiplicity of infection = 1.
[c] Number of PFU of Vaccinia developed in CHF after 24 h of infection. Multiplicity of infection = 1.
[d] Number of PFU of Poliovirus developed in HEp-2 after 24 h of infection. Multiplicity of infection = 1.
[e] Number of PFU of A/PR/8/34 developed in MDCK after 24 h of infection. Multiplicity of infection = 1.

## Lymphocyte proliferation

PCF/01 augments the mitogen or antigen induced T-cell proliferation of lymphocytes obtained from $C_3H/HAJ$ or $C_3D_2F_1$ spleens. At doses ranging from 0.1 to 10 µg/ml it also enhances the proliferative response of human peripheral blood lymphocytes to PHA or ConA at these same doses. In contrast the PWM and LPS induced proliferation of lymphocyte derived from Balb/c spleens was strongly suppressed with as little as 1 ng/ml. Preliminary evidence suggests a lymphokine mediated activity *in vitro*.

## Lymphocyte differentiation

PCF/01 has been tested in the Komuro and Boyse T-cell differentiation assay. Briefly, lymphocytes from nu/nu Balb/c mice were purified by density gradient, the θ negative fraction was separated and tested for viability (≥95%); cells were then washed and resuspended for 90′ at 37°C in the presence of concentrations of PCF/01 ranging from 0.1 to 10 µg/ml; thymic hormones were used as positive control and saline as negative. The expression of antigen was then evaluated with the trypan blue exclusion test after incubation with anti-θ monoclonal antibody plus complement. Results are summarized in Figure 2 from which it is clear that PCF/01, together with other hypoxanthine derivatives [4, demonstrates thymomimetic activity.

## Phagocytic activation

PMN-L from normal donors were tested in the luminol chemiluminescence assay [7]. PCF/01 induced a dramatic increase in the granulocyte respiratory burst in the presence of unopsonized Zymosan. This has been observed with doses higher than those used with lymphocyte targets (30 to 60 µg/ml). The phagocytic enhancing activity was comparable to that of Tuftsin, which has been described elsewhere in detail [8, 9].

## Pharmacologic activity in vivo

PCF/01 has been tested in two *in vivo* models:

1. Cytoxan-immunosuppressed Balb/c mice challenged with bacterial intraperitoneal (i.p.) inoculum;
2. Balb/c mice grafted subcutaneously with CE-2 sarcoma.

## Bacterial challenge

Experiments have been performed in order to verify the capability of PCF/01 to protect animals challenged with a lethal i.p. inoculum of Pseudomonas Aeruginosa (Table 4). Briefly Balb/c mice were injected 5 days before the bacterial challenge with Cyclophosphamide at various doses (50–200 mg/kg) and treated for 5 days with PCF/01 subcutaneously at various doses (from 10 to 60 mg/kg).

The survival rate was then evaluated and showed protection of animals treated with PCF/01 (40–50 mg/kg). Animals treated with lower doses did not survive. When Gentamicin and PCF were added at unprotective doses (5 mg/kg and 10 mg/kg respectively) only the animals treated with both drugs survived showing a clear synergism between antibiotic and immunomodulator.

## Tumor challenge

The model described by Forni et al. was used [10]; briefly CE-2 sarcoma cells were injected in Balb/c mice subcutaneously $(1 \times 10^4$ cell/animal). PCF/01 was parenterally injected at 40 mg/kg a day for 10 days. Control animals were injected with saline for the same period of time.

Table 4.

| No. experiment | Mice | Cyclophosphamide (day-5) | PCF/01 40 mg/kg (day-5/0) | MS/T[a] | D/T[b] |
|---|---|---|---|---|---|
| 1 | Balb/c | 50 mg/kg | − | 5 | 6/8 |
|  |  |  | + | − | 1/8 |
| 2 | Balb/c | 100 mg/kg | − | 2 | 7/8 |
|  |  |  | + | − | 1/8 |
| 3 | Balb/c | 200 mg/kg | − | 1 | 8/8 |
|  |  |  | + | 6 | 2/8 |

[a] Mean survival time (days).
[b] Death over total.

Table 5. Graft of CE-2 sarcoma induced by methylcholanthrene in Balb/c.

| Groups | Surviving (%) | Latency time (days) | Surviving time (days) |
|---|---|---|---|
| CE-2 | 0/10 (0%) | 14.7±2.4 | 22.5±4.1 |
| CE-2+PCF/01 | 8/10 (80%) | 30.1±1.0 | 35.9±2.6 |
| CE-2+PCF/01 + lymphocytes[a] | 0/10 (0%) | 16.7±2.8 | 23.0±1.9 |

[a] See. G. Forni [10].

Preliminary results (summarized in Table 5) show a clear protection of animals treated with the immunostimulant. Moreover a remarkable extension of the latency time was also observed in mice treated with the immunomodifier.

## Discussion

Like chemotherapy in its formative years, therapeutic utilization of immunomodifiers of various origins still meets with considerable skepticism in the oncological research community. This is largely due to some frustrating and disappointing clinical experiences following premature and over-optimistic conclusions. The belief that pharmacologic modulation of the immune system is likely to have a significant role in cancer therapy is based on the progress achieved along several independent lines of research (see [11] for review). It is clear, however, that because of our poor understanding of natural immune mediators and of various effectors of both specific and non-specific responses to neoplasia, attempts to pharmacologically modify such a complex system are in a relatively neonatal stage. Although considerable research has focused on synthetic immunomodifiers which bear the inosine or hypoxanthine structure, the eventual role for such compounds is unclear.

Data presented in this paper indicate that modifications of the N-9 side of inosine or hypoxanthine yield compounds with immunopharmacologic properties. The modification which was originally made by our research group involves the substitution of the inosine ribose moiety with one or several aminoacids bound with a simple polycarbon chain to the purine moiety. The prototypic structure of this series, here indicated as PCF/01, has potentiative effects on lymphoproliferative responses similar to isoprinosine [1]; it shares with other N-9 hypoxanthine derivatives a thymomietic activity [3] and also has stimulatory effects on granulocytes which are similar to those of Tuftsin [9].

*In vivo* this compound clearly protects animals immunosuppressed with high doses of cyclophosphamide from a lethal bacterial challenge (P. Puccetti and C. Riccardi, unpublished); it also protects the same animal strain grafted with CE-2 sarcoma (G. Forni, unpublished).

Beneficial effects observed *in vivo*, may not be directly attributable to the immunologic modifications observed *in vitro*. PCF/01 appears to act through physiological mechanisms and lacks the toxicity of other hypoxanthine derivatives. Compounds of this series also lack carcinogenic properties and are remarkably free of effects on other tissues. For this reasons further basic and preclinical research of these compounds is warranted.

## Acknowledgements

Many of the experiments reported in this manuscript are still unpublished. I warmly thank for that R. Stradi, Institute of Chemistry, University of Milan; C. Riccardi, Institute of Pharmacology, University of Perugia; P. Puccetti, Institute of Microbiology, University of Perugia an G. Forni, Institute of Microbiology, University of Turin.

I am also endebted to L. Delfino for her secretarial assistance in the preparation of the manuscript.

## References

1. Hadden JW, Giner-Sorolla A: In: Augmenting Agents in cancer Therapy, Current Status and Future Prospects. Chirigos M, Hersh E (eds). Raven Press, New York, 497, 1981.
2. Hadden JW, Delmonte L, Oettgen HF: In: Comprehensive Immunology and Immunopharmacology. Hadden JW, Coffey RG, Spreafico F (eds). Plenum Publishing Corporation, New York, 279, 1977.
3. Simon LN, Hocker FK, McKenzie DJ, Hadden JW: In: Biological response Modifiers in Human Oncology and Immunology. Klein T et al. (eds). Plenum Press, New York, 241, 1983.
4. Hadden JW: The immunopharmacology of purine related compounds. EOS 4:131–133, 1984.
5. Tsang KY, Fudenberg HH, Galbraith GMP: In vitro augmentation of IL-2 production and lymphocytes with the TAC antigen marker in patients with AIDS. N Engl J Med 310:987, 1984.
6. Cornaglia-Ferraris P, Stradi R: Int J Immunopharmacol 4:340, 1982.
7. Babcock GF, Phillips JH, Nishioka J: Tuftsin: a naturally occurring immunostimulating agent. Proc 4th Int Congr Immunol, 1980.
8. Cornaglia-Ferraris P, Melodia A: L-Arginine and L-Arginine derivatives identified as activators of human PMN-L Leukocyte in vitro. Biochim Clin 8:233, 1984.
9. Cornaglia-Ferraris P, Melodia A: Sensory neuropeptides (Substance P) and 4–11 SP enhance human neutrophils chemiluminescence as Tuftsin; the role of L-Arginine. Int J Immunopharmacol, submitted.
10. Forni G, Giovanelli M, Santoni A: Lymphokine activated tumor inhibition in vivo. J Immunol 134:1305–1311, 1985.
11. Mihich E: In: Biological Response in Cancer. Vols 1,2. Plenum Press, New York, 1984.

# 23. Antineoplastic *drugs modulating c-myc expression* in K562, induce erythroid differentiation and modify, with IFN, susceptibility to NK cell mediated lysis

GIAN PAOLO TONINI

## Introduction

The majority of antineoplastic drugs interact with DNA or DNA metabolism. Usually, the *in vivo* goal of polychemotherapeutic protocols is the complete destruction of neoplastic cells. Nevertheless drugs do not distinguish between the DNA of normal human leukocytes and the DNA of the tumor cells [1]. The effect of anticancer drugs on DNA should be reviewed in view of the latest information regarding the molecular biology of genes involved in tumors, in particularly viral oncogenes (v-onc) and cellular oncogenes (c-onc) [2, 3]. In fact, in recent years different research groups have discovered that several human neoplasias show rearranged, amplified or highly expressed, activated proto-oncogenes [2, 4].

There are indications that nucleotidic sequences of c-onc and their related products are involved in cell proliferation and differentiation [5, 6]. C-onc activation and its correlation with cell metabolism suggest that these genes and their products are strongly involved in the neoplastic process [4, 7, 8]. In contrast, there is also evidence for a relationship between cell differentiation and malignant transformation; neoplastic cells in several tumors are undifferentiated cells with a proliferative block. In order to better understand the action of antineoplastic agents on the oncogenes and their correlation with the differentiation of neoplastic cells, the level of c-myc oncogene expression has been evaluated in the human leukemia cell line K562, during erythroid differentiation induced by antineoplastic drugs and IFN.

## Materials and methods

### Cell structures

The K562 cell line was cultured in RPMI-1640 complete medium at a

$5 \times 10^5$ cell/ml. The cells had a doubling time of 22–30 h and were studied in the exponential phase of growth.

*Antineoplastic drugs and IFN*

Adriamycin (A), daunomycin (D), methotrexate (MTX), oncocarbide (OC), aracytin-C (ARA) and 1000 U/ml gamma IFN were dissolved in the culture medium separately; the cells were cultured in the presence of these agents for 5 days.

*Viability and morphology*

The viability and the morphology of the cells was checked every day with the trypan blue exclusion test and May-Grunwald staining respectively.

*Benzidine staining*

Erythroid differentiation was scored by benzidine staining as described by Rowley *et al.* [9].

*Cytotoxicity assays*

Chromium release assays were performed as described by Gronberg *et al.* [10]. The cytotoxicity was expressed as percent of $^{51}$Cr release.

*RNA cytoplasmic blot hybridization*

Dot hybridization analysis was carried out with the lightly modified method described by White *et al.* [11]. The cytoplasmic RNA was isolated from cells by hypotonic lysis with NP40 and 7M Urea [12]; the RNA was extracted by phenol-chloroform and precipitated with 0.3 M Na acetate pH 4.8 and ethanol 99%.

After treatment of the RNA with 37% (v/v) formaldehyde and incubation at 65 °C for 15 min the RNA was spotted on a nitrocellulose filter (Millipore) in serial dilutions.

*RNA gel electrophoresis and transfer*

RNA gel electrophoresis was performed in 1% agarose and 2.2 M formaldehyde (37% Fisher) and was run o.n. at 70 V with continous buffer recycling. RNA to be hybridized with a nick-translated fragment specific probe labeled with $^{32}$P was transferred from agarose gel to nitrocellulose filters (BRL, Bethesda) by the procedure of Northern blot with minor modifications [13].

*Hybridization of the RNA filters*

A 3′exon human c-myc probe was gently provided from Dr D. Watson, Laboratory of Molecular Oncology, NCI, Frederick, USA. It was labeled with $^{32}$P according to the procedure of nick translation kit (BRL, Bethesda). After hybridization in $5\times$ SSC buffer containing 50% formaldehyde, the filter was dried and exposed at $-70\,°C$ to Kodak XO-MAT AR5 X-ray film.

## Results

The drugs show cytotoxic or cytostatic effects at different concentrations. For the experimental conditions, we chose a cytostatic dose for each drug. During the first 24 h in the presence of the different antineoplastic drugs the cells showed morphological changes with an increase of the cellular volume and the appearance of two or more nucleoli. The benzidine test was positive after 96 h (Table 1). The IFN did not induce differentiation to erythroid lineage and the cells did not show morphological change. The susceptibility to NK cell mediated lysis was slightly reduced in drug-treated cells in com-

*Table 1.* Percentage of benzidine positive cells after 72 and 96 h of culture in presence of drugs (control 7%).

| µg/ml | A | | D | | MTX | | OC | | ARA | |
|---|---|---|---|---|---|---|---|---|---|---|
| | 72 | 96 | 72 | 96 | 72 | 96 | 72 | 96 | 72 | 96 |
| 1 | ct | ct | ct | ct | 40 | nd | ct | ct | ct | ct |
| $10^{-1}$ | CT | CT | CT | CT | 40 | nd | CT | CT | 25 | 58 |
| $10^{-2}$ | 22 | 40 | 30 | 65 | 28 | 41 | CT | CT | 23 | 55 |
| $10^{-3}$ | 7 | 7 | 13 | 19 | 12 | 11 | 24 | 50 | 31 | 47 |

ct = cytotoxic; CT = cytostatic; nd = not determined.

*Table 2.* Percentage of K562 cells susceptible to NK cell mediated lysis after 96 h in continuous presence of drugs (control 37%).

| µg/ml | A | D | MTX | OC | ARA |
|---|---|---|---|---|---|
| 1 | ct | ct | nd | ct | ct |
| $10^{-1}$ | CT | ct | nd | CT | 28 |
| $10^{-2}$ | 23 | 27 | 30 | CT | 29 |
| $10^{-3}$ | 39 | 34 | 37 | 24 | 27 |

See Table 1 for the abbreviations.

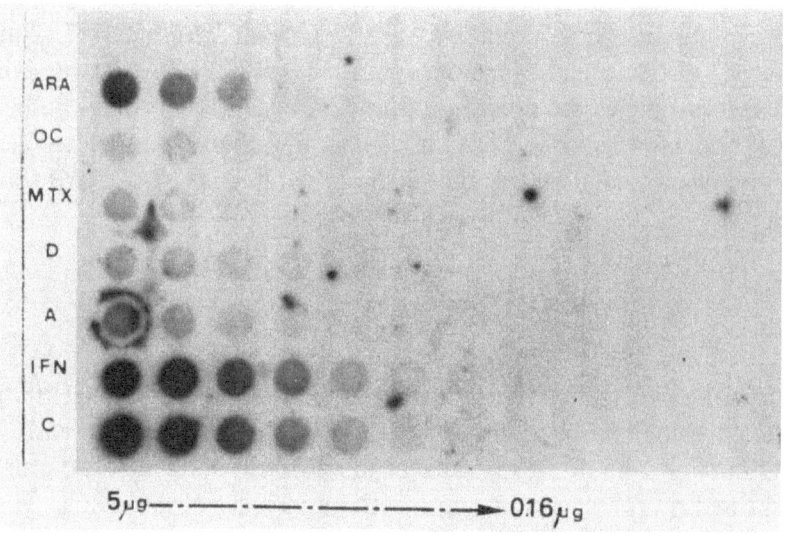

*Figure 1.* Dot blot analysis of cytoplasmic RNA of different drug-treated cells hybridized with 3' exon c-myc probe. For the abbreviations see text 'Materials and methods'.

parison to IFN treated cells which became resistent to NK activity (Table 2). The $^3$H-Thymidine incorporation was reduced progressively within 96 h while the $^3$H-Uridine incorporation was maintained 80% or more with respect to untreated cells (data not showed).

The level of c-myc expression at 48 h was dramatically reduced by D, MTX, and OC at $10^{-2}$ µg/ml. Furthermore, we observed a decrease for ARA ($10^{-1}$ µg/ml) and A ($10^{-2}$ µg/ml) to 16% and 25% of the control respectively, while the IFN does not affect the c-myc oncogene expression (Figure 1).

The same results have been obtained by Northern blot analysis where it was demonstrated that a c-myc mRNA transcripts as 2.4 Kb fragment (Figure 2).

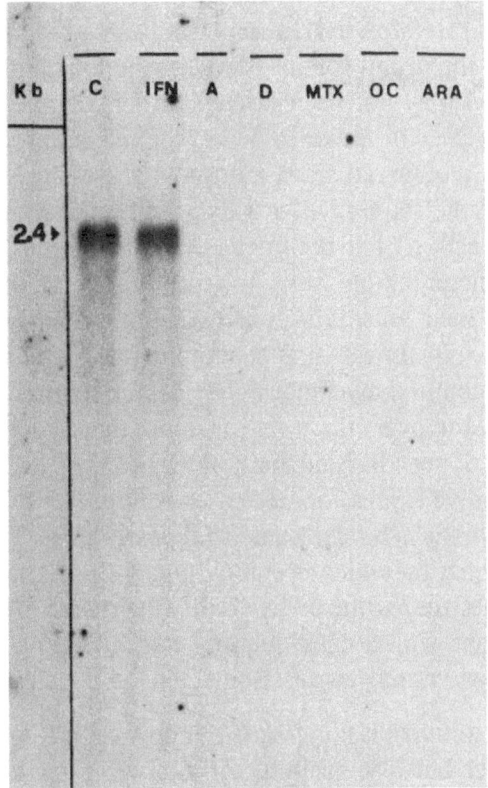

*Figure 2.* Northern blot of the same cytoplasmic RNA shown in Figure 1.

## Discussion

Antineoplastic drugs interact with DNA or its metabolism in different ways. On this basis we thought that the action of drugs would have modified the RNA transcription of several genes. In particular, in this work we studied the expression of c-myc and its role in cell differentiation. The model used *in vitro*, is a human leukemic cell line K562, derived from a pleural effusion of a patient with Chronic Myeloid Leukemia in terminal blast crisis [14, 15]. The K562 can be induced by several chemical substances to erythroid differentiation [9, 16]; furthermore this line was reported to be highly sensitive to natural killer cell mediated lysis [10]. Recently amplified c-abl [17, 18] and c-myc (C. Croce, personal communication) oncogenes have been detected.

A decrease of c-myc expression was observed during differentiation induced by a vitamin D metabolite of the human myeloid leukemic cell line HL60 [19]. On the other hand it has been reported that different oncogenes, such as c-myc and c-fos correlate with the state of differentiation and maturation of the cell [5]. Moreover, recent studies show that the c-myc gene product plays an important role in normal hematopoiesis although its physiological function may not be restricted to hematopoietic cells [4]. When different antineoplastic drugs are added to the cell culture at cytostatic doses or just below it, we observed a fast morphological change. The cells become positive to benzidine staining after 3 days and a reduction in the susceptibility to NK cell activity has been detected. The drugs at these doses act as promotors of differentiation while the IFN does not. However, the IFN treated cells lose their sensitivity to NK cell mediated lysis.

The treatment with drugs should demonstrate *in vitro* the relation between the expression of c-myc, morphological differentiation and haemoglobin production. Moreover, these results show that at lower doses of these drugs inhibition of cell division may occur without loss of other cellular functions. The c-myc expression decreases within 48 h of continuous exposure to drugs. This can be considered an 'early effect'. It is followed by erythroid differentiation which occurs within 4–5 days as a 'late effect'.

We can hypothesize that the drugs modify the transcriptional capability of the c-myc oncogene with a consequential cell differentiation.

Thus, these observations suggest some general conclusions:

1. the dose of an antineoplastic drug is not only critical for its cytotoxic and cytostatic effect but also to induce the erythroid differentiation of the K562 cell line;
2. chemotherapeutic drugs modulate c-myc expression not only by a direct action (intercalating agents) on DNA but also through the metabolic pathway of the cell;
3. the decrease in c-myc transcription observed in drug-treated cells precedes cell differentiation and points out the relationship between the two phenomena;
4. the action of anticancer drugs seems to have a certain selectivity on gene expression because there is an *ex novo* haemoglobin production and altered c-myc transcription;
5. the K562 system could be a useful experimental model *in vitro* both to investigate the antineoplastic drug interaction with DNA and to clarify the mechanisms of neoplastic cell differentiation.

## Acknowledgements

This work has been developed in the Laboratory of Molecular Immunoregulation, Immunology Section, NCI, Frederick MD, USA. The support was provided by American-Italian Foundation Cancer Research and G. Gaslini Research Institute.

The author thanks Dr L. Varesio, Head of Section, Dr E. Blasi, Dr A. Gronberg, Dr D. Radzioch for their technical advice and collaboration in the realization of this research. We also thank Miss L. Delfino for typing the manuscript.

## References

1. Sartorelli C, Lazo JS, Bertino JR: Molecular action and targets for cancer chemotherapeutic agents. Academic Press, New York NY, 1981.
2. Bishop JM: Cellular oncogenes and retroviruses. Ann Rev Biochem 52:301–354, 1983.
3. Bush H: Onc genes and other new targets for cancer chemotherapy. J Cancer Res Clin Oncol 107:1–14, 1984.
4. Muller R, Verma IM: Expression of cellular oncogenes. Current Topics in Microbiol Immunol112:74–105, 1984.
5. Mitchell RL, Zokas L, Schreiber RD, Verma IM: Rapid induction of the expression of Proto-oncogene fos during human monocytic differentiation. Cell 40:209–217, 1985.
6. Thiele CJ, Reynolds CP, Israel MA: Decrease expression of N-myc precedes retinoic acid-induced morphological differentiation of human nephroblastoma. Nature 313:404–406, 1985.
7. Weiss RA, Marchall CJ: Oncogenes. Lancet, Nov. 17, 1138–1142, 1984.
8. Hartmut L, Parada LF, Weinberg A: Cellular oncogenes and Multistep Carcinogenesis. Science 222:771–776, 1983.
9. Rowley PT, Ohlsson-Wilhelm BM, Farley BA, La Bella S: Inducers of erythroid differentiation in K562 human leukemia cells. Exp Hematol 9:32–7, 1981.
10. Gronberg A, Kiessling R, Masucci G, Guevara AL, Eriksson E, Klein G: Gamma-interferon produced during effector and target interactions renders cells less susceptible to NK-cell mediated lysis. Int J Cancer 32:609–616, 1983.
11. White BA, Bancroft FC: J Biol Chem 257:8569–8572, 1982.
12. Gorman CM, Merlino GT, Willingham MC, Pastan I, Howard BH: The Rous sarcoma virus long terminal report is a strong promoter when introduced into a variety of eucaryotic cells by DNA-mediated transfection. Proc Nat Acad Sci USA 79:6777–6780, 1982.
13. Maniatis T, Fritsch EF, Sambrook J: Molecular Cloning. Cold Spring Harbor Laboratory, Cold Spring Harbor, NY, 202, 1983.
14. Andersson CL, Nilsson K, Gahmberg CG: K562 – A human erythroleukemic cell line. Int J Cancer 23:143–147, 1979.
15. Lozzio BB, Lozzio CB, Bamberger EG, Feliu AS: A multipotential leukemia cell line (K562) of human origin (41106). Proc Soc Exp Biol Med 166:546–550, 1981.
16. Cioe L, McNab A, Hubbell HR, Meo P, Curtis P, Rovera G: Differential expression of the globin genes in human leukemia K562(S) cells induced to differentiate by Hemin or Butyric Acid. Cancer Res 41:237–243, 1981.
17. Collins SJ, Groudine MT: Rearrangment and amplification of c-abl sequences in the human chronic myelogenous leukemia cell line K562. Proc Nat Acad Sci USA 80:4813–4817, 1983.
18. Selden JR, Emanuel BS, Wang E, Cannizzaro L, Palumbo A, Erikson J, Nowell PC, Rovera G, Croce CM: Amplified c-lambda and c-abl genes are on the same marker chromosome in K562 leukemia cells, Proc Natl Acad Sci USA 80:7289–7292, 1983.
19. Reitsma PH, Rothberg PG, Astrin SM, Trial J, Bar-Shavit Z, Hall A, Teitelbaum SL, Kahn AJ: Regulation of myc expression in HL60 leukemia cells by a vitamin D metabolite. Nature 306:492–494, 1983.

# 24. *In vivo* treatment with recombinant interleukin-2 (IL-2) stimulates the differentiation of natural killer (NK) precursor cells

CARLO RICCARDI, GRAZIELLA MIGLIORATI,
ANTONIO GIAMPIETRI, LORENZA CANNARILE,
EMIRA AYROLDI and LUIGI FRATI

## Introduction

One of the most interesting problems in the field of natural immunity is represented by those regulatory mechanisms possibly involved in determining spontaneous reactivity [1, 2]. Natural killer (NK) cells have been shown to be influenced in their levels of reactivity by soluble factors such as prostaglandins and a number of lymphokines [3–8]. Interferon and interferon inducers have also been shown to be able to augment the spontaneous levels of NK activity both *in vivo* and *in vitro* in different species, including mouse and man. In addition, macrophage-like, null cell-like or T-cell-like suppressor cells have been shown to influence the levels of NK activity [9, 10].

A potentially useful approach to examine the possible modulating role of cells and factors on NK function is to study the influence of the above cited factors on the development of NK cells from their stem cell precursors. To achieve this we developed an NK stem cell assay which involves the transfer of syngeneic bone marrow cells into lethally irradiated recipients depleted of endogenous NK activity. The generation of NK cells was then analyzed by measuring splenic NK activity at different times after lethal irradiation and bone marrow graft. We also used a second experimental model in which the NK activity of infant mice was tested. Infant mice have been demonstrated not to have NK activity nor boosting susceptibility to IL-2, IFNs or IFN-inducers [2]. In this case mice were treated after birth with IL-2 and their NK activity tested at different times until day 30 when high reactivity is measurable in untreated controls.

## Results

*IL-2 modulates the NK cell maturation of infant mice*

To analyze the possible regulatory role of IL-2 on the maturation of immature progenitor NK cells we studied the NK maturity of infant mice in which the NK activity is virtually absent after birth and then matures between the third and the fourth week of age. In Table 1 are reported the data of a representative experiment in which the splenic NK activity (expressed as lytic units/spleen) of untreated or IL-2 treated mice was measured. Infant mice do not show significant levels of NK activity until day 21. In contrast, mice treated with IL-2 (10 U/day from day 0 through day 7) show high NK activity at day 15 after birth which reaches the levels of young-adult mice on day 18. These data clearly indicate that IL-2 is able to induce a pre-maturation of the NK activity of infant mice. This effect is not associated with a decline of suppressor cell activity, previously described to be present in the spleen of infant mice, and does correlate with an increase of the number of splenic large granular lymphocytes (LGL) (data not shown).

*IL-2 is able to modulate the growth of bone marrow progenitor NK cells*

We also studied the possible influence of IL-2 on the *in vivo* growth and differentiation of bone marrow progenitors of natural killer cells. For this purpose B6D2F$_1$ mice were lethally irradiated and then transplanted with syngeneic bone marrow. At different times (4, 7, 9, 11, 14 days) after irradiation and bone marrow graft mice were sacrificed and the splenic NK activity was evaluated in a 4-h $^{51}$Cr-release assay against the NK-sensitivity YAC-1 tumor line. In Figure 1 are reported the data of a representative experiment in which we evaluated the possible modulating effect of recombinant IL-2 on the *in vivo* development of bone marrow progenitor cells

*Table 1.* Effect of IL-2 administration on NK maturation of B6D2F$_1$ infant mice.

| Age (days) | IL-2 treatment[a] | NK activity[b] |
|---|---|---|
| 5 | − | 10 |
| 10 | − | 8 |
| 15 | − | 5 |
| 18 | − | 10 |
| 25 | − | 120 |
| 5 | + | 8 |
| 10 | + | 20 |
| 15 | + | 130 |
| 18 | + | 120 |
| 25 | + | 140 |

[a] IL-2, 10 U/day/mouse ip from day 0 through day 7.
[b] NK activity is expressed as lytic units$_{20}$/spleen.

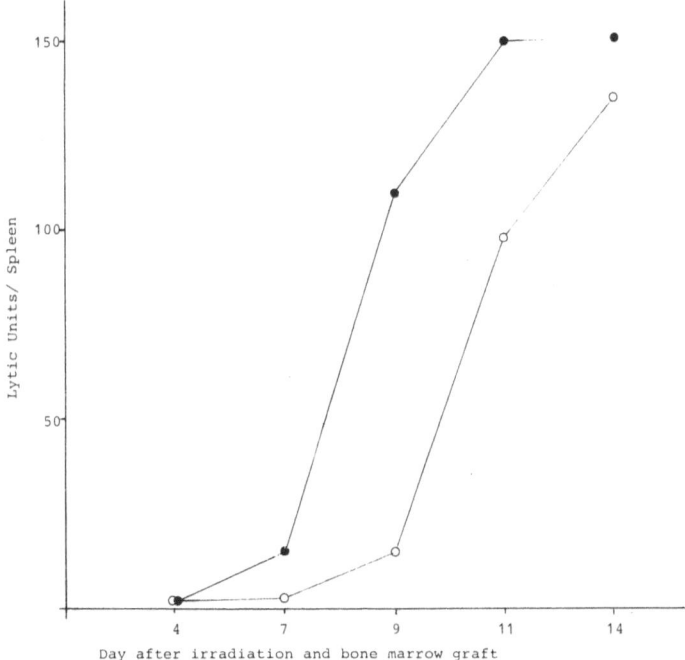

*Figure 1.* Reconstitution of splenic NK activity (expressed as LU_{20}/spleen) of lethally irralieted (1000 rads) and bone marrow grafted ($10^7$ cells iv) B6D2F$_1$ mice o-o medium injected controls; •-• IL-2 injected animals (IL-2 10U/day/mouse ip from day 0 through day 3).

responsible for the NK regeneration. As shown in the figure different groups of B6D2F$_1$ mice were treated, after lethal irradiation (1000 rads) and bone marrow graft ($10^7$ cells/mouse iv), with recombinant IL-2 (10 U/mouse/day) or media alone from day 0 through day 3. The NK activity of all the groups of mice is strongly depressed after lethal irradiation (day 4 and 7) and then progressively regenerates reaching the level of untreated control mice, in the case of the media-injected animals, on day 12. On the other hand in the case of IL-2-treated mice, valuable levels of activity appear on day 7 and 9 after irradiation and bone marrow graft. These data demonstrate that IL-2 is able to enhance the *in vivo* generation of NK activity by bone marrow progenitor NK cells and confirm the results of our previous *in vitro* experiments indicating that IL-2 is able to induce the growth and differentiation of progenitor NK cells [7, 11].

## Discussion

The data here reported clearly show that the *in vivo* administration of recombinant IL-2 is able to induce the maturation of immature precursors of NK cells to differentiated effector cells. Since progenitor cells present in the bone marrow are susceptible to the IL-2 signal *in vivo*, treated animals are reconstituted in a shorter time and reach higher levels of reactivity as compared to medium-injected controls. The treatment with recombinant IL-2 results in a prematuration of splenic NK activity in terms of *in vitro* cytotoxicity against YAC-1 cells and also in an augmentation of the whole number of spleen cells so that this results in a dramatic increase of lytic units/spleen.

Similar results are also obtained when mice are reconstituted with bone marrow which has been depleted of more differentiated cells by *in vitro* treatment with antisera (i.e. Anti Thy.1 or Anti-Asialo GM-1) and complement or by *in vivo* pretreatment with cytostatic drugs such as 5-fluorouracil (5-FU) or hydroxyurea (HU) (data not shown). These data indicate that the target of IL-2 is a non-differentiated precursor cell of the NK lineage unsusceptible to treatment with 5-FU or HU and which does not express Thy.1 or GM-1 antigens on its surface.

Infant mice represent an interesting model of NK activity maturation. Mice after birth do not have any NK cells nor boosting-susceptible pre-NK cells. After 3 or more weeks of age NK activity appears, reaching the levels of young-adult mice within the fourth week. Using this experimental model we have confirmed that IL-2 *in vivo* stimulates the growth and differentiation of progenitor NK cells so that the NK activity of treated mice appears after 2 weeks of age.

These data are not surprising as it has been shown that the IL-2 receptor is expressed on fetal cells and undifferentiated adult thymocytes [12, 13]. In this report we have shown that infant or bone marrow progenitor NK cells are susceptible to IL-2 stimulation. Most interesting is the fact that IL-2 appears very important in the process of maturation of the NK lineage. This model may also have a more general relevance in that it indicates that it is possible, *in vivo*, to modulate the process of growth and maturation of a particular cell lineage. Study of growth and differentiation factors should be pursued in an attempt to study the possible *in vivo* relevance of these agents and their regulatory role on different cell lineages. Their possible role as agents potentially able to treat different lymphohematopoeitic disorders remains to be elucidated.

### Acknowledgement

This work was supported by Contracts 84.00762.44 and 84.02484.56 CNR, Italy.

# References

1. Herberman RB: NK Cell and Other Natural Effector Cells. Herberman RB (ed). Academic Press, New York, 1982.
2. Herberman RB, Ortaldo JR, Holden HT, Djeu JY, Mattes J, Brunda M, Riccardi C, Santoni A: Natural killer cells. Regulation of activity and in vivo role. In: Thymus, Thymic Ormones and T lymphocytes. Aiuti T, Wizgell H (eds). Academic Press, New York, 165–172, 1980.
3. Ricardi C, Giampietri A, Migliorati G, Guadagni F, Herberman RB: Age dependent variation of natural killer (NK) cell activity: role of TCGF and interferon. First International Congress of the Italian Society of Immunopharmacology, October 10–11. Perugia Italy, 66, 1983.
4. Riccardi C, Barlozzari T, Santoni A, Cesarini C, Herberman RB: Regulation of in vovo reactivity of natural killer (NK) cells. In: NK Cells and Other Natural Effector Cells. Herberman RB (ed). Academic Press, New York, 549–556, 1982.
5. Trinchieri G, Santoli D, Dee RR, Knowles BB: Antiviral activity induced by culturing lymphocytes with tumor-derived or virus-transformed cells. Identification of the anti-viral activity as interferon and characterization of the human effector lymphocytes subpopulation. J Exp Med 147:1299–1313, 1978.
6. Herberman RB, Ortaldo JR, Bonnard GD: Augmentation by interferon of human natural and antibody dependent cell-mediated cytotoxicity. Nature 277:221–223, 1979.
7. Riccardi C, Vose BM, Herberman RB: Modulation of IL-2-dependent growth of mouse NK cells by interferon and T-lymphocytes. J Immunol 130:228–232, 1983.
8. Riccardi C, Vose BM, Herberman RB: Regulation by Interferon And R cells of IL-2 dependent growth of NK progenitor cells: a limiting dilution analysis. In: NK Cells and Other Natural Effector Cells. Herberman RB (ed). Academic Press, New York, 909–915, 1982.
9. Cudkowicz G, Hochmann P: Do natural killer cells engage in reguleted reactions against self to ensure homeostasis? Immunol Rev 44:13–42, 1979.
10. Riccardi C, Santoni A, Barlozzari T, Cesarini C, Herberman RB: Suppression of Natural killer (NK) activity by splenic adherent cells of low NK-reactive mice. Int J Cancer 28:811–818, 1901.
11. Riccardi C, Migliorati G, Herberman RB: Partially restorative role of T-cells for low interleukin-2 dependent growth of NK cells progenitors from nude mice. In: Natural Immunity and Cells Growth Regulation. Lotzovà E (ed). S. Karger AG, Basel, 7–21, 1983–1984.
12. Raulet DH: Expression and function of interleukin-2 receptors on immature thymocytes. Nature 314:101–103, 1985.
13. Boehmer H, Crisanti A, Kisielow P, Haas W: Absence of growth by most receptor-expressing fetal thymocytes in the presence of interleukin-2. Nature 314:539–540, 1985.

# 25. Immunopharmacology studies related to *in vitro* infection with HTLV-I

C. GRANDORI, G. GRAZIANI, C.F. PERNO, C. D'ONOFRIO
and E. BONMASSAR

## Abstract

Ficoll-separated mononuclear cells from human umbilical cord blood (cord blood lymphocytes, CBL) or adult peripheral blood (peripheral blood lymphocytes, PBL) were treated with two immunomodulating agents (i.e. human beta interferon, IFN, or PCF-39) for 16 h at 37°C. The cells were washed and tested for their cell-mediated natural cytotoxicity (CMNC) against NK-susceptible K562 targets or a variety of HTLV-I positive lymphoblasts, using a 4-h 51Cr-release assay. Part of pretreated lymphocytes were also co-cultivated with irradiated virus-donor MT-2 cells, and later tested for non-specific or MT-2 specific cytotoxicity, and for virus infections monitored by cellular expression of HTLV-I P19 protein. The results show that the agents increased immune functions in selected experimental conditions and reduced virus infection by increasing target cell resistance, and decreasing MT-2 infectivity. Limited or no influence of the agents on virus transmission has been found when target leukemic instead of immunocompetent cells were used in the donor-recipient co-cultures.

These preliminary results suggest a possible role of immunological functions and immunomodulating agents on *in vitro* HTLV-I infection. While the use of agents such as interferon or synthetic immune modulators has had limited clinical application to date, the increasing incidence of diseases such as AIDS suggest that immunopharmacologic approaches may be relied upon to a greater extent in the future to treat both adult and pediatric disorders.

## Introduction

Attempts to isolate retroviruses putatively responsible for human leukemias and lymphomas led to the discovery that a type-C retrovirus was associated with a form of adult T-cell leukemia (ATL, 1). The virus, known as human T-cell leukemia/lymphoma virus, type I (HTLV-I) has subsequently been isolated from other patients with mature T-lymphocyte malignancies and from clinically normal family members of leukemic patients in different parts of the world including Japan, the Caribbean, Africa, South America, Israel and the USA [2–6].

Since the first isolations of HTLV in the United States and other countries by Dr Gallo and colleagues [1–6], other investigators confirmed these findings independently, either in Japan [7, 8], or the USA [9], Holland [10] and London (Greaves *et al.*, in preparation).

The HTLV-I morphology shows the typical pattern of a type-C retrovirus with budding from the cell membranes. The virus contains reverse transcriptase [11], high molecular weight RNA [12], and envelope and internal core proteins including the serologically-defined P15, P19 and P24 proteins [13, 14].

Other subgroups of HTLV have been more recently identified. HTLV-II has been isolated from a patient with a T-cell variant of hairy cell leukemia, but does not appear to be the etiological agent of the more common B-cell hairy cell leukemia [15].

HTLV-III has been isolated from a number of patients with acquired immunodeficiency syndrome (AIDS), and has been proposed as one of the main causative agents of this disease [16]. Recently an increasing number of pediatric cases of AIDS have been reported.

Extensive studies on the HTLV family showed that these viruses share several well defined biological, immunological and nucleic acid characteristics. The most important biological features of HTLV's can be summarized as follows: (a) they are isolated from mature T cells, so that these agents are defined as T-tropic retroviruses [17]; (b) HTLV's are infectious predominantly for OKT-4 positive lymphocytes although they can infect T cells carrying other OKT markers [18], non-T cell targets [19], or even cells of non-lymphoid origin [20]; (c) *in vitro* infection with HTLV-I is easily attained by co-cultivating virus-positive donor cells and recipient targets. In addition, cell-free transmission *in vitro* has been achieved using the HTLV-III type or high concentrations of HTLV-I virus particles [17].

*In vitro* transmission into human T lymphocytes using efficient HTLV-I donor cells can be accomplished with adult or newborn umbilical cord blood (CB) T cells as recipient lymphocytes. The data presently available point out that adult lymphocytes are less susceptible to virus infection than CB cells. Moreover it has been demonstrated that bone marrow mononuclear cells are similar to CB lymphocytes in terms of HTLV-I susceptibility, being rapidly infected *in vitro* by co-cultivation with irradiation virus-positive donor cells [17].

These observations suggest the hypothesis that the stage of maturation of immunocompetent cells present among recipient lymphocytes could play a significant role in conditioning their susceptibility to HTLV-I transmission. Further support for this point of view is provided by recent findings of our laboratory showing that peripheral blood lymphocytes (PBL) of leukemic donors with impaired immune functions are more susceptible to *in vitro* HTLV-I infection than normal PBL (Graziani G *et al.*, in preparation).

If immunosurveillance mechanisms are involved in the control of horizontal *in vitro* transmission of HTLV-I, it is conceivable that immunomodulating agents would be capable of influencing the rate and extent of target infection. Therefore studies have been performed with human beta-interferon (IFN, kindly furnished by Sclavo S.p.A., Siena, Italy) and with a recently synthesized N-9 arginil hypoxanthine derivative PCF-39 (kindly furnished by Sigma-Tau S.p.A., Pomezia, Italy).

The immunomodulating effects of IFN are well-known [21]. This agent is capable of increasing substantially either natural resistance and cytotoxicity, or antigen-driven elicitable responses.

The hypoxanthine derivative PCF-39 was found to increase lymphoproliferative responses, the synthesis of interleukin-1 and 2 by human lymphocytes, the expression of theta antigen of lymphocytes of nude mice, and to protect mice from bacterial infection and growth of immunogenic tumors (Cornaglia Ferraris P. *et al.*, in preparation).

The results of the present study point out that both agents are capable of influencing natural cytotoxicity and cell-mediated responses in experimental models of *in vitro* co-cultures leading to HTLV-I transmission. Moreover IFN and PCF-39 were found to affect virus infection in selected experimental conditions.

## Experimental methods and results

### Effect of human beta-interferon (IFN) on immune functions related to HTLV-I infected lymphoblasts

Adult peripheral blood lymphocytes (PBL), or newborn cord blood lymphocytes (CBL) were obtained following centrifugation of heparinized blood on Ficoll-Hypaque gradient. After washing in RPMI-1640 medium supplemented with 10% heat-inactivated fetal calf serum, glutamine and gentamycin (Adv. Biotech., Bethesda MD, USA), hereafter referred to as 'complete medium' (CM), PBL and CBL were incubated with CM alone or CM containing IFN (Sclavo, Siena, Italy) 1000 U/ml, in a 5% $CO_2$ incubator at 37°C, for 16 h. After washing, control of IFN-treated PBL or CBL were tested for their cell-mediated natural cytotoxicity (CMNC) against 51Cr-labeled human target leukemic cells.

The targets included the standard NK-susceptible K562 line, three cultured cell lines (i.e. Mjd, TK and MT-1) obtained from HTLV-I positive donors [17] and two cord blood lines (i.e. MT-2, and C5/MJ) infected *in vitro* with HTLV-I [17]. The cytotoxic assay was performed by mixing 0.1 ml of target cells ($5 \times 10^4$/ml) previously labeled with 100 uCi of 51Cr (Amersham, England) for 1 h at 37 °C, with 0.1 ml of effector cells at different effector: target (E:T) ratios in 96-well round bottom microtiter plates (Limbro, Flow Labs., McLean, VA). The plates were then incubated in a 5% $CO_2$ incubator at 37 °C for 4 h, and 0.1 ml collected from each well and the radioactivity read in a gamma-scintillation counter (Packard Mod 6401). Percent specific lysis (SL) was calculated as follows:

$$\% \, SL = \frac{S - AC}{TC} \times 100$$

where S is the counts per minute (cpm) of the sample, AC the cpm of the autologous control (i.e. of target cells incubated with non-labeled target cells), and TC the cpm of the total count (i.e. 50% of the cpm of the labeled target cells used).

The results of a representative experiment illustrated in Table 1 show that IFN pretreatment substantially increased CMNC against all lines tested, including the HTLV-I positive cells, essentially non-susceptible to basal CMNC activity.

Further studies were performed by co-culturing CBL with *in vitro* irradiated (10,000 R from a Cesium source) MT-2 cells, using the experimental

Table 1. Effect of IFN on CMNC of adult PBL or cord blood lymphocytes (CBL) against K562 or HTLV-I positive leukemia cell lines.

| Target cell[a] | Effector cells[b] (% specific lysis) | | | |
|---|---|---|---|---|
| | PBL | PBL/IFN | CBL | CBL/IFN[c] |
| K562 | $26.0 \pm 0.9$[d] | $62.8 \pm 1$ | $16.6 \pm 0.7$ | $70.4 \pm 1.2$ |
| Mjd | $0.1 \pm 1$ | $10.5 \pm 1.2$ | NT[e] | NT |
| TK | $3.1 \pm 0.6$ | $6.7 \pm 0.8$ | NT | NT |
| MT-1 | $3.0 \pm 1$ | $63.6 \pm 1.3$ | NT | NT |
| Mt-2 | $3.6 \pm 1.1$ | $24.0 \pm 0.8$ | $2.1 \pm 1$ | $30.4 \pm 0.9$ |
| C5/MJ | $5.6 \pm 0.4$ | $36.8 \pm 0.5$ | NT | NT |

[a] Mjd, TK and MT-1 are cell lines obtained from HTLV-I positive donors; MT-2 and C5/MJ are CBL infected *in vitro* by co-culturing with HTLV-I donor cells [17].

[b] Effector cells (E) were tested against target cells (T) at E:T ratio of 100:1.

[c] PBL/IFN or CBL/IFN, effector cells pretreated with IFN (1000 U/ml) for 16 h at 37 °C.

[d] Mean ± standard error (SE).

[e] NT, not tested.

*Table 2.* Effect of IFN on cell-mediated cytotoxicity of CBL, co-cultured with irradiated (10,000 R) HTLV-I donor MT-2 cells, tested against CMNC-susceptible K562 or MT-2 target cells at 1, 2 or 4 weeks of coculture.

| Effector cells[a] | Target cells | % Specific lysis (mean ± SE)[b] at | | |
|---|---|---|---|---|
| | | 1 week | 2 weeks | 4 weeks |
| CBL | K562 | 5.6 ± 0.3 | 9.5 ± 0.5 | 4.0 ± 0.4 |
| CBL/IFN | K562 | 24.7 ± 0.7 | 18.7 ± 1.0 | 14.4 ± 1.4 |
| CBL | MT-2 | 7.8 ± 0.4 | 18.2 ± 0.9 | 4.1 ± 0.6 |
| CBL/IFN | MT-2 | 25.3 ± 1.3 | 31.7 ± 0.7 | 12.6 ± 0.6 |

[a] Effector cells, $2 \times 10^6$ cells co-cultured with irradiated MT-2 cells ($4 \times 10^5$) in 2 ml wells (24-well Limbro plate). CBL/IFN, CBL pretreated with IFN (see table 1) before co-culturing with irradiated MT-2 cells.
[b] % specific lysis at E:T cell ratio of 50:1.

design adopted for *in vitro* transmission of HTLV-I from infecting virus-producer cells and recipient lymphocytes or lymphoma cells (i.e. $2 \times 10^6$ recipient cells admixed with $4 \times 10^4$ irradiated infecting cells in 2 ml of CM in presence of 10% TCGF (Cellular Products, Buffalo NY), in 24 well Limbro plates). Untreated or IFN-pretreated CBL were used as recipient cells, and their non-specific or antigen-specific cytotoxicity was assayed against target K562 or MT-2 cells respectively, at 1, 2 or 4 weeks of co-culture. The results (Table 2) showed that IFN pretreatment enhanced both specific and non-specific cytotoxicity of CBL up to 4 weeks of co-culture.

*Effect of PCF-39 on immune functions related to HTLV-I infected lymphoblasts*

Non-treated PBL or adult lymphocytes pretreated *in vitro* with 1 or 100 µg/ml of PCF-39 were co-cultured with irradiated MT-2 cells, using the same conditions described for CBL. Their non-specific cytotoxicity was tested against K562 targets on day 0 before admixing with MT-2 cells, or on day +7 of co-culture.

The results described in Table 3 show that (a) significant inhibition of CMNC (P < 0.05 according to student 't' test analysis on the original cpm's) was afforded by 100 µg/ml of the drug used for PBL pretreatment, either on day 0 or day +7; (b) when the drug was added to the PBL + MT-2 co-culture instead, a significant increase of cytotoxicity was found on day +7 (P < 0.01).

The effect of PCF-39 on specific cell-mediated cytotoxicity (i.e. against the 'infecting' as well as 'stimulating' allogeneic MT-2 cells) was tested by pretreating recipient (i.e. 'responder') PBL, or HTLV-I producer MT-2 cells, or by adding the drug to the co-culture. The results (Table 4) show that (a) the cytotoxic response of control PBL against MT-2 cells was essentially zero in this experimental condition (i.e. responder (R): sensitizer (S) ratio of 5:1), whereas high responses can be obtained at R:S of 40:1 (data not shown); (b) pretreatment of effector cells did not induce any CMNC against

Table 3. Effect of PCF-39 on CMNC against target K562 cells, of adult PBL before or 1 week after co-culture with irradiated HTLV-I donor MT-2 cells.

| Effector cells[a] | PCF-39[b] (μg/ml) | % Specific lysis (mean ± SE)[c] | |
|---|---|---|---|
| | | Day 0[d] | Day +7 |
| PBL | none | 34.5 ± 2.1 | 24.4 ± 1.0 |
| PBL/PCF-39 (1) | none | 30.3 ± 3.8 | 30.4 ± 0.9 |
| PBL/PCF-39 (100) | none | 11.9 ± 2.7 | 20.1 ± 0.6 |
| PBL | 1 | – | 26.6 ± 2.6 |
| PBL | 100 | – | 35.8 ± 1.8 |

[a] PBL were non-pretreated, or preincubated with PCF-39 for 16 h at 37 °C, before testing on day 0 or co-cultured with irradiated MT-2 cells (PBL, $2 \times 10^6$ cells, + MT-2, $4 \times 10^5$ cells, in 2-ml wells, 24-well Limbro plate).
[b] Added to PBL + MT-2 cell co-cultures on day 0.
[c] E:T ratio, 50:1.
[d] CMNC assay performed before co-culturing PBL with MT-2 cells.

Table 4. Effect of PCF-39 on cell-mediated cytotoxicity against target MT-2 cells, of adult PBL before or 1 week after co-culture with irradiated HTLV-I donor MT-2 cells.

| Effector cells[a] | Sensitizer cells[b] | PCF-39[c] (μg/ml) | % Specific lysis (mean ± SE)[d] | |
|---|---|---|---|---|
| | | | Day 0[e] | Day +7 |
| PBL | Mt-2 | None | 0.4 ± 0.5 | 0.9 ± 1.1 |
| PBL/PCF-39 (1) | MT-2 | None | 0.7 ± 0.2 | 7.5 ± 1.1 |
| PBL/PCF-39 (100) | MT-2 | None | 0.6 ± 1.0 | 10.7 ± 1.4 |
| PBL | MT-2 | 1 | – | 10.4 ± 1.1 |
| PBL | MT-2 | 100 | – | 7.6 ± 0.4 |
| PBL | MT-2/PCF-39 (1) | None | – | 8.9 ± 1.6 |
| PBL | Mt-2/PCF-39 (100) | None | – | 9.9 ± 1.0 |

[a] See table 3.
[b] Irradiated (10.000 R) MT-2 cells, non-treated or pretreated with PCF-39, 16 h at 37 °C, before co-culture with PBL (see Table 3), MT-2/PCF-39 (1), PCF-39 1 μg/ml; MT-2/PCF-39 (100), PCF-39 100 μg/ml.
[c] Added to PBL + MT-2 cell co-cultures on day 0.
[d] E:T ratio, 25:1.
[e] The cytotoxic assay was performed before co-culturing PBL with MT-2 cells.

MT-2 on day 0; (c) any schedule of PCF-39 treatment produced detectable cytotoxic responses on day +7.

*Effect of IFN or PCF-39 on the expression of P19 viral protein following co-culture of recipient cells with irradiated, HTLV-I producer MT-2 cells*

The presence of P19 core protein in lymphocytes or tumor cells exposed to HTLV-I producer cells provides an excellent indication of successful virus transmission [17].

Positively for P19 antigen was tested using an indirect immunofluorescent assay. Cells to be tested were washed twice with phosphate buffered saline, (PBS pH 7.1) and resuspended in PBS at the concentration of $10^6$ per milliliter. Twenty microliters of cell suspension were spotted on a slide, air dried and fixed in acetone and methanol (1:1) for 30' at room temperature. Ten microliter of a 1:500 dilution of mouse monoclonal antibodies (MoAb) recognizing the core protein P19 of HTLV-I, were applied to the fixed cells and incubated for 45' at room temperature. The slides were washed for 1 h in PBS and 10 µl of 1:50 rabbit anti mouse F (ab) IgG conjugated with fluorescein isothiocyanate (FITC, Cappel lab. Cochranville, PA) were added for 45' at room temperature. Slides were then washed in PBS extensively overnight before microscope examination. The slides then were embedded in glycerol and examined under the microscope with ultraviolet illumination (Nikon Inc. Japan; HBO 100 w filter 450 nm NCB10; magnification × 1000).

Untreated or IFN-pretreated (1000 U/ml for 16 h at 37 °C) CBL were co-cultured with irradiated MT-2 cells, and the percentage of P19-positive cells was tested 2 weeks later. The results of four experiments, illustrated in Table 5, show that IFN pretreatment of recipient lymphocytes reduced markedly their susceptibility to P19-productive HTLV-I infection.

*Table 5.* Effect of IFN pretreatment of CBL on expression of P19 viral protein following 2 weeks of co-culture with irradiated virus-infected MT-2 cells.

| | % P19-positive cells | |
|---|---|---|
| Experiment number | Untreated CBL | CBL pretreated with IFN[a] |
| 1 | 13.5 | 5.0 |
| 2 | 42.0 | 11.0 |
| 3 | 42.0 | 22.0 |
| 4 | 29.0 | 4.5 |

[a] IFN 1000 U/ml for 16 h at 37 °C, before co-culture with MT-2.

These results were supported by DNA blot analysis of co-cultures, which showed a significant decrease in the amount of integrated HTLV-I proviral DNA in IFN-pretreated co-cultures on day $+10$ of culture (data not shown).

Table 6. Effect of IFN pretreatment of infecting MT-2, or recipient MOLT-4 leukemia cells, or of IFN added to infecting+recipient co-culture on HTLV-I transmission.

| Group number | Pretreatment[a] with IFN of | | IFN added to MT-2+MOLT-4 co-culture (μg/ml) | % P19 positive cells[b] |
|---|---|---|---|---|
| | Infecting MT-2 cells (μg/ml) | Recipient MOLT-4 cells (μg/ml) | | |
| 1 | 0 | 0 | 0 | 18.0 |
| 2 | 10 | 0 | 0 | 15.7 |
| 3 | 100 | 0 | 0 | 12.3 |
| 4 | 1000 | 0 | 0 | 13.8 |
| 5 | 0 | 10 | 0 | 22.0 |
| 6 | 0 | 100 | 0 | 20.7 |
| 7 | 0 | 1000 | 0 | 20.0 |
| 8 | 0 | 0 | 10 | 17.2 |
| 9 | 0 | 0 | 100 | 24.2 |
| 10 | 0 | 0 | 1000 | 21.6 |

[a] See Tables 1 and 2 for IFN pretreatment and co-culture conditions.
[b] Tested after 4 days of co-culture.

Table 7. Effect of PCF-39 treatment of infecting MT-2, recipient CBL or MOLT-4 leukemia cells, or of PCF-39 added to infecting-recipient co-culture on HTLV-I transmission.

| Group number | Pretreatment[a] with PCF-39 of | | PCF-39 added to the co-cultures (μg/ml) | % P19 positive cells[b] | |
|---|---|---|---|---|---|
| | Infecting MT-2 cells (μg/ml) | Recipient cells (μg/ml) | | MOLT-4 | CBL |
| 1–2 | 0 | 0 | 0 | 18.1 | 20.7 |
| 3–4 | 1 | 0 | 0 | 12.8 | 1.8 |
| 5–6 | 100 | 0 | 0 | 13.2 | 8.3 |
| 7–8 | 0 | 1 | 0 | 21.3 | 9.4 |
| 9 | 0 | 100 | 0 | 14.0 | NT[c] |
| 10–11 | 0 | 0 | 1 | 16.8 | 21.9 |
| 12–13 | 0 | 0 | 100 | 14.4 | 12.9 |

[a] See Table 3 for pretreatment and co-culture conditions.
[b] Tested after 4 days of co-culture for MOLT-4 cells, or 14 days of co-culture for CBL.
[c] NT, not tested.

When MOLT-4 T-cell lymphoma was used as HTLV-I recipient (Table 6), IFN pretreatment of MOLT-4 cells (groups 5–7), or IFN added to the co-culture (groups 8–10) did not impair, but rather slightly increased the efficiency of virus infection. A limited inhibition was instead observed when the HTLV-I donor MT-2 cells were pretreated with the agent (groups 3–4).

Preliminary data obtained on the influence of PCF-39 treatment on HTLV-I transmission *in vitro* to MOLT-4 or CBL recipient cells are illustrated in Table 7. The results point out that the drug is capable of reducing the infectivity of MT-2 donor cells, expecially when recipient CBL were used (groups 4). Limited impairment of HTLV-I transmission seems also to occur when CBL but not MOLT-4 cells were pretreated with the drug (groups 7, 8), whereas PCF-39 added to the culture does not seem to affect substantially the outcome of virus infection, except for the culture with a high concentration (i.e. 100 µg/ml) of the agent (group 13).

## Conclusion

The results of the preliminary studies illustrated in the present report confirm that immunomodulating agents such as IFN and PCF-39 can augment natural and antigen-elicited cell-mediated cytotoxicity in selected experimental conditions. The boosting of CMNC produced by IFN renders effector lymphocytes capable of lysing a variety of HTLV-I positive leukemia cells, non-susceptible to the cytotoxic effects of intact lymphocytes. In addition both agents are capable of increasing the cytolytic response of viable immunocompetent cells admixed with HTLV-I infecting cancer cells, in co-culture conditions of *in vitro* virus transfer. If immune reactivity of HTLV-recipient lymphocytes would play a role in virus transmission, it is reasonable to hypothesize that immunomodulating agents would interfere with *in vitro* (or possibly *in vivo*) infection. Actually the results obtained on P19 expression of recipient lymphocytes suggest that IFN and possibly PCF-39 would augment the resistance of target cell to virus transmission. Both agents seem to be capable also of reducing the infecting ability of HTLV-I donor leukemic cells. Since no evidence was obtained for a direct effect of the drugs on virus transmission when present in MT-2 recipient cell co-cultures (except for high concentrations of PCF-39), it could be suggested that IFN and PCF-39 would reduce HTLV-I infection through their effects on the immune system and on the infectivity of HTLV-I donor lymphoblasts. However the data presently available are largely preliminary and must be confirmed by further studies in various experimental conditions.

318

## Acknowledgement

This work was supported in part by Progetto Finalizzato Contr. Malattie da Infezione, UO Bonmassar, CNR, Rome, Italy.

## References

1. Poiesz BJ, Ruscetti FW, Gazdar AF, Bunn PA, Minna JD, Gallo RC: Detection and isolation of type C retrovirus particles from fresh and cultured lymphocytes of a patient with cutaneous T-cell lymphoma. Proc Nat Acad Sci USA 77:7415–7419, 1980a.
2. Poiesz BJ, Ruscetti FW, Reitz MS et al.: Isolation of a new type C retrovirus (HTLV) in primary cultured cells of a patient with Sezary T cell leukaemia. Nature 294:268–271, 1981.
3. Kalyanaraman VS, Sarngadharan MG, Nakao Y, Ito Y, Aoki T, Gallo RC: Natural Antibodies to the structural core protein (p24) of the human T-cell leukemia (lymphoma) retrovirus found in sera of leukemia patients in Japan. Proc Nat Acad Sci USA 79:1653–1657, 1982a.
4. Gallo RC, Kalyanaraman VS, Sarngadharan MG, Sliski A, Vonderheid EC, Maeda M, Nakao Y, Yamada K, Ito Y, Gutensohn N, Murphy S, Bunn PAJr, Catovsky D, Greaves MF, Blayney DW, Blattner W, Jarrett WFH, zur Hausen H, Seligmann M, Brouet JC, Haynes BF, Jegasothy BV, Jaffe E, Cossman J, Broder S, Fisher RI, Golde DW, Robert-Guroff M: Association of the human type C retrovirus with a subset of adult T-cell Cancers. Cancer Res 43:3892–3899, 1983a.
5. Popovic M, Sarin PS, Robert-Guroff M, Kalyanaraman VS, Mann D, Minowada J, Gallo RC: Isolation and transmission of Human retrovirus (human T-cell leukemia virus). Science 219:856–859, 1983b.
6. Sarin PS, Aoki T, Shibata A, Ohnishi Y, Aogagi Y, Miyakoshi H, Emura I, Kalyanaraman VS, Robert-Guroff M, Popovic M, Sarngadharan MG, Nowell PC, Gallo RC: High incidence of human type-C retrovirus (HTLV) in family members of a HTLV-positive Japanese T-cell leukemia patient. Proc Nat Acal Sci USA 80:2370–2374, 1983a.
7. Miyoshi I, Kubonishi I, Yoshimot S, Akagi T, Ohtsuki Y, Shiraishi Y, Nagato K, Hunuma Y: Type C virus particles in a cord T-cell line derived by co-cultivating normal human cord leukocytes and human leukemic T-cells. Nature 294:770–771, 1981a.
8. Yoshida M, Miyoshi I, Hinuma Y: Isolation and characterization of retrovirus from cell lines of human adult T-cell leukemia and its implication in the desease. Proc Nat Acad Sci USA 79:2031–2035, 1982.
9. Haynes BF, Miller SE, Palker TJ, Moore JO, Dunn PH, Bolognesi DP, Metzgar RS: Identification of human T-cell leukemia virus in a Japanese patient with adult cell leukemia and cutaneous lymphomatous vasculitis. Proc Nat Acad Sci USA 80:2054–2058, 1983a.
10. Vyth-Drees FA, De Vries JE: Human T-cell leukemia virus in lymphocytes from a T-cell leukaemia patient originating from Surinam. Lancet 2:993, 1982.
11. Rho HM, Poiesz BJ, Ruscetti FW, Gallo RC: Characterization of the reverse transcriptase from a new retrovirus (HTLV) produced by a human cutaneous T-cell lymphoma cell line. Virology 112:355–360, 1981.
12. Reitz MS, Poiesz BJ, Ruscetti FW, Gallo RC: Characterization and distribution of nucleic acid sequences of a novel type C retrovirus isolated from neoplastic human T lymphocytes. Proc Nat Acad Sci USA 78:1887–1891, 1981.
13. Kalyanaraman VS, Sarngadharan MG, Poiesz BJ, Ruscetti FW, Gallo RC: Immunological properties of a type C retrovirus isolated from cultured human T-lymphoma cells and comparison to other mammalian retroviruses. J Virol 38:906–915, 1981b.

14. Robert Guroff M, Ruscetti FW, Posner LE, Poiesz BJ, Gallo RC: Detection of the human T-cell lymphoma virus p19 in cells of some patients with cutaneous T-cell lymphoma and leukemia using a monoclonal antibody. J Exp Med 154:1957–1964, 1981.

15. Kalyanaraman VS, Sarngadharan MG, Robert-Guroff M, Miyoshi I, Blayney D, Golde D, Gallo RC: A new subtype of human T-cell leukemia virus (HTLV-II) Associated with a T-cell variant of Hairy cell leukemia. Science 218:571–573, 1982b.

16. Popovic M, Sarngadharan MG, Read E, Gallo RC: Detection, isolation, and continuous production of Cytopathic retroviruses (HTLV-III) from patients with AIDS and Pre-AIDS. Science, 224:497–500, 1984.

17. Gallo RC: Human T-cell leukaemia-Lymphoma virus and T-cell malignancies in adults. Cancer Surv 3:113–159, 1984.

18. Markham PD, Salahuddin SZ, Gallo RC: In vitro cultivation of normal and neoplastic human T lymphocytes. Clin Haematol 13:423–445, 1984.

19. Mann DL, Clark J, Clarke M, Reitz M, Popovic M, Franchini G, Trainor CD, Strong DM, Blattner WA, Gallo RC: Identification of the human T cell lymphoma virus in B cell lines established from patients with adult T cell leukemia. J Clin Invest 74:56–62, 1984.

20. Clapham P, Nagy K, Cheingsong-Popov R, Exley M, Weiss RA: Productive infection and cell-free transmission of human T-cell leukemia virus in a nonlymphoid cell line. Science 222:1125–1127, 1983.

21. Djeu JY, Heinbaugh AJ, Holden HT, Herberman RB: Augmentation of mouse natural killer cell activity by interferon and interferon inducers. J Immunol 122:175–181, 1979.

# Index